Louis Gifford
Aches and Pains

Book One

Aches and Pains 1-14

CNS Press, Aches and Pains Ltd., Kestrel, Swanpool,
Falmouth, Cornwall, TR11 5BD, UK

Email:info@achesandpainsonline.com
www.giffordsachesandpains.com

A CIP catalogue record for the book is available from the British Library.

First published 2014
Reprinted 2015, 2016 (thrice), 2017 (twice), 2018 (thrice), 2019 (twice), 2020 (thrice),
2021 (twice)

ISBN 978 1 7399486 0 3

Louis Gifford Aches and Pains

Book 1 Aches and Pains Sections 1-14. Book 2 Aches and Pains Sections 15-20.
Nerve Root 1-5. Book 3 Graded Exposure 1-4. Case Histories 1-4.

Louis Gifford MApplSc FCSP

Editing	Philippa Tindle, Mick Thacker and Paula Ross
Typesetting and	
Figures redrawn by	Harriet Gendall and Julian Tredinnick
Printed and bound by	TJ Books Limited, Padstow, Cornwall, UK.

To Philippa, Ralph and Jake

Foreword 1

I was deeply honoured when Louis asked me if I would consider writing a forward to his book(s); originally he thought it would be a single volume but as he started to write he realised just what a massive amount of knowledge he had to share with the interested reader. He asked me to be honest and forthright without being too 'nice'; his modest demeanour not comfortable with what he knew I could and should write about him and his work. I am writing in the past tense, sadly Louis didn't get to see the publication of his books. I can therefore say what I want to without fear that I will embarrass him by telling the truth.

Louis and I go back a good few years from the earliest days of the physiotherapy 'pain revolution'. It was a long, tough journey but one that has ultimately been highly successful. Louis was always at the centre of the movement, motivating, teaching and supporting those around him. His modesty and lack of ego made him the perfect person with which the everyday clinician could most easily relate. Louis was always motivated by the need to answer clinically based questions, although his fierce intellect allowed to him to read and grasp all aspects of the basic science, psychology and philosophy of pain. Louis had a fantastic, well-rounded knowledge of pain in all its domains, developed by hours and hours of self-directed study. Above all Louis was the embodiment of a clinical scientist.

This collection of books demonstrates exactly that; they draw on this massive knowledge and bring together his thoughts, observations, reading and ideas, all presented from a clinician's perspective. This makes these books unique; there are no other books like this on the topic of pain. In addition they are, especially in the first book, autobiographical. They demonstrate the honesty and integrity of one of our professions' greatest practitioners and thinkers.

Louis literally jumps off every page, the humour, wisdom, clarity of expression and deep affection for people are all here. For those of us lucky enough to know him they will produce a warmth of feeling difficult to describe unless you spent time in his company; for those who will get to know him only through these books, enjoy the journey with him, you will soon grow to love him too! The only things missing here are his lovely Cornish lilt and the twinkle in his 'blueys'.

Throughout his career he sought out, read and communicated with the brightest minds in the fields he was interested in, including most notably, Geoff Maitland and Professor Patrick Wall. He details some of their interactions in book one. He was able to hold his own with the very best because he had confidence in his own knowledge; a knowledge that was acquired from having the most inquisitive of minds and the ability to readily grasp the crux of a concept or argument.

For 15 years Louis taught the courses he and Philippa developed as part of "achesandpains". There were three main courses. The Clinical Biology of Aches and Pains, the Nerve Root and Graded Exposure. The material from these courses has been extensively updated by Louis and forms the bulk of these books. In addition, he includes extensive updates and explanations of his three major theses; The Mature Organism Model, The Shopping Basket Approach and the 'Toblerone' Recovery Model.

The Mature Organism Model (MOM), first published in 1998 in the Physiotherapy Journal is a classic model of pain, and built upon in the first book in the Topical Issues in Pain series. Here is what Pat Wall said:

"I was particularly impressed by the chapter by Gifford on the 'Mature Organism Model' which places pain in an integrated context without any permission to accept the old dualistic split that pain must be either in the body or in the mind."

Without overstatement, I think it has been and remains, the most influential and best-understood model of pain within the physiotherapy profession and has wide utility outside of our profession also. Both those new to it and those well versed in its key concepts will find a state of the art update and the most extensive discussion of it in anywhere in Book 1 section 10.

The influence of the MOM cannot be understated; I believe it is now as widely used as the gate theory in British Pain Management Programmes. Many of the models proposed by widely accepted experts have it at their heart. I personally include it in almost every lecture I deliver.

Equally impressive in their simplicity and useability are The Shopping Basket Approach and the 'Toblerone' Recovery Model. Again, both are brought up to date and expanded upon in these volumes.

Throughout these volumes Louis offers clinical examples and specific case studies to highlight how his ideas can be applied in the clinic. The patients he discusses, will, I am sure, become well known in their own rights thanks to the warmth and humour Louis uses to detail their problems and his solutions for/with them.

I think these books are a fitting legacy to him and will continue the already huge impact he has made in ensuring that patients all over the world are treated more wisely and with more respect because of the ideas and insights he offers. Ideas he gives freely and generously without a hint of self-importance or ego.

Before I finish, I have to mention the love, support and dedication shown to Louis over the years from his family - Philippa, Ralph and Jake. They gave him the space and freedom to develop his ideas and offered the necessary distractions from getting too immersed in work. They helped him keep a healthy perspective and not to take it all too seriously. They are all wonderful people who have played a massive part in bringing this to fruition. Philippa has worked tirelessly to get these books published and there was no one who Louis would trust more with his ideas, work and to do the right thing with them than *his* Philippa.

To conclude, I have had the amazing privilege to have proof read all 450,000 words of these books. They are without exaggeration a masterpiece; they have reignited my interest and passion for pain. Most fortunately for me, this process allowed us the opportunity to have the most amazing discussions and the excuse to talk for hours at a time, not just about the book but about life and Louis' experiences. I will cherish these precious times forever. I loved him very much and miss him more than words can describe. I know by the time you have read them for yourself, you will feel that you knew him too and feel you have a new friend standing beside you in the clinic, offering the right sort of help and support and I know that would have made him very happy.

Mick Thacker

March 2014

Foreword 2

Louis Gifford's Aches and Pains series are truly fantastic. I cannot recall any other textbooks which cover the subject of pain with such an overarching, integrated depth of knowledge, clarity and honesty – a true biopsychosocial masterpiece! Louis accompanies the reader on an amazing and skilfully guided journey of learning and monumental discovery through the history of pain science, particularly over the last 20 years. Most importantly for clinicians working with patients with pain, are the gold nuggets of clinical information imparted here by a consummate practitioner who has worked at the clinical 'coal face', helping people manage and recover from their pain for more than two decades. Scientific discovery is great but what all clinicians really want and need to know is, 'How can this knowledge help me to help my patients?' Explaining and outlining this is exactly what Louis does best and it's what he succinctly and superbly achieves here.

This is a brave body of work, unafraid to question old and new concepts alike, some of which have been 'held dear' for years and even become 'accepted truth' within the physical therapies. The review of available evidence is undertaken with an appropriate dose of open ended and healthy scepticism, with helpful direction to the high quality scientific evidence or lack of it. Pain myths are unmasked and the ridiculous is playfully exploded. This all happens in a refreshing conversational style that exudes the essence of Louis. Reading these books feels like the author could be sitting alongside you in the room, deep in conversation, suitably relaxed in an easy chair, glass of wine in hand.

Helpful case histories demonstrate how the author approaches many common clinical scenarios encountered when treating people with pain. It is a rare and bold thing for any clinician to openly discuss not just 'what' they are thinking but 'why they are thinking what they are thinking'. This open access to Louis thinking during patient examinations allows the reader to fully understand and appreciate what lies behind the author's highly skilful clinical reasoning and decision making. The patient-centred biopsychosocial approach is central here; Louis' own 'mature organism model' provides a wonderful demonstration of neurobiology in practice and a deep understanding of the 'human condition' and how this influences all of our pain states. I cannot emphasise enough how important I feel the mature organism model is to understanding human pain states and the opportunities it provides both clinicians and patients engaging pain.

Whether the reader already has an in-depth knowledge of pain science or whether they are new to the subject area, there is much of interest to be found in this series for anyone interested in pain. Complex pain biology is broken down and presented in accessible, understandable sections with many 'minor detours' provided to further enhance the readers understanding and interest of the topic.

This series represents Louis lifetime of learning and knowledge, poignantly detailing the true and extraordinary story of pain science. These books aptly demonstrate why Louis is so highly regarded as a world class educator, thinker and clinician. Louis' unique approach towards helping us understand pain is done with humility and humour, containing many 'laugh out loud' moments along the way. This is a journey that is never dull, always interesting and absolutely inspiring.

Steve Robson

Northumberland, UK

March 2014

Foreword 3

I was lucky enough to meet Louis in September 1978. We sat next to each other on our first day of the three year physiotherapy course at Sheffield City Polytechnic. We were part of a large intake of about fifty students – the majority eighteen year old school leavers. We were considered 'mature', both having done first degrees in zoology. Our surnames were at either end of the alphabet which meant that we were in different sets and we never went on student placements together. I never really saw much of Louis in the first two years of our training. But we all met in the Poly café and discussed our experiences and frustration at not having a consistent method of assessing and treating patients when we went out to the different teaching hospitals around Sheffield. We couldn't believe the variation of approaches we witnessed from our mentors, the senior physiotherapists. We tried to copy their approach only to be told to do things differently by another teacher. We really didn't have a clue what we were doing. We moaned and groaned at our tutors to 'show us the right way'. Robbie Blake had just been to Bad Ragaz in Switzerland to learn the 'Maitland' approach and he, plus, Ted Morgan Jones were a great influence in our final year. At last a method we could follow.

Louis and I got together in January 1981, our graduation year, (it wasn't the easiest of starts as we both had to leave other partners). Fellow students, Pete Lawlor, Lesley Bird (and many more) plus our school principal Norma Brook and Ann Parry were very supportive. We passed our exams, moved to our first jobs in Liverpool and our careers began. Thanks to Peter Lageard, Steve and Nicky Profitt (nee Birch) we had a ball. Getting places on the 'Maitland' course in Adelaide was the ultimate goal and we attended the Manipulation Association of Chartered Physiotherapy study days and gained entry to the MACP via the viva voce.

I realised early on in our life together that I was with a man who was very self-sufficient, (I was very impressed. He could repair and service my old mini and also cook 'ground nut soup', a West African dish). Louis was slightly obsessive when he got interested in something and taught himself new skills via buying and reading the latest books on the topic. Over the years we have accumulated libraries of; how to windsurf – tricks and racing; guitar playing – the blues (a spell of saxophone playing too); sail trimming and racing rules; all the Spine articles from 1978 onwards...; ballroom and Latin American dancing; the novels of Charles Dickens and many of the Classics; mushroom identification; British wildflowers; sea and trout fishing and the best rods; the Angler and how to fly tie a 'Woolly bugger'; GOLF; woodworking for the beginner and beyond; how to service your motorbike; atheism – every book supporting and criticising it; running lore; the cycle routes of Cornwall; circular walks in the south west; bread-making and Jamie Oliver; crosswords and the thesaurus. The list does go on (Amazon may now be feeling the pinch!). And I could tell by the pile of books, papers and notes beside his bed what the latest interest was. He was a quiet achiever. Sometimes he dipped into a number of topics at once!

I remember the first time I heard Louis speak publicly. He was presenting his dissertation paper on, 'Circadian Variation in Human Flexibility and Grip Strength' to the Australian Manipulation Association in Melbourne in 1987. Brian Edwards and Geoff Maitland shared the floor for one of the sessions, so it was quite a prestigious conference. I remember turning to my neighbour as Louis started his presentation and saying, 'Where did this come from?' He was very confident, (slightly cocky!), funny, full of information, clear, understandable, enthusiastic and brilliant! I was amazed as I had seen the nervous character beforehand. But he knew his stuff. Over the many years that I helped to organise his teaching programme and the times I sat in on his talks and courses I never lost that excitement of hearing Louis speak. I think it is rare to find someone you can listen to all day, who makes complex subjects understandable and gives the audience something to take to the clinic the next day. I was proud to be promoting him. But he never lost the nervousness he had before any presentation. It was a performance that he made look effortless but it took many hours of reading, writing and preparation to get to the level of seemingly easy lecturing.

This nervousness even carried over into the clinic, as he always spent the start of his day reading all his patients' notes, however long it took, so that he was fully prepared for the patient encounter. He was always confident with the detail of each patient he saw, whether they be a complex chronic patient sent by the Pain Clinic consultant, or the old farmer from up the road who had a stiff shoulder. Everybody was treated with equal care and consideration and Louis worked hard with every patient.

Way back in about 1994 I remember receiving a request from a physiotherapist for Louis to lecture one of his two day courses. This physio made some disparaging comments about the cost of the course. I don't believe I could put a price on the hours/days/weeks/months and years that Louis thought, read, wrote and worked to try and make sense of the patient and their problem in front of him. Louis would have liked to; not charge for his courses; offer free treatment to patients and give away his books!

But Louis would ask one thing. If you find some of his material and ideas resonate with you and your practise he would be thrilled. If you want to use his words or ideas then simply acknowledge your source – very simple and very easy to do. Louis tried throughout his whole professional life to give credit to what and who stimulated his thoughts. Once he had an amazing relationship with a friend, a colleague, who was like another brother. This friend air-brushed Louis out of his life and made claim to many ideas. Louis was hurt beyond words.

Our career travels have been written about elsewhere: Sheffield, Liverpool, London, Adelaide and from March 12, 1988 Falmouth, Cornwall UK. Back to the womb! We returned to the Gifford family home. And for the last 26 years we have been dividing our time between running a small, local, private physiotherapy clinic, running Louis' teaching programme and book publishing.

In late April 2007, just after running the Scillies marathon for the second time, Louis was diagnosed with advanced metastatic prostate cancer. He was just 54. His prognosis wasn't great. One of our sons was travelling in New Zealand and the other was doing his GCSE's. We took the diagnosis/prognosis on board and chose to get on with living and to keep our private life to ourselves. We were lucky. Louis outlived his original prognosis and life has been full, active, fun, and fantastic to wake up to every day. Louis decided to stop lecturing (I know his last course was a Graded Exposure programme in Nottingham in early April 2007). But he continued working and seeing and treating patients in our clinic until May 2013.

Louis received some treatment for bone pain at the end of May 2013, (after returning from 3 weeks snowboarding in Colorado – thanks Bern and Ellen). The treatment and disease have been a pain since June and Louis has had to take up 'sitting down hobbies!' In his own remarkable way Louis had the most productive summer of his whole life. Over the last 6 months he has written these amazing books. They are funny and readable; full of 'tips from the coal face'; and constructed to make some difficult concepts and topics understandable and hopefully useful to the whole physiotherapy profession.

At the beginning of this piece I said I was lucky enough to sit next to Louis all those years ago – I really mean it with all my heart.

Philippa Tindle

January 2014

Louis died on 9th February 2014. He knew that I would publish his words. I have stayed true to him and not altered his style at all. He would have liked to have added a few more case histories and he would have 'polished' some of his explanations because he was very thoughtful and careful with his words. I have tried to be consistent and to hear him talking through the text – the dashes and exclamation marks are all there for you to take a pause with him! I can do no more.

I know that Louis has given each section and chapter a 'Read what I've read' addition. I hope you enjoy my 'Read what Louis was reading' list – the books and papers that were stacked on Louis' bedside table in February.

1   *Noe, A. (2010) Out of Our Heads: Why You Are Not Your Brain, and Other Lessons from the Biology of Consciousness. Hill and Wang, New York.*

2   *Nutt, D. (2013) Drugs Without Hot Air. UIT Cambridge Ltd. UK.*

3   *Jablonka, E. and Zeligowski, A. (2006) Evolution in Four Dimensions Genetic, Epigenetic, Behavioural and Symbolic Variation in the History of Life. The MIT Press, Cambridge Massachusetts.*

4   *Zheng,Z. Paterson,C. Ledgerwoood,K. Hogg,M. Xue,C. Arnold,C. (2013) Chaos to Hope: A Narrative of Healing. Pain Medicine 2013:14: 1826-1838. Wiley Periodicals, Inc.*

5   *Pain & Rehabilitation, Journal of the Physiotherapy Pain Association, Cormac, R (ed.) Winter 2014 Issue 36.*

6   *Gifford, L. (2005) The Nerve Root. Aches and Pains Ltd Course Workbook.*

7   *Francis, R. (2012) Epigenetics: How Environment Shapes Our Genes. W.W.Norton Company Ltd. New York.*

8   *Cheney, Michael. (1984) A field guide to the Insects of Britain and Northern Europe. Collins, London.*

9   *Sapolsky, R. M. (2006) Monkeyluv And Other Lessons on Our Lives as Animals. Vintage Books, London.*

10   *Wilson, E. (1992) The Diversity of Life. Harvard University Press, Massachusetts.*

11   *Grayling, A.C. (2013) The God Argument: The Case against Religion and for Humanism. Bloomsbury, London.*

12   *Hitchens, C. (2007) The Portable Atheist: Essential Readings For the NonBeliever. Da Capo Press.*

13   *The Twenty-Fourth Pan Book of Crosswords (1975), Burgess,L.W. (ed). Pan Books Ltd. London. The Daily Telegraph: Cryptic Crossword Book 62 and 24.(2008). Pan Books Ltd. London.*

14   *Vonnegut, K. (1985) Galapagos. Dell Publishing, New York.*

15   *Carey,N.(2012) The Epigenetics Revolution. Icon Books Ltd. London.*

16   *The Romantic Poets: An Anthology; Wordsworth, Coleridge, Byron, Shelley and Keats. Published in 1987 for the great Writers Library by Marshall Cavendish Partworks Ltd. London.*

17   *Singh, S. & Ernst, E. (2008) Trick or Treatment. Alternative Medicine on Trial? Corgi Books, London.*

18   *Damasio, A. (2000) The Feeling of What Happens. Body, Emotion and the Making of Consciousness. Vintage, Random House, London.*

19   *Dennett, D. (1991) Consciousness Explained. Penguin Books Ltd. London.*

20   *Rose, S. (2005) The 21st Century Brain. Explaining, Mending and Manipulating the Mind. Vintage Books. London.*

21   *Beattie, R. (2007) 101 Golden Rules of Fishing. Wiles, Wit and Wisom to Inform and Entertain. Ebury Press.*

22   *Vaughn, A. & Ladle, M. (1988) Hooked on Bass. The Crowood Press Ltd. Wiltshire.*

23   *The Holy Bible. Oxford University Press.*

24   *Leakey, R. (1994) The Origins of Humankind. Orion Books Ltd. London.*

25   *Screwfix. June 2013 catalogue*

26   *Goleman, Daniel. (2013) Focus The Hidden Driver of Excellence. Bloomsbury, London.*

27   *The Biology of Brain: From Neurons to Networks. In Llinas, RR. (Ed) Readings from Scientific American Magazine. (1977-1988). W.H. Freeman and Company, New York.*

28   *Dudai, Yadin. (1989) The Neurobiology of Memory Concepts, Findings, Trends. Oxford University Press.*

29   *Fields, R. D. (2011) Powerhouses of the Brain. In Scientific American Mind, May/June 2011: 54-59*

30   *Kandel, E.R, Schartz,J.H, Jessell,T.M (Eds) (1995) Essentials of Neural Science and Behaviour. Prentice Hall International Inc.*

From me to you forever
Philippa Tindle
January-March 2014

Acknowledgements

At Sheffield City Polytechnic, where I trained, I'd like to thank Robbie Blake and Ted Morgan-Jones, both passionate physiotherapists and teachers. Thanks in particular to Robbie for teaching me basic Maitland principles and mobilisation techniques and also for being so supportive over the years.

On my various placements as a student, I'd like to thank Akram at Doncaster Royal Infirmary for teaching me how to handle and manipulate spines and necks and not be fearful. He used 'feel' and he taught it to me. He also made me realise how problematic the rules of the Maitland approach were by showing me how easy it was to manipulate spines that would be designated 'high severity' and 'high irritability' under the 'SIN' system.

I'd also like to thank Asoka Jaywardena, who continued to teach me all the Maitland skills he could and helped me with patients when I was on placement at Mansfield Hospital. We had a lot of fun and I still have great memories.

After qualifying my first job was at Walton Hospital Liverpool – the hospital next to the jail! Two amazing physiotherapists there were, Paul Chadwick and Shirley Orme. I loved every minute with the two of them and couldn't get enough of their wisdom. I also enjoyed working on the neurology and neurological diseases unit – no one in particular to thank, except the patients with their rare neurological presentations. I learnt more about assessing and diagnosing neurological conditions in a few weeks on rotation there, than I did in the whole of the rest of my career. I also had one of my first astonishing 'pain' experiences...

It was about 4 pm and I was doing some simple passive movements on an old fellow who'd had a mild stroke about three or four days previously. An Irish Doctor happened to be up at the head end checking on the various monitors that were beeping away. We were ignoring one another as we quietly got on with our work. Then, quite calmly the Doctor looked up and caught my attention, 'His heart's stopped, do you know how to do cardiac massage?'... 'Er, yes'... 'Off you go then.' Within seconds I was pushing away on the old fellow's chest. 'A bit harder can you?' says the Doc. 'Well, I'm not sure his old ribs will take it...' was my response. 'It's his ribs or his life fella'… Calm as you like, harder I went. Crack, crunch, scrunch went the ribs as they were breaking under my pressures… 'Got him' said the Doc… 'He's coming back quite well now, keep going a while more can you…' On I went, the rib cage was sickly soft and compliant now, but I carried on. 'Hang on there a minute can you, we'll see how he manages on his own for a few minutes now, if I'm still having trouble we'll get the crash team…' Relaxed as you like, the two of us just sat and watched; we watched the monitors and we watched his chest rise and fall. After about ten minutes the Irish Doctor said I might as well go because there was little more I could do.

I left the ward a little shaken. I said 'fuck' a few times, like you do and then went off to see the next patient.

The next day the first thing I wanted to do was go and see the old fellow; for one thing—was he still alive and for the other—what was his rib pain like!

'Hi, Louis isn't it?'

'It is. Hi Bert, how are you today?'

'Fine.'

'Breathing alright?'

'Seem to be.' He took a deep breath.

'No problems? Can you give me a cough by any chance?'

He gave a big cough and then spat the muck into a plastic cup.

'Is that OK?'

'Absolutely, I'll come and see you later…'

I left the ward rather dazed. I said 'fuck' a few times, like you do and then went off to see the next patient.

'You know, I bust his ribs yesterday and he's fine today, how weird is that…?'

After Liverpool Philippa and I got jobs in London; Philippa went to work at Roehampton and I was lucky enough to get a job working for Peter Wells at St Stephen's Hospital. Here, my manual therapy skills came on in further leaps and bounds. Thanks, in particular, to Peter for teaching me so much and for his friendship and nurturing in a wonderful department. Thanks, in particular, to Joan Blair for her wonderful sense of humour and Scottish no-nonsense approach – a great manual therapist. Agneta Lando, also a great manual therapist – soft sure hands, plus having to deal with my naughty cheekiness; what great times we had. I know I was a bit of a nuisance. Thanks also to Rosemary Keer and Kate Sheehy.

The Adelaide course in 1985 was a manual therapy high point, as were the two years that followed. Huge thanks to Geoff Maitland with whom I worked for a couple of years after the course. I felt very close to him. I have always realised how special he was, despite the criticisms of his approach and of manual therapy in general that are in this book. I was very lucky to be there, in that it showed me what manual therapy could achieve and also its weaknesses. Thanks also to my teachers on the course:

Patt Trott, Mary Magarey, Helen Ruebenach and Ruth Grant. I also learnt a great deal and had a great many laughs with fellow course participants in 1985: Rob Burgess, Libby Fardy, Ali Bell, Dave Butler, Mark Jones, Anton Harms, Rosa Ng and Ellen Guth.

Back in the UK I'd particularly like to thank those responsible for the cohesiveness and fantastic energy of the Physiotherapy Pain Association in the 1990's and early 2000's. It was great to be involved and a huge learning curve that still goes on. I have a great admiration for and gratitude to the following colleagues: Heather Muncey who was the founder of the PPA; also Jan Williams, Sue Mickleburgh, Vicki Harding, Paul Watson and Lorraine Moores. Also, thanks to two very special CBT physiotherapists who taught me so much – Suzanne Brook (nee Shorland) and Liz Macleod.

The 'Topical Issues in Pain' volumes wouldn't be what they are without the dedication, knowledge and input of all the authors involved. Not only was it a pleasure editing your work, it was also hugely enlightening and educating – so, a massive thank you. I have never stopped enjoying reading and re-reading them and have come to realise that it's unlikely that they'll ever need much updating. I hope the books and all the work in them continue to thrive for many years to come. They seem to mark a very important era in the development and 'shift' of modern musculoskeletal physiotherapy.

David Butler and Juliet Gore gave us the impetus to self publish the TIP books. And I remember the collaborative years with David when we shared everything with honesty and respect.

Special thanks to all at Physiofirst (formerly OCPPP). Your committee members, 'In Touch' editors and many members have always promoted, published and supported me.

To the many UK course organisers and participants – who invited and welcomed me, listened and challenged me nicely, thank you!

I have had wonderful support from some key physiotherapists in Switzerland, Holland, Denmark, Belgium and Norway. Big hugs to Hugo Stam and Kees Rigter. Thanks to Eric Thoomes, Filip and Kristof, the 'Ingers', the 'Jeroens', Harry VP and Chris Drummond for inviting me to your countries. And many, many more, whose names allude me, but I will always be grateful.

In the USA, Adriaan and Colleen Louw have recently shown massive support to myself and Philippa. They encouraged me to 'tell my story', write my blog and get these books out. Thanks.

Nicky and Andy Hunter, great hosts and people.

To Louise Nicholettos, for coming to work with Philippa and I – the 'oldies'. And for our lunches together!

Harriet and Tessa Gendall, Julian Tredinnick and Paula Ross – for getting down to the nitty-gritty and helping Philippa make these books happen.

Lastly, there are a few individuals who I'd like to thank for their support and closeness and what they've taught me over many years:

Pete Lawlor and Pete and Mary Cooper – who welcomed Philippa and I and gave me a home a long time ago.

Viv Gleave – physio extraordinaire and life-long friend whom we first met in Liverpool and then in London at the Royal Free Hospital's five day Robin Mckenzie course over thirty years ago. And who came on the very first Dynamic Nervous System course Dave Butler and I did in Aberstwyth around 1996.

Ellen and Bernie Guth, from the US, for being there and knowing what I went through with   David . Your love and support over the years has been both immense and touching.

Heather Muncey – for being a great friend, an amazing physiotherapist and my Hero. I love you to bits.

Paul Watson – for being in the right place at the right time for me. Paul, there can't be many on the planet like you, or who have such admirable knowledge, logic and thinking. Another Hero! Paul has done so much for the profession.

Steve Robson from Prudhoe, north of Newcastle, thanks for reading some of this and all the feedback. Thanks too for thinking like me! In particular, thanks for the support you've given me over the years, but especially recently when times haven't been so easy for me. It was an honour to have collaborated on some of our writing projects and I'm so pleased you agreed to write one of the forewords.

Ian Stevens – for keeping me informed so well; for your sustained and correct scepticism and for supporting my case from time to time.

Mick Thacker who I love to bits. The most 'pain' informed physiotherapist on the planet, for whom I have the deepest respect. As a profession we are lucky to have you and I am especially lucky to have had some of your time over the years. Together we have pondered much and it's been so interesting. If only we had more time. Lastly, I truly haven't the words to thank you for helping me edit this and for writing a foreword. With you and Kath we have had the best of times.

My Philippa, my greatest supporter, my deepest critic and my best friend. We have been to some wonderful places and we have shared some amazing moments together. You have urged me to get this book done for many years and I finally made it – just! Thanks for being the biggest help of all; thanks for lifting me from the gloom; thanks for bringing me down to earth; thanks for putting an inappropriate swear word to bed; thanks for enjoying the freedom with me and thanks for being there – you are nearly always right!

Louis Gifford

January 2014

Preface

I want the reader to enjoy reading this book. That's why it's three books, three smaller books rather than one huge one that you have to sit at a desk to read. It's three – each of which you can hold in your hand, with chapters that don't take too long to read.

Several years ago I read Bill Bryson's book, 'A Short History of Nearly Everything.' Bill Bryson wanted to know more about the world and about science and remembered being totally disillusioned by the dry and turgid writing he found in his school science textbooks. So, he took three years of his life and read, studied and wrote about the science that interested him. He also interviewed a vast variety of scientists, many of whom were great characters and had wonderful stories to tell and wonderful explanations for difficult concepts. He wrote the book in a style he would have enjoyed when he was at school; a style that asked the questions that he would have asked and which he would have loved to have had understandable answers to; a style that made the topics covered full of wonder, amazement and fascination.

While this book of mine has been gathering itself for a great many years, it is only in the last year that I have really settled to it. I have to say that I am grateful for having a progressive and terminal illness to give me time off work in order to really concentrate on it! But my point here is that Bill Bryson's approach and style for his book has been in the back of my mind throughout. I hope you find that the read you get here is a little more than just another one dimensional, boringly written pain science text that fails to answer all the clinical questions you have. In a rather selfish but fun way, like Bill Bryson, I have written this book in the way that I would have loved to have read about pain when I was a young and maturing physiotherapist.

Unfortunately, a book like this would not have been possible when I first trained, because back in the late 1970's and early 1980's a great deal of what is in this book wasn't widely known about or was only just being found out! How lucky then, to have lived through times of such great discovery and been there when it was more generally available. In retrospect, I guess the best thing I ever did, was to climb out of the confined and restrictive 'burrow' that contained the standard declarative knowledge base provided by physiotherapy training and all the subsequent post-graduate courses and take a look around! I expand on this theme in the chapter Graded Exposure 2.7, but all I need to say here is that once I started to look down into other disciplines' 'burrows', I realised that there was a massive body of knowledge that was of relevance to physiotherapy and the way the profession analysed and dealt with pain.

The big driving force throughout my career has been, 'I want a better explanation… I want to be able to give my patient honest and useful answers to their questions and I want to help them understand their problem in a much more realistic and helpful way.' I hope those who read and absorb what is in this book will be able to give far better and more rational information and explanations to their patients. Throughout the book I give clinical examples of how the material can be used and explained. Far better the clinician reads, understands and later, given a fair amount of 'seeding, watering and growth' of the material – they independently generate their own explanation and information- giving style.

So, it's not a textbook. It's a book about real pain, the patient's pain; it's about me and my professional journey to try and fathom what I saw in the clinic and then be more effective and relaxed with it. It's also my misery, my anger, my angst, my elation, my rants, my discoveries, my fun, my scepticism, my humour, my swearing and my naughtiness and political incorrectness. It's partly memoir – where I came from, what happened, who influenced me and who annoyed me, what made me think and marvel, what made it all seem to make sense and fall into place and most of all, what satisfied me and made me a better listener and clinician. It's all about my patients and how their suffering and narrative made me think and appeal for better answers, much better answers. My patients took me on the voyage from which I was able to produce these three volumes and they are what make the books to be enjoyed by clinicians. I set out to make it clinical and relevant and I hope I've done that.

One hope when I first began writing, setting fingers to keyboard, was for those who have heard me speak be able to go, 'I can hear Louis talking out from the page.' That notion freed me from the confines of scientific writing and that constraining feeling that every little thought or clinical speculation had to be backed up by heavy referencing to make it credible. The reader has to trust me and trust that over the last 35 years I have read a vast amount of material and thought about it a great deal in relation to clinical presentations and problems. The result is that my 'reference list' has become a simple 'Read what I've read' list. Some of the books and references are dated; to me this is not a problem because a great deal of what was written 15-20 years ago cannot be bettered. It is my belief that the significant threads of this book will still be relevant for a great many years to come, if not always and, that on-going research will keep adding more and more wonderful insights into and onto what we already know.

These three books are loosely based on the three courses I used to teach, 'The Clinical Biology of Aches and Pains', 'The Nerve Root' and 'Graded Exposure'. Books 1 and 2 cover the Aches and Pains and Nerve Root courses plus a lot more! Books 3 and 4 cover the Graded Exposure course material, plus a section of patient case histories.

Last thing, whenever I used to start any of the courses, I used to say something like this:

'Feel free to stand up and wander round, lie down, walk out... go to the loo... smoke a fag... To save embarrassment, it's a good move to switch your phone off. Feel free to ask questions anytime as I go along, but try not to be one of those annoying, nerdy guys who keeps asking questions every two minutes – when you're not the slightest bit interested in the answer, just in showing off to everyone else how much you know...'

This usually brought on a bit of a laugh and lots of people nodding their heads going...'Yeah we know those guys, they often spoil the course...' After a short pause I go on...

'Now, good science is all about challenging and criticising; it's all about applying logical evidence based reasoning and applying it to the questions of the day to try and find solutions. This course embraces those sentiments and the method of science. In physiotherapy we have a great many 'guru' based treatment approaches that unfortunately don't take kindly to criticism and try to bury challenging evidence. So, the contents of this course and my interpretation of the science I tell you about, isn't dogma – feel free to challenge it and offer alternative perspectives. That's good science and it's welcome. My advice is to listen with an open mind, take what you like and leave what you don't.

These books have been written with the same spirit and sentiments as my lectures were delivered. I hope you have as much fun reading them as I have had writing them!

Louis Gifford

December 2013

Contents

Section 1

EARLY DAYS

Chapter 1.1
Karen's sciatica

'Desolation Row' (5th verse)

Einstein, disguised as Robin Hood
With his memories in a trunk
Passed this way an hour ago
With his friend, a jealous monk
He looked so immaculately frightful
As he bummed a cigarette
Then he went off sniffing drainpipes
And reciting the alphabet
Now you would not think to look at him
But he was famous long ago
For playing the electric violin
On Desolation Row

Bob Dylan, 1965 from the album 'Highway 61 Revisited'

I hadn't a clue what I wanted to do for a career so I went off to college and studied Zoology. I enjoyed the natural world; I loved trout fishing and felt at ease outdoors. I liked to know the names of things; I collected butterflies, I bird spotted and had learnt a bit about wildflowers and mushrooms too. All that sounds a bit wet really – but I also liked Jimi Hendrix, The Stones, Bob Dylan, Pink Floyd, Led Zeppelin and some light psychedelic enhancement from time to time.

Zoology kindled my interest in entomology (useful for my fishing exploits), as well as cell biology, genetics and evolution which later became invaluable in my quest and struggle to understand pain.

But a zoology degree didn't really give me a huge 'job' option other than teaching biology in a secondary school. I completed college, decided to do VSO (Voluntary Service Overseas) and ended up teaching biology in a teacher training college in Sierra Leone, West Africa for two years. I made a massive collection of snakes, ants and butterflies and got to know quite a bit about tropical rainforests, Yamaha Enduro motorcycles and touch-typing on an old mechanical typewriter – at the same time teaching the college students human biology and botany. And there was also this very cheap stuff called 'happy-leaf'.

As the second year came to an end I realised that I didn't want to return to the UK and become a biology teacher. I thought about physiotherapy, both my parents were physiotherapists – they had their own practice in Falmouth, Cornwall and seemed to enjoy their work and I had met a physio in Sierra Leone who talked non-stop about her work in the local hospital in Freetown. I observed physiotherapists and occupational therapists working with post-surgical leprosy sufferers and came to realise that some people could achieve incredible things with often quite dramatic disabilities. I also touched quite a lot of lepers in one day and didn't notice any ill effects.

After coming home in the summer of 1978, I went on to start my physiotherapy training at Sheffield City Polytechnic that autumn.

It's not like what the books or the teachers say...

In the UK, physiotherapists training and working in the National Health Service (NHS) hospitals, see patients with musculoskeletal pain conditions in physiotherapy out-patients departments. The 'out-patient' case-load that I experienced when I trained was in the main difficult, chronic, agonisingly complex and had already had a great deal of unsuccessful treatment. In those days, in the late 1970's and early 1980's, we were taught 'things to do to patients'; how to apply short wave diathermy (SWD), ultrasound, passive movements, massage, proprioceptive neuromuscular facilitation techniques (PNF), infra-red; and thanks to Robbie Blake, one of the tutors at Sheffield City Polytechnic where I trained, we learnt some basic 'Maitland' manual therapy reasoning and skills too.

I remember struggling with 'out-patients' terribly – I hadn't a clue what was going on. I couldn't understand the reason for asking all the questions that I was told to ask. I had no 'diagnostic guidance' to pigeon-hole patients into so that their condition could be identified, discussed and then treated. Some of us complained to our tutors of this difficulty and as a result we were rewarded with a few lectures on Cyriax's 'differential diagnosis' methods (see Cyriax 1977, Cyriax and Russell 1978). This sounded good; you take a history and in so doing, find out where the pain is located or referred. You stress the appropriate tissues with static isometric tests for muscles and passive stretch tests for joint and ligamentous tissues, then quickly work out the structure responsible for the pain. We also learnt about the potential of deeper structures and nerves to refer pain 'segmentally' along dermatomes. We learnt the clinical characteristics of various musculoskeletal syndromes, diagnoses and injuries – the 'accepted' presentations that are still very much in use today.

Karen's sciatica

Armed with these basic diagnostic skills and some rudimentary ideas of the 'Maitland' approach, I was now looking forward to my next out-patient clinical placement. Remember this was around 1979-80.

My first patient, Karen, was a 28 year old lady who was due to get married in three weeks. Her problem was given as 'sciatica' – which she had had for only two weeks. Two things favourable here I thought; firstly, a relatively fresh problem, being only two weeks duration, and secondly, Karen was young, she had no previous history of back pain and lacked the usual historical complexity of the classic NHS 'out-patient'. But, her pain was severe, she hadn't slept properly, the painkillers didn't have any effect and the physiotherapy treatment she had been having (short wave diathermy or SWD) was aggravating it for several hours after the sessions and overall she was worsening. She had been coming for treatment three times a week and was becoming upset and desperate to feel better for her wedding. She couldn't comfortably stand for more than a few seconds and walked stooped in flexion.

During the assessment I soon found her 'sciatica' didn't fit into the S1 dermatome as the Cyriax books and my notes describe—it was all over her lower back—radiating bilaterally into her buttocks and thighs. The pain was most intense down the back *and front* of her right thigh, she had severe *anterior* knee pain and she had generalised paraesthesia over the *whole* of her lower leg and foot. Why wasn't it over the lateral border of the foot into the little toe? Why wasn't it down the back of her leg? How could it be down the back and the front too? Was I dealing with some horrible pathology that was attacking all the nerves of the leg?

Why wasn't it like the book said it should be? Was I dealing with something unknown to science and medicine? It felt like it.

She could hardly stand for the examination – all her movements hurt her intensely and she could only get acceptably comfortable, lying on her right side with her legs bent up. For me to do the supine examination she kept having to flip back on her right for a few minutes to ease things up. It all took so long in the limited time.

Her right straight leg raise test (SLR) was horribly painful everywhere (right leg, both buttocks and all the pins and needles too) at about 25 degrees, her reflexes were fine though and all muscle tests just gave way and produced pain and groaning. Everything I touched seemed to hurt. So much for my healing hands! I can recall feeling hopeless and very anxious, my fresh and renewed confidence from the 'Cyriax' lectures so quickly and cruelly dissolved.

This was awful. Not just because of the intensity of the pain and the suffering of the patient, but also because all the tests I performed were positive! How could everything I tested be so badly 'wrong' like this? My feelings were made even more intense when I did my palpation testing (she just about managed to be able to get into prone lying). Gentle postero-anterior pressure over lumbar vertebra 5 (L5) with the tips of my thumbs (Maitland – grade II)[1] produced massive tension and the patient reported searing pain into the whole back, the buttocks and right thigh.

'Ahhh, phew, found it... *this* is the source of the problem' I thought. But then I repeated on L4 – same response, L3 – same, L2 – same but slightly less – all the way to thoracic 9 which was 'OK'. Repeat palpation, now unilaterally, on each side of the vertebrae – same, vast reaction to all pressures. Sacro-iliac area pressure on right – again, same thing, all the pains and a big increase in tension. Even mild pressure over the *left* buttock brought on all the pain in the back and the *right* leg. Pressures on the painful areas of the right thigh sparked the back and the whole leg off, pins and needles included.

What the heck was going on?

I was now angry inside. And frustrated with the 'Cyriax' differential-diagnosis that we had been taught and at the people like Cyriax, who wrote the text books who didn't seem to have listened to the patients they described. That stuff didn't fit this patient and this patient's sciatica was definitely not in any of the texts. In fact even NOW, there is still no text that I have ever found that adequately records or explains this type of very common presentation. I decided long ago that 'experts' who write books on medical presentations don't see patients, or at least stopped long ago and didn't listen even then. I hope bits and pieces in this book go some way to addressing the deficit and maybe even spur someone on to listen and record what's really happening in an unbiased way.

That aside, I now had to deal with Karen, I had to do something. I made an excuse to get out of the cubicle...

'I just want to have a word with the physiotherapist who was seeing you last week before we start treatment,' was my nervous excuse.

I went outside and longed for a crafty cigarette. I was overwhelmed with information and cursing the lecturers in college for not telling me about this type of awful presentation. I decided on two things. One, was to use my recently acquired manual therapy 'Maitland' skills, where the technique selection logic ran, pain highly irritable, severe in nature, dominantly right sided – dictates a low grade 'unilateral'

---

1 - Refer to Maitland 1978 and 1986 for details of techniques if you're interested. Grade II is a very gentle oscillating pressure.

technique (grade I or II, i.e. super gentle). Then re-measure the SLR as my objective sign. The other was to have a quick word with the physiotherapist who had been treating Karen with SWD. I nervously managed to entice the physio away from the patient she was working with and tried to explain my findings. She butted in... 'Look, she's screwed up about marrying the guy and she's using this as an excuse to put the whole thing on-hold, SWD's helping her heaps anyway.'

That was the first of many experiences of therapist/Dr rigid thinking, narrow-mindedness and blaming the patient for lack of progress and the state they are in.

So, was I to listen to and believe the patient, or the physiotherapist? I felt even sicker. Was this the job for me? Could this really be made-up so she could get out of a wedding? How could I take this physiotherapist seriously when the patient had told me that the pain was getting worse with the SWD? I was now angry with the physiotherapist as well as the college lecturers and the textbooks. I could just as easily have been cross with the patient for not complying with the perspective of the lecturers, the textbooks and the therapist, but strangely I wasn't. I felt quite strongly that I was on her side; she was just reporting what she happened to be feeling at the time.

I went back into the cubicle, explained to the patient that I was going to try a different tactic than the last physiotherapist by using a joint mobilising technique to 'mobilise and free up the joint next to the sore nerve.' I felt I had to explain something, even though I felt it was utter rubbish. I said it with as much belief and enthusiasm as I could muster. The treatment I decided to opt for was a Maitland grade I lumbar rotation with the patient lying on her comfortable side (right). This I performed for 30 seconds and then I got her over onto her back and re-assessed her SLR with my home made inclinometer placed on her tibia. The 'range-to-pain' increase had improved by five degrees! YES! (punch the air Louis...). With that I ushered her up off the couch and ended the session. I recall wondering what she might be thinking after such a long history-taking and examination session (one hour) followed by only a 30 second treatment input. How on earth could doing so pathetically little, to such a seemingly massive problem, have any effect at all? This just could not be correct? On the other hand the SLR was improved and I enthusiastically offered to see her the next day. She was grateful and I relaxed a bit as I watched her rather sadly and awkwardly shuffle away.

This is not an early physiotherapist success story like you get in most 'my therapy' books, but more an early eye-opener that profoundly set the scene for thoughtful and continuing scepticism throughout my career.

I treated her every day for the two week placement and carried on in a similar vein – assessing her SLR, which did improve on a sessional basis, but overall was fluctuating between only 25-30 degrees and 45 degrees! In the end she moved back to the 'SWD-giving' physiotherapist who mustered a sneery smirk when I handed over. I don't think I helped her pain one jot and I never found out how the wedding went or what may have eventually happened.

I now know that she was presenting a whole host of features indicating that she, her tissues and her nervous system, were already in a highly sensitised state; that there was unlikely to be anything hugely wrong and that she was ripe for developing into a chronic pain state. Or, she was just in the slow process of going through a ghastly and very slow 'nerve-root-related-to-disc-extrusion' natural history, before eventually recovering. A main priority for her was far better pain control, something she wasn't getting at all.

Later on in the book there will be discussions of how I have come to feel comfortable and understand many of the puzzling things that Karen's problem revealed. For example: why a deeper understanding of nerve irritation/injury and pain helps make sense of the reality of her pain presentation; why pain can spread so far out of 'classic dermatomes' and why tenderness and sensitivity can be so marked and so widespread; why passive treatment 'modalities' are OK but there is far more to good physiotherapy management; why finding the cause and location of a problem is not always necessary or hugely productive – but that understanding natural history and giving an explanation that makes sense and reassures the patient can be very productive; why seemingly pathetically little input/treatments can have a huge effect in some and not at all in others and so on.

Throughout my professional life patients' presentations have thrown up question after question for me and in those early days, most of them were unanswerable. There was no satisfactory clinical literature to shed any reasonable light on those clinical puzzles and even now it's very sparse. As I have already said, I still wonder if anyone really listens to their patients or hears what they are telling them in an unbiased way. A great deal of this book is about my patients and my observations about them and the best answers I have been able to find to the puzzles and questions that have bothered me along the way. If you have had patients like Karen and felt quite inadequate then I hope some of this can help you!

I want to try and provide the answers that I would like if I were the patient and that I would have liked to have been taught as a keen and budding young physiotherapist.

Chapter 1.2
Vivien in the Volvo

'Science is a broad church full of narrow minds, trained to know ever more about even less.'

Steve Jones, Geneticist and Biologist;
from 'Coral. A pessimist in paradise,' p 6

In the middle of my training I came home to Cornwall and spent six weeks relaxing and enjoying the summer. One Saturday morning the physiotherapy clinic phone rang and my Mum answered the call...

'Yes, yes, right no problem, bring him in now, my son will see him, he's brilliant and he's learnt all the latest techniques...'

My mouth dropped... 'Oh Christ Almighty, oh shit.'

Twenty minutes later I'm looking out the practice window with my white smock top on and this big Volvo estate pulls up with a lady driving.

I thought the patient was going to be a bloke? I opened the entrance door of the clinic and this very posh accent met me.

'He's in the boot dear.' She whipped round to the back of the car.

'Come and see if you can help, he's slipped his disc out again picking up Trago's saddle.' I peer round the back of the car.

'Louis, my name's Vivien, buggered the 'back-to-front', worst ever.'

The dread was now big and real. I could kill my Mum for doing this to me. I've never seen an 'acute back' in my bloody life. (Yes, I'd seen Karen with sciatica for two weeks and I didn't help her). In the NHS there isn't this kind of patient with this kind of pressure. Acute back pain is not on the NHS planet at all. I was secretly wishing I was called Jesus Christ Almighty so I could hold his hand, kiss him on the forehead and say you're cured and then somehow take the money.

Ten minutes later, with the help of Constance (his wife), we managed to get Vivien out of the Volvo and into the treatment room. He wasn't happy. He was panting with pain and rocking about from one side to the other as he stood answering my awkward and seemingly irrelevant questions.

'How's your general health?'

'Do you take steroids?'

'Have you an upper respiratory tract infection?'

I rolled all the questions off because I'd learnt them rote from that little green book we were all advised to get. They were meaningless to me; I hadn't a clue why I was asking them. And so the time rolled on...

'Have you ever had this problem before?' I asked.

'Every bloody season and I always forget to be careful, look can I lie down on the bed a minute.'

'Yes, yes, no problem, how many pillows...' I fumbled around.

To my relief, he settled and relaxed.

'So the pain in your back comes on when you cough and sneeze?'

'It comes on when I fart, when I wink, when I move my foot, when I lift my head, when I bloody think about it.'

I was writing furiously, everything had to be recorded... I daren't tell him to slow down.

'So when do you get it?'

I realised my mistake as he frowned at me.

'Sorry, I meant, how long have you had it for?'

'Since I lifted the nag's saddle this morning ker-pow right to the front.'

'To the front?' I puzzled.

'Yup, feels like my back is pushing my bladder half out of my Todger and half out of my navel.'

(Yet more 'text book stuff' I sarcastically thought).

Eventually I'd dried up with all the questions and asked him to take some things off so that I could see what was going on.

... More struggling and grunting, finally he was perched on the side of the plinth and panting. Gut hanging, sweaty armpits, saggy air-holey pants with much of the tragic contents unaware they were out and about...

... More frowns, more pain and distress.

What to do?

Start simple, 'Can you bend forward at all Vivien?'

He looked at the floor but didn't otherwise move.

'No,'

'Oh, right, backwards?'

His eyes rolled up...

'No.'

'What about side to side like this?'

'Doubt it, hang on... No.'

And so it went on. No back movements at all and plenty of refusals to move – just like his bloody horse 'Trago' I thought to myself. Head flexion increased the pain, so did foot dorsiflexion, so did farting no doubt if we'd had chance to test it.

Why was I getting cross internally with the guy?

He lay down on his side, the pain was all over his back. And, just like with Karen, everything hurt and, just like with Karen, I felt cross – with my Mum, with my training, with the textbooks, with the whole thing, it was all crap.

Back to Maitland rules and the famous 'SIN': this was the diagnosis for me, 'SIN' – with all the capitals spelling 'Severity', 'Irritability' and 'Nature'. This had the lot. I felt like jumping on him and running away, but no, calm it Louis, the rules were that when SIN is high you should use low force.

'You've really fired up your back I think. Let's see if I can get it going for you.'

'Do what you like Louis, I'm shooting tomorrow with a crowd from the office.'

I then got him on his side and did 30-45 seconds of grade I lumbar rotation, (by now my favourite/fall-back technique). I wanted to close my eyes and try and send some magic force into him, some kind of hand prayer but I couldn't bring myself to. I did what I was taught – ask about the symptoms as I gently wobbled his pelvis and his back.'

'Where's the pain now Vivien?'

'Todger,' he informed me.

'Right.'

20 seconds later... 'still Todger?'

'Todger and navel now.'

20 seconds later, I stopped.

'Let's have a look now, come and stand again.'

Up he came, grunt-groan-wince-whine. There he perched once more.

'Right, can you try a bend?'

His eyes rolled down...

'No.'

'Backwards?'

'No.'

'How's the pain now?'

'Same.' He frowned.

That word was so harsh, so abrupt. Such a flat monotone, that seemed to be accompanied by a huge dagger attached to it that sort of cut into pieces and minced and messed up your whole career, (together with its bloody airy-fairy ethos and fragile and naive psychology).

It's not supposed to be the same, the rules and the fancy patient histories in the Maitland book say it should have changed. I thought and wished.

'Right, that's all I'm going to do today, let's see you again tomorrow morning before the shoot if you can make it.'

He looked shocked. The look said, 'If you want me to pay for that, you're out of your mind.'

I opened the door and together with Constance we bundled him carefully into the back of the Volvo again.

'Take it easy I think is best,' I offered.

The door slammed. I felt crap. That was 100% hopeless. That was my first private patient experience!

The next day the car pulled up, Sunday morning, 8.30am. He was driving! Vivien jumped out the car, strolled up to me and gave me the £12.00 fee from the day before.

'I don't know what the bloody hell you did to me yesterday, but within an hour I was 50% better and this morning it was gone.' There was a pause and then he said with a smile, 'Miracle man!'

I smiled, relieved more than anything, but in truth I was deeply puzzled – hey, that guy who walked on water did things like this.

Well great, he thanked me, but how on earth did the pathetic little bit of jiggling I did to him make the pain go away like that?

Rather than think I was all powerful (which probably would have been a lot easier), or the patient was 'psychological' (as many Drs might think), I wanted a better explanation and they do exist.

Thoughts...

Early experience with patients like Karen and Vivien provided the seeds for a reasonably rational, but life-long, medical scepticism and, mistrust of famous 'guru' practitioners and 'authorities' that physiotherapy and medicine in general, seems to be saddled with. I'm suspicious of practitioners who make unbending rules about treatments that are taken as proven truths and woe betide anyone who perks up with any kind of challenge.

Down with their dogma and up with reasoning based on sound scientific findings and well reasoned theories! But keep an open mind to any possibility!

For me the best thing about science is the scepticism component of it. For this reason I would like you to feel quite comfortable to be critical and sceptical about the contents of this book. Say what you like, think what you like. As I used to say on all my courses – take what you like and leave what you do not. If some of this book makes you think, helps you understand and ask better questions, helps you explain something to your patient or to answer their questions well, or helps you to be a more proficient and understanding practitioner, then my purpose in writing is fulfilled. While pain can be horrid for the sufferer, the reasoning and unravelling of it can be fun for the practitioner. Most pain sufferers improve and we can help their journey to recovery be a more efficient one – without too much of the bull-shit.

My early experiences with patients like Karen and Vivien left me wanting to know more, for example, about:

- Sciatica and nerve root pain – is it always so crazy, where did the authors of the standard texts get their information about nerve root pain from?

- Why does pain spread so far?

- Why tissues that look and feel quite normal can be so sensitive and hurt so much?

- Why everything can hurt very badly and how this situation can rapidly change?

- Why doing 'little' treatments can sometimes have a huge effect yet at other times do virtually nothing or even make the situation worse?

- Why pathetic little pressures can produce a massive amount of pain and a massive spread of pain?

- The effect of pain on the individual?

- The reason why I had to ask so many questions and what the information meant for me and for the patient?

- What the various physical tests meant in terms of the tissues tested and what I could do in terms of treatment?

In addition to a growing list like that above, I also realised that I wanted to be able to:

- explain the problem to patients and be able to answer any question they asked with confidence

- give the patients an understanding of their recovery process

- feel comfortable with anything that I was presented with.

But back then it was early days; I still had to get more proficient with patients; I had to learn more skills – in particular physical examination skills and manual therapy skills and manipulation, because at the heart of physiotherapy then was confident touch and handling. So to finish this section, setting the scene, there's one more patient story about manipulation. It's also a story about my late Dad who had great hands and liked to manipulate everything. He was brilliant at diagnosis, what today we call identifying red-flags, he was also brilliant at giving patients confidence – that they were OK to move, that they could move and that it was good to move. He died before I started my physiotherapy training but he knew what I was going to do.

Chapter 1.3
Wersey's manipulation

'Is that hurting you Boss, I can't feel a thing!'

Vernon Gifford (1918-1978), while performing a technique on a patient. He was a Physiotherapist and a human, human.

'Your Father used to tell you this filthy joke and while you were laughing he'd flick your neck around and there'd be this almighty ripple of cracks—for some reason it made you want to say 'Hang on I wasn't ready for that'— but it was all over with. There was always laughter in that place.'

A patient of my Father's recounting experiences
with him at Falmouth Hospital (c.1970)

While doing relatively little in the way of treatment to Vivien and having a huge success might have left many practitioners feeling really good about what they had done, it left me, as I said, feeling pretty uncomfortable. I couldn't get away with doing that again. People come for treatment and expect something to be done. Surely it's more logical that you have to do something big to achieve something big?

Manipulation of the neck and making huge cracks and clicks is something big. It takes a lot of guts to do a technique to a human's neck that for centuries has been used by gamekeepers to quickly dispatch rabbits. Never fear. If others do it, so could I!

In those early days, because I'd already witnessed Wersey's manipulation (more of his story in a moment), I liked the idea of learning an impressive skill and being able to confidently apply it to patients. I look back now and I realise that as soon as I felt I could get away with full-on-manipulating from my college tutors and the senior staff responsible for me, I got carried away with it, but I'm grateful. If you don't try something you cannot comment on it and you cannot reach any conclusions. Manipulation of the spine has been around for centuries and people keep doing it and having it done, so it must be of some value? I must admit that back then I had the impression that 'clicking' a joint, especially a spinal joint, produced miracle results. We've all heard it, 'I walked in bent double – had my disc put back in and I ran out!'

Years of subsequent experience, and listening to patients, has made me realise that this 'miracle' is far nearer the fictitious than the fact.

I have my late father to thank. Sadly he died too young at 59 years old back in 1978. He was a physiotherapist who had learnt manipulation from bone-setters and osteopaths long before there was ever any formal training in it and when, for the most part, it was frowned upon by the physiotherapy profession. Dad was a natural, flamboyant operator who cracked jokes and joints and communicated with an infective ability which resulted in a profound relaxation and trust—the 'art' of physiotherapy and the effective artist—brilliant. He was my Hero and still is.

When I was seventeen I witnessed him manipulate a fellow's neck in a local pub. The man, Wersey, a Cornishman, approached my Dad and said simply,

'You're Mr Gifford from the hospital aren't you? Well, I've had this horrible neck pain for three years, look.'

He pointed to his neck, and moved it stiffly about ten degrees right and left, and winced. Moments later the fellow was on the floor and my Dad was kneeling above him with his neck and head in his hands. The pub had gone silent; all eyes were on the show.

Wersey's eyes closed and my Dad worked his neck slowly and smoothly, right and left, until after a few moments there was a rapid flick and a loud click which made the guys in rest of the pub gasp. Wersey's legs shot up and then down again. 'Shit!' he cried and laughed at the same time. Immediately my Dad said, 'Who's farted?' And the whole pub screamed in laughter and then the crack went the other way just when we all didn't expect it. 'You bastard!' Wersey yelled and the pub just kept on laughing. The fellow rolled over, tears of laughter in his eyes and my Dad sat back down. He could have bowed for the performance, I was open-mouthed, but that wasn't it. The fellow gradually got to his feet and slowly and repeatedly turned his head right and left, each time a little more than the last time until, with the pub cheering and clapping he almost put his chin on his shoulder.

Well, what was that? Gross professional mis-conduct, no doubt! Dad asked no questions, he did no special tests, he just relaxed the guy and cracked his neck off – just like millions of Indian barbers do to millions of their clients after cutting their hair, day-in-day-out, without any report of adverse reactions that I have heard of (now there's a good research project!).

So why didn't I put Vivien on his side, crank him over into full rotation and give his back a quick flick and a crack? And what a huge contrast; me, with Vivien spending around an hour questioning and examining and then doing a little bit of flesh wobbling; and my Dad, no questions and no examining, bar feeling Wersey's neck tension as he massaged and moved it about, and then two almighty cracks. Both got better via vastly different paths. With Vivien I did what I had been taught to do and conformed to the indoctrinated SIN that I'd been taught. With the experience of Vivien and Karen, and the memory of my Dad with Wersey, I knew I was going to have to be a bit of a rebel. However, I still wanted to be a good manual physiotherapist and I was prepared to study hard and sponsor my own education.

In Sheffield, Robbie Blake had introduced me to the 'Maitland' approach to treating painful musculoskeletal problems and I practiced all the techniques I was shown and others I learnt from any manipulation book I could find[1]. As a student I was lucky to learn more manual therapy from Asoka Jaywardena on my 'out-patient' rotation at Mansfield City hospital. Asoka, like Robbie, had been learning manual therapy by doing the various Maitland based 'Manipulation Association of Chartered Physiotherapy' courses. It was he who told me about Paul Chadwick and Peter Wells – two UK physiotherapists who had been to Australia and done the 'Manips' course in Adelaide – learning from Geoff Maitland himself. In the following three years after qualifying I was lucky enough to get work with these well known physiotherapists and learn first-hand some of what they had been taught.

Also, while a student I learnt how to do 'proper' Wersey style manipulations from a physiotherapist called Akram who was the head of physiotherapy 'out-patients' at Doncaster Royal Infirmary. Like my Dad, Akram had those magic manipulation hands. He 'whopped' virtually everything and so did I while I was there. It was fun and it taught me that even when a problem can be deemed to have very high 'SIN' in Maitland terms – it can still take a nicely performed manipulation. That was one rule shattered and I hadn't even qualified! The sense of freedom working and learning with Akram was uplifting.

---

1 - I still have copies of my Dad's Alan Stoddard and James Mennell books –
see 'Read what I've read' at the end of the chapter.

Section 1
Read what I've read

Cyriax J. (1978) Textbook of Orthopaedic Medicine Volume 1. Bailliere Tindall. London.

Cyriax J., Russell G. (1977) Textbook of Orthopaedic Medicine Volume 2. Bailliere Tindall. London.

Maitland G. D. (1978) Vertebral Manipulation (1st Ed). Butterworths. London.

Maitland G. D. (1986) Vertebral Manipulation (2nd Ed). Butterworths. London.

Mennell J. (1952) The Science and Art of Joint Manipulation. Vol 2. The spinal column. J&A Churchill Ltd. London.

Stoddard A. (1969) Manual of Osteopathic Technique. Hutchinson Medical. London.

Stoddard A. (1977) Manual of Osteopathic Practice. Hutchinson Medical. London.

Section 2

BEFORE AUSTRALIA

Chapter 2.1
Treatment formulas, whims and force. Cyriax v Maitland

Faith is the great cop-out, the great excuse to evade the need to think and evaluate evidence. Faith is belief in spite of, even perhaps because of, the lack of evidence.

Richard Dawkins

Experiences with my Mum and Dad before I trained, then, while training with tutors Robbie Blake and Ted Morgan Jones and on placements with Akram and Asoka Jaywardena eventually faired me well for my early out-patient manual therapy experiences. I was getting the hang of the Maitland system at last and I was learning and practicing loads of techniques.

But it went like this at first: take a prolonged history/subjective exam, do a prolonged physical exam (45-60 minutes go by in a flash), then quickly whip out of the cubicle to grab the battered copy of 'Maitland's vertebral mobilisation' book and check out the case histories in the back. If any sounded anything like the patient I'd note the techniques used and then whip back into the patient and perform the technique. What I really wanted was to find a nice list of signs and symptoms neatly laid out so as to define the problem (the disease/the pathology/the fault/the cause)... and then to provide the appropriate treatment approach or technique. This of course, is the essence of a 'biomedical approach' and it is formulaic:

1. Symptoms plus physical signs/findings
   = describes the injury, disorder or disease.

2. Identification of the injury/disorder/disease is then done by looking up the symptoms and signs in an appropriate medical text which usually goes on to provide details of the treatment required.
   Every diagnosis gets more or less the same treatment.

3. Sometimes there are competing treatments and each clinician's decision is governed by 'what works best for him.'

It didn't really work though, as I've already shown in section 1 none of the patients in Maitland's (or Cyriax's) books were anything like the ones I saw in the UK NHS system, or even in the private system (Vivien!) and the occasional ones that were somewhere near it never responded in the way Maitland described. The case histories all seemed so bitty, with no common features or common linking patterns which I was sure there had to be. Looking back I now realise that this was when it was beginning to dawn on me how magnificently 'unreliable' pain could be.

In reality the results I had with treatment were quite random and unimpressive. But at the time, doing something to a patient and then observing an immediate increase in a few degrees of pain-free range during the re-examination, was the thrill that made it all worthwhile and made you think you had to be helping. The thing that frustrated me for a very long time was that I hadn't a clue as to what was going on in the vast majority of patients. In particular, I couldn't answer their perfectly reasonable but very awkward questions!

I amassed tons of information from the history and physical examination and then merely applied the simple Maitland treatment formula derived from SIN, the laterality of the pain (was it one sided or evenly distributed from one side to the other) and a 'comparable sign' (some structure not in the area of pain, but which could refer to it, and which was found to 'just maybe' have a bit more stiffness or be a tad more tender than it 'should' be). What was the point of all that information? I got it all because it was on the list of what to get.

The whole Maitland thing was formulaic too, but didn't seem quite so tightly controlled as in the treatment and management of purer 'medical' problems, e.g. for diabetes the treatment is – this and only this. The Maitland system, as I interpreted it, applied a treatment formula to pain of musculoskeletal origins without the requirement of a diagnosis or any notion of what was causing the problem and how long it might go on for – its natural history. I came to see this as quite shocking.

I often wondered if all that 'subjective' information was really required. If all you do is apply a 'SIN/laterality/comparable sign' formula, surely all that is required is that you ask where the pain is located, find out how severe and reactive it is, check the facet joints proximally, have a feel and do a few little movement tests and then apply the appropriate direction and grade of manual treatment from there.

Well – yes! It should also mean that for any one problem, when then passed around several different Maitland trained therapists, that they should all end up doing more or less the same thing. The cynic in me doubts that this would ever happen and I don't know of anyone brave enough to do the simple piece of research required (called 'pass the patient!'). Even back then, with these sorts of naughty thoughts, I also tended to feel that the outcome of the treatment technique would be more a result of; who was doing it, how they got on with the patient and how well the treatment was done – *as far as the patient was concerned*.

Wersey and many of Akram's patients were somewhere in the back of my mind most of the time. They were treated without any reference to 'severity,' 'irritability' and 'nature', in fact the amount of questioning was minimal and why wouldn't it be – if the operator does virtually the same thing to every patient! When you go to the barber's you get a haircut. When you go to Akram, he'll handle you nicely until it cracks-off. Many patients that Akram saw may well have been deemed to have highly reactive pain but were tackled using end-range-high-velocity, but beautifully done, techniques, and yet they still survived and apparently did well! If the rules could be broken, what was the point of them? Akram wasn't inhibited by knowledge, listening and reasoning-generated fear.[1]

The contrast in force used between what the proponents of the Maitland approach advocated (gentle) and those using Cyriax's methods was startling. In his books Jimmy Cyriax has pictures of himself 'tractioning' a patient's neck, using as much pulling force of his quite large frame as he could muster and then doing a rotation manipulation to 'reduce' a disc (Cyriax 1977 and 1978). Two physios or nurses often held the patient to stop them sliding off the couch! Interestingly, these were the techniques that Robin McKenzie advocated to reduce 'derangements' when his exercises failed to work and that I witnessed him do when I did his courses in London in 1983.

---

1 - IMPORTANT: *The experienced, the inexperienced and those who haven't been trained in the use of 'high velocity' manipulation should be aware of the dangers. Edzard Ernst, well known for his high quality research in the area of alternative medicine, has published a systematic review of chiropractic manipulation causing death. See:* Ernst E 2010 Deaths after Chiropractic: A review of published cases. Int J Clin Pract 64(10):1162-65. *His conclusion: 'Numerous deaths have occurred after chiropractic manipulations. The risks of this treatment by far outweigh its benefit. I strongly recommend an internet session using the research term: 'death by chiropractic adjustment.' Stick to 'death by chocolate.'*

My gathering thoughts back then were: firstly, that the human back and neck are incredibly strong, even when they hurt quite badly and secondly, that notions of 'mechanical' faults, presumed from diagnosis then required strong forces in order to have any impact with treatment. How on earth could a gentle Maitland grade I or II technique (remember Karen and Vivien in the Volvo) impact on a 'cervical disc' disorder? The logic and reasoning here is that a degree of force is a significant requirement?

This seemed to be a field of medicine/therapy that was, almost worryingly, biased towards guesswork, whims and weird personal belief systems, rather than anything rational or reasonable. I still plugged on with it though – there wasn't anything else on offer!

After qualifying in summer 1981, I was lucky enough to get my first basic grade (junior) rotation post at Walton Hospital in Liverpool. Paul Chadwick worked there. Paul also worked with Liverpool football club and was nurturing his private practice. Good stuff, we smoked cigars in the 'crutch' cupboard at break times and I learnt yet more 'Maitland'. Paul had been over to Adelaide in South Australia and done the 'Maitland' post graduate manipulation course with the great man himself. I was now getting it nearly first hand! Paul had big, strong, soft hands and used a lot of manipulation and his mobilisations always felt good. He seemed far more confident and clued in than many of the others. I knew then that it was important for me to go to Adelaide if I could.

Paul ran regular in-service training sessions with the staff and we learnt heaps. He started teaching us about syndromes. This was interesting, at last, recognisable patterns of symptoms that had some kind of explanation. But I still wanted to know more about causes and most of the time those syndromes were still best left on the piece of paper they were written on.

In our profession syndromes are more often attached to a bit of anatomy, for example, piriformis, carpal tunnel, T4, phantom limb, cervical disc, cervical root... syndromes. Then there's a pain clinician's favourite – complex regional pain syndrome (CRPS) and on it goes. The key thing is that there's usually no clear connection to proven pathology with syndromes – so it's OK to challenge them if you want.

Chapter 2.2
Mary, Sue and then me.

'Recovery is the project of heart and mind. The person, not his or her autonomous brain, is the agent of recovery.'

Sally Satel and Scott Lilienfeld from the book 'Brainwashed' 2013

I quite liked basic grade rotational physiotherapy. You get to see loads of different conditions, you learn about their presentations and, you never forget. I learned to love physiotherapy 'rehab' at Walton Hospital, Liverpool. Rehabilitation is the most basic and fundamental thing that's special to physiotherapy, I think we need to appreciate it more.

Thanks to Shirley Orme, the senior orthopaedic physiotherapist, who, among a great many other things, showed me how to teach a young orthopaedic patient quadriceps exercises; get him confident and then get him up and out of bed for his first walk for four weeks, without him giving even a wimper. It was then that I realised the importance of simple communication, quiet encouragement and physiotherapist confidence. For example, you can't get anywhere unless *you know*, and the *patient knows*, it's safe to proceed. Also, you can't get anywhere until the patient wants to.

No wonder applying someone else's formula is unlikely to succeed!

Mary's story

What follows is a success story.

On Shirley's orthopaedic ward it was often easy to observe other physios at work.

Mary was in her mid 60's and was due to be mobilised after a right hip replacement. Sue was the student physio, about to do this task and I was just across the aisle outside a cubicle waiting for my next patient, Hilda, to finish on a bed-pan.

Sue was very nervous. She fumbled about Mary's bed; she didn't make good eye contact; she banged about with the zimmer frame and forgot to draw the curtains round properly. I could see Mary was frowning.

Sue started... 'I've checked your notes and talked to the Dr and they say your knee operation was a great success and it's time to get up and try a bit of a walk with me.'

'I'm Mary Ferris,' said Mary with a very stern voice... then... 'What ... and who... are you supposed to be?'

Mary Ferris was really quite a posh 'la-de-dah' type for Liverpool!

Sue was bright red and managed to blurt... 'I'm Sue and I'm a student physiotherapist, sorry, I should have introduced myself.'

There was a pause and a bit of a smile followed by a frown.

'Did you say get up because of my knee operation just now?'

'Yes, I did.'

'Whose notes have you been reading then?'

'Yours, of course Mrs Ferris.'

'Wonderful, well the knee operation has completely healed up and is doing fine.'

She pulled up her night gown to reveal her normal knees.

'It's my hip. I've had a new hip dear... '

Sue blushed more horribly red and I winced and looked the other way. After another 2-3 minutes of apologising and squirming, Sue got back to the need for a walk. Mary dug in...

'That's the first I've heard... the maestro said it would be three days before I'm about ready and that he'd need to check it first.'

There was a pause and then she went on,

'Look dear, I can't even bend it, how am I going to walk if I can't bend it?'

'We've got to have a go otherwise you'll get clots, which could even kill you.'

I couldn't believe what I was hearing. And at the same moment Sue was pulling Mary's legs over the side of the bed and rotating her round to sit with legs dependent.

Mary now looked scared stiff and Sue was quite oblivious, she was almost chatting away to herself...

'That's right, deep breaths, try and relax, slide forward now and hold the frame, feel the floor, you'll be fine...' Sue was pulling at her.

Mary was gripped with fear and her whole being was tensed and resisting.

'Look love, put me back, I'm going to faint.' She gargled a bit and was moaning as I quickly came over to help and we got her safely back and comfortable.

Sue thanked me and said to Mary she'd come again the following morning and have another go. I went back over to Hilda and I spied Mary with a little tear in her eye.

Later that morning, Shirley asked if I could have a go at getting Mary up in the afternoon. 'Spend some time chatting with her and examine and move her leg before you do any standing, see if you can reassure her.'

Hmm, she's already anti-physio I thought. I read her notes at length and had a look at all the x-rays.

I went to see her with low expectations, just have a chat and see how things developed, any problems and I'd call my Shirley-the-cavalry in.

I wandered over.

'Mrs Ferris, I'm Louis, I met you this morning after you felt a bit faint, are you a bit better now?'

'I'm fine dear.'

'Can I sit down?'

'Help yourself.' There was a pause and she eyed me up and down.

'You don't look like a student.'

'I'm not, but I've only just qualified. I'm a bit older because I've done a bit of travelling before my physio training.' We talked a bit about my West Africa adventures and about Cornwall too. It turned out that she'd spent some time in Bude, North Cornwall and she'd enjoyed the great coastal walks.

After a while I said, 'How did the operation go?'

She said she liked the 'maestro' and that he must have done a good job, but that she was still at a bit of a loss to understand how the operation he'd done on her hip was going to help her thigh and knee pain. It turned out that she'd never had any pain around the hip area.

'Can you explain to me why he didn't operate on the knee Louis?'

'Well Mary, I've had a good look at your notes and x-rays and the main thing is that your hip had quite bad arthritis, yet, your knee looks very good. Also, all the observations and physical tests that the Drs have done repeatedly show that your hip was responsible for the pain.'

'What do you mean observations and physical tests?' she said.

'Well, when they observed you walking, you rolled from side to side a bit which is typical of a hip problem, not a knee. I got up and said, 'You may have walked a bit like this.' I proceeded to walk round the bed with a typical OA hip roll. She smiled. 'You've got me exactly!'

'Also, when they moved your hip to feel it, you'd get your thigh and knee pain. It's called referred pain – meaning, where you feel the pain isn't where it's coming from.'

Mary sighed.

'Why didn't someone tell me all this before?'

I expect someone probably had, but the key thing was that she hadn't heard it or taken it on-board.

I just raised my eyebrows to acknowledge her point and then said, 'Well, if they got it right you're going to be better when you get going again.'

She acknowledged my point and we chatted on and pretty soon we were doing some leg exercises together. She was now bending the leg well to about 30-45 degrees and I then told her that the surgeon, her maestro, was keen for her to get some weight through the leg and start walking today – he'd written the request in her notes.

'Well, why did he tell me that he'd see me and I'd be up in three days not two?'

'I think he said that because he thought you might be a pit poorly after the operation, but because you're so well, he's keen to get you moving.'

Mary nodded and smiled.

'Stop me dying of some blood clot, eh?' she quizzed with a little smirk.

I smiled, and stage by stage we went about the process of sitting up, grabbing the zimmer and standing. With lots of chat and giggles she gradually got going and then walked well with the frame. She was so pleased with what she'd done.

I winked at her and she pulled me close and whispered, 'I think I'm going to do well, thanks.'

I gave her a little hug and a peck on the cheek. 'Yes you are... '

Brilliant, little did I know it then, but years later I was to realise that Mary's walk, her 'rehab', held just about all the vital elements of all good pain treatment and management processes.

For now, see that the interaction process is likely a very natural one. Any caring person who acts naturally with someone who is not able or is not well, will tend to talk and discuss, listen and empathise, explain and encourage, and take the time required – before they start 'doing' anything with them. For the last few years I have been calling it, **'top-down before bottom-up'**, simply meaning, deal with the person (top-down) before performing any physical process like rehab or treatment (bottom-up). Bottom-up without top-down gets poor results, often makes patients worse and rarely helps get them better. Sue's attempts with Mary and my wish to fit the patient to the case history in Maitland's book are good examples of bottom-up without top-down.

Later chapters will look at top-down and bottom-up in more detail.

Walton hospital gave me plenty of good early basic-grade physio experience, but from the pain perspective I came to realise that there were two important things:

1. That purely to treat pain you don't have to know what is wrong or where the pain is coming from, even though you like to think you do. As unnerving as this may seem, it still holds true today, some thirty plus years on. I often say at the beginning of my lectures that if one patient with some form of musculoskeletal pain went to ten different practitioners they'd get ten different diagnoses, ten different forms of advice and ten different treatments, all of which could well be successful. True? Maybe? I reckon it is and it's a good research project perhaps, all you have to do is find a few willing volunteers to go to the ten different practitioners.

    The point, in some ways, is that Maitland's famous 'brick wall' has it all. On one side of it are the signs and symptoms; what the patient tells you about their problem and about their pain; combined with what you find out about it during the physical examination and this is what you treat. On the other side of the 'brick wall' is all the theory, things like the pathology, the pathophysiology, the syndrome, the disease, the biomechanics and the anatomy. Things that Maitland acknowledged but fiercely argued should not drive treatment decisions. Having said that he did say that his 'brick wall' was permeable – in other words information from one side can diffuse across to the other and influence it. Exactly.

    Very wise stuff and still appropriate to a degree today so long as you're not mucking about with someone who has something seriously wrong and you've missed it, or you're failing to give the patient an opportunity at a medical approach that has a proven track record. My current spin on pure pain relief treatment, so long as what you do is safe and not ripping the patient off, is this: **if it works, do it!** Try not to be cornered and stymied by your own narrow beliefs and prejudices towards your favourite treatment method and the (usually) questionable/untested theories that surround it.

Since it seems that pain can sometimes be helped by almost anything, being a one technique/one exercise approach/one management approach pain therapist may be missing a great deal. But the biggest point of all, which I didn't really come to appreciate until a little later on in my career, was that just focusing on pain relief, is nowhere near enough for the patient in pain. As we now know and will be discussed further later on, it can be a totally wrong thing to do with some patients.

Mary, my hip patient above, we didn't even mention pain, we just got on with getting her moving, standing and walking! Think about it – two days before I did all this the surgeon had cut her leg half off, sawn through her greater trochanter and thrown away the neck and head of the femur, bored a hole down through the shaft of the femur that was left, filled it with glue and then banged home a 'new' metal one... Now if that isn't nociception! What's all this crap about severity and irritability and nature in this scenario? Bonkers!

2. That I wanted to know more about the theory. Why? Because if something is wrong with me, I want to know about it. I want to understand it and be well informed and above all I want it to make sense. I want an explanation and this is what I believe many patients want too; they want the feeling of being in control somehow. Knowledge can, very powerfully, help a patient feel more in control. Mary for example wanted it, she had her questions, and it helped her to get going feeling confident; but Wersey wasn't at all concerned, he just trusted my Dad who had a reputation and who could have done anything! We are all different and as therapists we need to be able to adapt to whoever we meet as patients.

So, I wanted to make sense of a great many seemingly impossible pain presentations that I had already witnessed. I believed that somewhere there had to be some kind of rational explanation. 'A facet joint' or a 'trapped or stuck nerve' was just not good enough. This desire to find out more and explain it better was to dominate much of my professional career.

After about eight or nine months in Liverpool, Philippa and I moved to London. Philippa got a post at Queen Mary's Hospital in Roehampton and I got one at St Stephen's Hospital where Peter Wells was superintendent of the physiotherapy department. I was over the moon; it was the hot summer of 1982 in Chelsea on the Fulham Road! Back then and for many years after I left, St Stephen's was one of the big strong-holds of manual physiotherapy in the UK and there were lots of MACPs (Manipulation Association of Chartered Physiotherapists). I was in amongst them! Peter had been over to Adelaide, as Paul Chadwick had done, and was widely regarded as an outstanding manual therapy teacher. I was lucky to get the job and it was great. I learnt so much from Peter, as well as from Joan Blair, Agneta Lando and Geoff Boyling who joined the staff after I did. We had plenty of in-service teaching and training and lots of help with difficult patients. I was now reading as much as I could by quietly borrowing articles and books from Peter's office as well as starting to look out my own in the hospital library. I also read Stoddard, Grieve, Maitland, Kaltenborn, Cyriax and much more.

This was also the time of the 'slump' and the early 'upper limb tension test' or 'the brachial tension test of Elvey' as it was called back then. It was a time when I learnt a great deal about the use of force and it was a time when I was starting to see patterns of clinical presentations emerging.

Chapter 2.3
Trevor's slump

'It is almost impossible to replace widely accepted medical dogmas, especially where the paradigm being challenged has to be replaced with a more complicated one!'

Pat Wall (1925-2001), Pain Scientist and a friend of
Physiotherapy and the Physiotherapy Pain Association

Up to now I'd believed that Cyriax used all the force and Maitland was gentle. Not anymore.

Here is a patient problem that crops up again and again: the young to middle-aged patient with a sciatica that has moved on from the horrid acute phase and left them with nagging leg ache, a bit of a lumbar shift and the inability to bend forward very far, and when they do, the back twists and there's often a deviation away from the midline. There may or may not be clear neurological signs but the key feature is a 'stuck' straight leg raise (SLR) that provokes the pain and a similarly positive slump test (Maitland 1979). Here, knee extension phase is markedly limited, and symptoms can often be increased or decreased by neck flexion/extension and foot dorsi/plantar flexion. The 'end-feel' of knee extension is of significant tightness and like the SLR it feels pretty much stuck solid. Adduct the leg during 'slump knee extension' or SLR and the pain gets much worse. Abduct it to ease it right out.

Trevor, with his on-going sciatica down the right leg, was in with me. This was the second treatment and the assessment and first tentative treatment I'd done had made little difference. I got him to undress and re-examined some of the physical 'asterisks'[1]. He stood with a slight shift to the right. Forward bending, he deviated towards the right leg and stopped, being barely able to reach his knees before his knees flexed; extension was reasonable but brought on a bit of buttock and calf pain, side bending to the left was markedly limited and pulled a bit in the leg, while to the right it tweaked the buttock pain. SLR on the right was 40 degrees and 'solid'. Pain response was increased by the 'tension' increasing manoeuvres of foot dorsiflexion and hip adduction. The slump test was similarly limited having lost about 40 degrees of knee extension. It was 'SOLID' too.

I began treatment with SLRs – me up on the couch with my right knee holding down his left leg while I pushed his SLR up with my left shoulder. I heaved it slowly up into a solid end-feel.

'How you doin'?'

'Right down me friggin' leg.' Trev was frowning.

'OK, push down on my shoulder with your foot, try and push against my pressure... that's it, harder if you can... hoooold... hooold... hooooold and... let go, relax now.'

I pushed on, we were up to about 55 degrees and he was groaning a bit.

'Once more Trev, hoooollddd it, puuuush, come on... haaaarder ... hooooold it... and... let go'

I pushed on to about 65 degrees and he didn't relax much. In fact his body was twisting against me and his left leg was trying to come up. We were both sweating and he's going...

'Uhhh, uhhh, shit, shit, uhhh...'

I come down an inch and we all relax.

---

1 - *Physical 'asterisks' is a term used by Maitland for physical test findings that are deemed important in management.*

There's a deathly silence from the surrounding cubicles. I quietly wish for a sound-proof room. I imagine that for the patients in the nearby cubicles it's like the feeling you get when you're in the birthing room with your wife, when she gets her first mild contractions and swears a bit under her breath and then there's this almighty agonising scream from the birthing room next door... 'Holy fucking Jesus, fucking, fucking, fucking, fucking Chriiiiiiiiiistttttttttttttttttttttt...................' Hearing other people in agony makes you feel really sick. In childbirth it's far easier to witness it and be involved a bit than be next door.

On I go regardless with Trevor, accept what they're all feeling, but I'm getting somewhere...

'Once more now let's go, then we'll stand up and see what's happening.'

He looked resigned to it. We repeated the whole thing twice more and then I got him up and looked at his forward bend.

'Yup, straighter and you're going further Trev.' I said.

'Yeah?' he retorted, a bit sarcastically I thought?

I was pleased he'd improved his forward bend by two inches.

'This is improving well. What I'd like to do now, is do the stretch while you're sitting in the slump position rather than lying, is that OK with you?'

'I guess so, if it has to be done', he said in a rather resigned sort of way.

I was pleased; this was my first strong 'slump technique' on my own patient. I'd only helped others in the department and seen what was needed. I leaned my head out of the cubicle curtains raising my voice a bit...

'Anyone got a minute for a slump...?'

Ten seconds later two faces appeared round the curtains from nearby cubicles and then quickly gathered round the sitting Trevor. He hadn't a chance. Joan jumped up on the couch behind him and pressed down on his shoulders holding him slumped, Jo got up next to his right leg and placed her knee on top of his leg and said, 'I'll time, how long to start?'

Joan piped in, 'First time?'

'Yup.'

'45 secs and see how we go?'

'OK, let's go.'

Joan pushed down on his shoulders and then pushed his head forward, chin more or less to chest. Jo checked her watch and I extended his leg into some good resistance.

'Alright Trev, let us know how you're doing or if you want to stop?' I said.

He just grunted and expired with a groan. We carried on... 25, 26, 27... 30, 31, 32 seconds...

I pulled and pulled, Trev groaned, the others hung on as Trevor was straining against them. Finally 45 secs was reached and they all leaped off and looked at him.

'Again?' Joan said.

'I'll re-test first.'

Up came Trev and forward he went. Brilliant: four inches below his knees, less deviation to the right until the last bit.

'Once more Trev?' I checked and Joan replied with a big friendly smile,

'Yes, come on you can do it, you're doing really well, won't take long, quick before you think about it too long...' then in her very Scottish way... 'This place isn't for wimps...'

Trev managed a frowning smile and let us go at him again.

Up he went, back on the plinth and again we pinned and jammed him into place. Pressure on. Then up with the leg. This time I got the knee fully extended. The tension in his body was staggering, another inch with his knee and he would have sprung us off him I'm sure. The human body's capacity to withstand force is incredible, even when it's in pain and not 100%. The nerve's capacity to withstand force is incredible too.

We gained about another inch and Jo and Joan dutifully went back to their own patients.

Trevor kept coming for about five weeks. I saw him twice a week. The range of movement maintained but never really got a great deal further than what was achieved at the end of that first session. Treatment stopped because progress had plateaued, yet I saw it as a success. Years later, when I had the chance to observe these sorts of problems over longer time frames (a year or more), I realised that expecting large changes so quickly was unnecessary as they generally gradually improved without the need for such force. I also thought to myself that there'd be no way, if it were me, that I'd let anyone stretch it like that! I'd rather live with the tight leg and the wonky bend and have my nerve still intact and it's my opinion that most do.

I will revisit nerve root problems in more detail in a later chapter (see Nerve Root section). For now, an important element of a pain presentation is having an understanding of natural history – the time frame of recovery. Sometimes recovery takes a long time. Think frozen shoulder for example. Stubborn SLR/slump limited presentations may take similar lengths of time and some are unlikely to ever get full range back.

I saw and treated many more patients like Trevor. I got confident about using plenty of force and came to appreciate that most humans, even when they are in a great deal of pain, are still very strong structures! One drawback, which I didn't come to realise until later, was that the view of pain at the time was very much dominated by 'mechanical' thinking and reasoning. For example, on-going sciatica was viewed as a stuck nerve and that freeing it by stretching and manipulation would solve the problem.

I agonised with what to do when patients presented with lots of pain, yet very little, if any, movement restrictions, and there's plenty of them. What do you treat? The answer back then was simply, that if you really looked you could always find something in about the right place that was 'stiff' in some way, and that was what you focused on treating. The gaping discrepancy that the stiffness was a pathetically small issue (and probably normal) compared to the vastness of the pain problem, never seemed to get a hearing. If I haven't quite got you here, think of the patient with on-going RSI or post-whiplash pain – who has a great range of movement (yes it hurts through range) – but complains that they can't sit, can't lie, can't walk and can't write for more than about five minutes and you're treating by mobilising a slightly stiff C5 facet joint on the left side. Come on!

While at St Stephen's I was lucky to have been taken under the wing of Peter Wells as he very kindly included me as an assistant teacher on some of his weekend courses. I studied hard and learnt a great deal, we got along well and had great times being wined and dined by the various course organisers.

Two last things from this 'mini' but 'major' era of my experience.

The first was a very slight but growing and evolving scepticism with some of the techniques we were taught and which I later came to teach on Peter's courses. For example, try as I might I couldn't believe that you could honestly feel anything of real relevance doing all the sacro-iliac movement tests. One thumb on the right PSIS, the other thumb on the spinous process of S1 and while standing on the left leg, the patient flexes their right. The PSIS is supposed to move downwards relative to S1 as the ilium supposedly rotates backwards. If it doesn't, it's stuck and can be mobilised or manipulated. So I read and so I was told – but I found it hard to believe – especially with the knowledge that the amount of movement in a mobile S-I joint is around 3 degrees and the amount of 'translation' about 2mm or less in the majority of people (Harrison et al 1997). The argument that is so often put forward is that when treatment is directed at the apparent movement impairment the pain improves. The fact that a similar result can be achieved by doing something quite remote, for example reflexology or cranial osteopathy, doesn't seem to be entertained in the reasoning by many in mainstream manual therapy. So, to my current way of thinking, just because a pain can be altered or relieved by a technique directed to a particular structure *does not necessarily mean that this structure is the source of the problem.* That the technique can have a significant impact on pain processing is not in doubt. I will revisit some issues relevant to this argument later on.

The second thing, was attending a five day McKenzie course with the man himself – one of his first courses in the UK back in 1983 at the Royal Free Hospital in London. This was a revelation – here was a simple diagnostic system, with convincing pathologically-based reasoning combined with a logical treatment protocol that seemed to work. I devoured the book and every back pain patient was examined with repeated movements and the appropriate exercises for their McKenzie 'syndrome'. This was the biggest relief of all because it was logical, enabled you to make a diagnosis, then explain it to the patient and finally, do something that made sense in terms of the diagnosis and the explanation you had given. It meshed and made things easy. This was how I wanted to work. You've just got to have a plausible understanding of what is going on in order to make the whole process of treatment make sense and work. Or at least, I had to. While I have had many problems over the years with the McKenzie system because of its dogmatism and the fact that it completely stopped working for me when I lost confidence in it. I cannot take away from the fact that it provided me, for the first time, with what I was yearning for as a young inexperienced physio – a system of pain diagnosis, pathology and treatment that meshed well – and was easy to explain and get patients involved in.

Go to my blog online to see the full 'Mckenzie debate':
www.giffordsachesandpains.com

After my second application to get onto the Adelaide Manipulation course I was accepted and Philippa and I left for Australia in early 1985.

Section 2
Read what I've read

Bourdillon J.F. (1982) Spinal Manipulation (3rd Ed). William Heinemann. London.

Cyriax J. (1978) Textbook of Orthopaedic Medicine Volume 1. Bailliere Tindall. London.

Cyriax, J., Russell G. (1977) Textbook of Orthopaedic Medicine Volume 2. Bailliere Tindall. London.

Hartman L.S. (1984) Handbook of Osteopathic Technique. NMK Publishers. Hadley Wood

Maitland G. D. (1978) Vertebral Manipulation (1st Ed). Butterworths. London.

Maitland G. D. (1986) Vertebral Manipulation (2nd Ed). Butterworths. London.

Mennell J. (1952) The Science and Art of Joint Manipulation. Volume 2 The spinal column. J&A Churchill Ltd. London.

Stoddard A. (1969) Manual of Osteopathic Technique. Hutchinson Medical, London.

Stoddard A. (1977) Manual of Osteopathic Practice. Hutchinson Medical. London.

Section 3

AUSTRALIA AND AFTER

Chapter 3
Australia and back

A Whiter Shade of Pale

We skipped the light fandango
turned cartwheels 'cross the floor
I was feeling kinda seasick
but the crowd called out for more
The room was humming harder
as the ceiling flew away
When we called out for another drink
the waiter brought a tray
And so it was that later
as the miller told his tale
that her face, at first just ghostly,
turned a whiter shade of pale...

Procol Harum (1967), lyrics by Keith Reid and Gary Brooker

Early 1985 and off to Adelaide with Philippa for the one year 'Post Graduate Diploma in Advanced Manipulative Therapy' course. If I passed I would become a member of the 'Manipulative Therapy Association of Australia'. I would get to meet Geoff Maitland himself and be taught by him. Fantastic. This was the next big step on my 'pain journey'. My chest was puffed up.

I not only met, got to know and work with Geoff Maitland in his practice, I also met and got to know David Butler and Mark Jones who were both on the course with me. David and Mark were later to become well-known innovators, writers and lecturers. We all became great friends, had great times, many laughs and we all worked very hard on the course. I was also taught by and got to know many other well-known manipulative physiotherapists, Patt Trott, Ruth Grant and Mary Magarey – who were brilliant teachers on the course – and also became great friends.

One year actually became three for us; as Philippa decided she would like to do the course too; applied and was accepted onto it for 1986. Pleasingly, I got on well with Geoff and he asked me to come and work in his practice. I also did some part-time teaching on the manips course!

Working at Geoff's practice was incredible. There were positives and negatives, and on reflection, I learned a great deal from both aspects.

I was lucky to have time to sit in with Geoff while he examined and treated patients. From the word go I found I was fascinated by his communication. I furiously made notes as I sat in the corner and what I wrote down most of all was his questioning – the way he asked questions and the emphasis he put on them. The effect was that he gained the attention of the patient completely yet they relaxed and talked spontaneously. Some of the main features were: the eye contact, the total interest in the patient's problem and the intense listening. There was no fear; the patient was given time to tell their story and never felt hurried to get-on-with-it or to shut-up or get-to-the-point. To me his natural 'communication' style was the best thing and possibly the biggest positive I took from working with him. He was interested in the slightest little thing that was of concern to the patient.

I liked his 'paralleling' idea, where, when interviewing the patient the clinician follows the line of thinking of the patient, but dips in occasionally to get clarification, or more details. It basically meant letting the patient talk more spontaneously and take a more random route into the details of their problem. This was quite a contrast to the more direct and orderly line of questions we were used to sticking to. The problems, when you start with this more chatty style of interviewing, are that you can lose control; one minute you're getting a bit of history, the next a bit about the pain site, then about what makes it worse, then a comment about the work situation, then what the Dr said, then what the bloke next door said and so on. However, as you get more proficient at it, you learn to control the patient by dipping in with another question or comment. I noted that the ability to dip-in without upsetting the patient was another huge skill. Geoff called these dip-ins *immediate response questions* – often they're essential questions required to clarify a point made by the patient, but also keep the patient on track and for the most part, in control. Geoff Maitland, from the point of view of gathering information and getting right into and fully understanding the patient's problem, was ahead of his time; he was very much a 'patient orientated' practitioner during the history taking and assessment stage of management. He listened and he didn't stop listening until he felt that the patient had told him all they wanted to tell and he'd heard all he needed to hear.

To this day, just about all the chronic pain patients I meet report that they just haven't been listened to properly. And that no-one has taken their time to help them understand anything about what might be going on, what the treatment given was, is or does; why they've heard different and very often conflicting things from different practitioners, what the drugs they've been given do and why, what the future holds, what they should do, etc..

Geoff was good at listening, but back then the explaining part of management was greatly lacking. To me the reason was because we simply didn't have sufficient knowledge of what we were doing or what was going on, to be able to do this in any kind of meaningful way.

I am not going to go into the 'Adelaide' three years in great detail, it's not necessary. What is necessary as far as my pain narrative is concerned, is to point out a few things that spurred my sceptical thinking on.

First: I witnessed more use of huge levels of force; on slump techniques with stubborn pains like I had seen at St Stephen's Hospital; with joints that were blocked and physically stiff and with joints that were not at all blocked or stiff. I witnessed a shoulder dislocation as a result of forceful manipulation of a frozen shoulder (I can still hear the screams of the patient in my head now). I witnessed a rib fracture in an elderly patient from a unilateral pressure applied to the prone patient. I witnessed the hardest upper cervical manipulation of a normal neck that I have ever seen (it was a demonstration on a student). I'm amazed the student didn't die there and then, a rabbit would have! I witnessed such strong upper limb tension tests that patients were left with median nerve dysfunction.

Three things from this:

1. Collagenous tissues do not elongate over very brief periods of time – they tear and rip. This includes nervous tissue, which, especially in the upper limb, has only modest natural protective mechanisms in response to elongation. For collagenous tissues to elongate, stretching needs to be done slowly over time and repeated regularly over a very long time. Even then, results may be modest.

2. The approach that uses huge force is based wholly on a notion that the problem is purely mechanical and that stretching it and getting its former tissue extensibility back will relieve the problem.

3. I didn't like the high force, it wasn't compatible with the biology I knew and understood. The patients didn't like it – and it wasn't worth the risk.

Because it often involves force, my second point above is linked to the first and made me realise that even here in Adelaide, no one had a clue as to what they were doing – it was 'hit and hope'. Geoff Maitland told us that it was often helpful to *find what hurts and hurt it* – especially if you were not getting anywhere! Imagine my puzzlement when I witnessed him spending about fifteen minutes with a chronic headache sufferer, finding out exactly where his pain was on top of his head, palpating around the area until he found a tender spot and then driving his thumbs into the painful spot as hard as he could for about five or six minutes! In the context of 'joint-based' therapy at that time, this was hard to feel comfortable with. However in years to come it was easy to. Physios (and of course humans for centuries) have used pain or 'intense sensory stimuli' to relieve pain for a very long time (think of repeated movements into pain, frictions, firm deep massage, trigger point manipulation and needling as just a few examples). The pain modulation mechanisms for this are clearly described now. If you're interested, pain scientists call it 'diffuse noxious inhibitory control' (DNIC).

'What sort of therapist would you say you are Louis?'

'I'm a very specialised 'D-NIC' clinician, not a therapist... and by the way it's 'D-nickers' collectively and the verb is D-nickering! All you have to do is become an expert in finding as many different ways of hurting people you can get away with – and make them better. It requires a masters degree and ten years of clinical supervision to become fully qualified.'

'Oh, I see, right...'

(I am only kidding!).

Another thing was finding out that if I really stood back and looked at the results of what I was doing, or anyone around me was doing, there actually wasn't much happening! Geoff's practice, where I worked for nearly two years after the manips course, was literally full of chronic pain patients – they were classic 'difficult' patients. In some ways it was very similar to the types of patients that I'd been used to seeing in the NHS in the UK. These were patients who had seen multiple practitioners, were long term unemployed/sick, on benefits and had very, very thick treatment files. Some of the patients came for treatment three or four times a week and had been for several years. It was incredible.

Patient appointments were forty minutes for a new assessment and twenty minutes a follow up. Treatments were purely manual 'Maitland' therapy. In the two years I was there, I can hardly recall a patient being given an exercise to do – the treatments were purely passive – and based on the simple *'observe a movement, do a technique and then re-observe the movement'*, to get a result and justify the next appointment.

The bigger picture of the patients' situation was just not there. I seemed to be wallowing in the pointless and never-ending coming and going of patients' pain, with no time or concern for anything else. It made me very despondent, to such a degree, I took a couple of weeks off and went and worked on a building site – I was burnt-out with physiotherapy and I was saddened that what I had dreamed about when going to Australia, just hadn't come true. I remember coming home to Philippa one evening and saying...

'I reckon I've helped 5% of the patients 1% this month and I don't reckon anyone else in the practice is doing any better either.' I meant that to include the great man himself, I'm afraid to say.

Astonishing as it may seem, the results were not impressive and not what the world of Maitland followers believed or were led to believe. There were no magic cures here. What there was – was empathy, understanding and the desire to help; which is hugely appreciated by patients who have problems that mystify medicine and which medicine has little, if any, interest in. I came to realise that the hardest patients to treat and manage *in the whole of medicine,* are the ones with 'on-going' pain who constantly hanker and demand treatment.

So, my thought with chronic pain for everyone is this: do the best you can with whatever tools you have (Geoff Maitland did – he cared a lot) and never feel bad that you do not help or that you fail. Even the best in the world fail with these patients. *Please don't go believing that the gurus of the world always help all of them. If they say they do, they're deluded, they're not listening, they're not doing any sort of long term follow up, and in this respect they're no better than faith healers. Or they may just be keeping a myth going because it's financially advantageous to do so!*

Chronic pain patients are incredibly difficult to help. They are often complicated as people; their lives are usually complicated; their beliefs are complicated and deeply entrenched and their problems are complicated. Even with all the understanding and tools we have at our disposal today, results do not come easy for anyone. At least now, with the type of knowledge and management approaches we do have, there is a much greater chance that these patients' difficult lives can be improved and changed for the better.

If this all sounds a bit depressing, all I can say is that I now believe that it is possible for some chronic pain patients to get rid of their pain – at least in theory – if not very occasionally, in practice. Later on in this book, I review the mechanisms and models that I believe are important to appreciate if this is to be the case. The other thing about chronic pain sufferers is that it is perfectly possible for a great many of them to be a great deal fitter, more active and more productive than they are, despite the pain. A great deal of this book shows you how it's possible to deal with this type of patient and how they can get there, but also how to deal with the more acute patient and prevent them from becoming chronic.

Yet another thing, the new 'adverse mechanical tension' (AMT) of the nervous system phenomenon was around then and even though I was a little tiny bit a part of it, it really didn't excite me too much. I couldn't make it work any better than doing any other manual technique; in fact I often found it made a good deal of patients quite a lot worse. I was realising even more, that you had to have belief in what you were doing to make anything work.

In the early and mid 1980's the new fad was the 'upper limb tension test'. Credit for its introduction to physiotherapists back then must go to the late Perth based physiotherapist, Bob Elvey, whose 'brachial plexus tension test of Elvey' was the first into the general physiotherapy literature and was soon being scrutinised in Adelaide. Here, Helen Rubenach made some modifications to it and then Dave Butler started blowing the world apart with lots of new tests, new names and new approaches to difficult problems. The tissues of the peripheral and central nervous system and their dynamics and testing became the latest fad and a great deal has since been written (see Nerve Root section for refs).

The terms shifted from AMT to ANT (adverse neural tension), which seems to have been maintained to the present day, even though the term 'nerurodynamic tests' is now much preferred in deference to the influence of pain science.

After the manips course, Dave Butler worked in a practice which had a huge number of patients with chronic repetitive strain injury (RSI) related pain. He and I used to get together and quite often on a Friday night after work, we discussed the trials and tribulations of the week in Dave's bathroom. (Philippa and I didn't have a bath in our flat so we used to have a 'special treat'– bath night – round at Dave's house!).

Back then the only upper limb tension test was the $ULTT_1$ – where the components of the test involved gleno-humeral abduction with a fixed scapula; lateral rotation, then elbow extension, followed by wrist extension... and then neck manoeuvres. The arm is basically out to the side of the body.

While sitting on the toilet (seat down!), talking to Dave, who was in the bath, I remember showing him this:

(Try it if you like!)

Sitting down in a slouchy posture on a standard dining room chair (or on the loo!); place your right hand palm down on your right thigh – the little finger is nearest the knee and placed on a line that demarcates roughly half thigh; have your right elbow out to the side so that the forearm and thigh are roughly at right angles; in this position the angle of the forearm to the horizontal is about 45 degrees. Now, without moving the trunk at all depress the shoulder so as to make the point of the elbow go down and out a little – allow the elbow to flex a bit... note what you feel?

You may not get anything, but I get a nasty ulnar nerve sensation at the elbow and a nervy pulling sensation with slight pins and needles in the little finger.

If you do not get this response – then you need to maintain the position; grasp the hypothenar side of the hand with your left hand and further pronate the forearm plus lift the hand so as to flex the elbow. For me, this is not pleasant and very nervy.

If I remember correctly, I think we both discussed how we'd been struggling with making sense of the standard upper limb tension test on RSI patients. We both agreed that RSI sufferers didn't have their arms out in abduction when they got their symptoms at the keyboard – they were down by their sides! Hence the standard ULTT was irrelevant to keyboard related pain, or so we reasoned, in the 'make features fit'– Maitland style.

The thing about what I had just demonstrated was that scapular depression was a very strong component and very much like the postures that typists and keyboarders maintain for long periods; 'slumpy' posture and depressed shoulder complex (thoughts about the opposite, i.e. elevated scapulae with increased tone in postural muscles didn't really enter our reasoning at the time – which of course it should have).

Dave tried it and I can't remember what else we discussed, but a few weeks later he showed me his new upper limb tension test – what has now come to be called $ULTT_{2a}$. Here the test is done with the patient diagonally across the couch with the shoulder over the edge, so that the operator can depress the shoulder with their thigh. The test is basically in a much more 'functional' position for a keyboarder.

I think what then happened is that we (Dave mostly, as he was much more enthusiastic about it all than me) started drawing nerves onto bodies and working out all sorts of neural 'tension' tests from there. Credit to David for coming up with what most current physiotherapists learn about upper limb tension tests and all the variations. The bibliography to this chapter has a list of good reading, as well as some of historic interest.

Even in 1985 the 'neural tension' thing was going mad! With Dave's new input it went even more mad! Students in Adelaide were researching the effects of ULTT in just about every position and variation possible. There was even a research project done on the effect of slump on the normal responses of the upper limb tension test! Yes, students were being slump tested and then having the upper limb tension test done to them or vice versa. Some individuals noted changes in their arm symptoms with changes in foot or even toe movements in the slump position! RSI patients were being slumped, upper limb tension tested and prone knee bent in all combinations with reports of success and the new excitement began to spread. Dave went on to write his book 'Mobilisation of the Nervous System' and it has since become a 'classic' physiotherapy text.

I tried it all with my RSI and whiplash patients in Geoff's practice and so did he and neither of us were really impressed by the results. From what I could see Geoff seemed to ignore the new fad and went on with what he knew best, but I kept going, wanting to learn and get better, but really getting ever more despondent with it.

Here are some of the problems I had with it back then:

1. The proposal was that there was some kind of problem with the dynamics of nerve movement or the nerves ability to absorb and undergo tension. With a stuck straight leg raise I could appreciate this – it felt stuck – the nerves ability to slide/elongate/sustain tension seemed to be compromised considerably. However, in the upper limb I never felt that same kind of resistance, nothing felt stuck, all there was, was an increased pain response and an increase in muscle tone (understandably!).

2. The ULTT's in all the variations and combinations never seemed to reproduce the pain the patient complained of. The only time now that I feel that it does reproduce the pain to a convincing degree is with a small population of nerve root problems (discussed later in the Nerve Root section), as well as with some clearly diagnosed peripheral nerve injuries. But what it did do with all those chronic RSI's and whiplash patients was to produce a hugely amplified response compared to the normal response during the test. Thus, it was horrid for them, but it was not the pain complained of. However, it often seemed to stir their pain up for a good while afterwards. A clinical paradox then – it didn't reproduce the pain but it had a huge potential to stir it up!

3.   Hence, my treatments using the ULTT techniques were more likely to provoke than relieve – but in a way, all the hands-on treatments I had been doing to these types of patients, had been anyway. For example, I can recall (I bet you can too!) stirring many RSI patients or whiplash patients up after doing modest unilateral neck mobilisations. The unilateral mobilisations didn't reproduce the pain either, they were just sore. We worked on them because they were found to be sensitive and hence deemed a Maitland style 'comparable' sign. So, ULTT tests became a useful examining tool for me but not a useful treatment tool. I tended to either shy away completely or try to break down the tension test into simple non-painful components. For example, doing passive scapular depression as a Maitland grade III – which really seemed like doing nothing. I reasoned that the patient probably shrugs their shoulders many hundreds of times a day without realising it – so how could my doing it to them with probably only 20 or 30 repetitions have any useful long term effect? Sometimes I could hardly bring myself to do it – it reminded me of the tissue wobbling I did with Karen and Vivien (back in chapter 1)!

What I liked about it though, was all the theory that went with it. Here was a structure in the body whose dynamics had been described in detail by Alf Brieg and more recently by Bob Elvey for the upper limb nerves during the upper limb tension tests. The nervous system moved and stretched in response to the body's movement; it adapted and still managed to keep sending its vital signals. All the anatomy of nerves, when reviewed from the perspective of movement and tension, revealed a great many beautiful adaptations to allow this to happen. Via his teaching and writing, Dave Butler reviewed all this new literature and brought it into the declarative knowledge base of physiotherapy. This was a major move away from the 'joint' of manual therapy and manipulation; this was softer; this had chemistry and physiology; it had circulation and communication; it was far more interesting.

Staying in Australia and working at the university and in Geoff's practice forever was not to be and Philippa and I returned to the UK in early March 1988.

We bought my Mum's house (Dad had died suddenly in 1978, sadly aged only 59) and her practice and we took over the business in mid March 1988. The family practice continued on! Importantly I was free to assess, think, examine, treat and reason in my own way, I could at long last be myself.

Section 3
Read what I've read

*Breig A. (1978) Adverse mechanical tension in the central nervous system.
Almqvist and Wiksell. Stockholm.*

*Butler D.S. (1998) Commentary: adverse mechanical tension in the nervous
system: a model for assessment and treatment. Adverse Neural Tension
reconsidered. Maher C. Australian Journal of Physiotherapy: 33-35.*

*Butler D.S. (2000) The Sensitive Nervous System. NOIGroup publications.
Adelaide.*

*Butler D.S., Shacklock M., et al., (1994) Treatment of altered nervous system
mechanics. Grieve's Modern Manual Therapy. Boyling J. D. and Palastanga N.
(Eds) Churchill Livingstone. Edinburgh.*

*Butler D.S. (1989) Adverse mechanical tension in the nervous system: a model for
assessment and treatment. Australian Journal of Physiotherapy 35: 227-238.*

*Butler D.S. (1991) Mobilisation of the Nervous System. Churchill Livingstone.
Melbourne.*

*Butler D.S. (1994) The upper limb tension test revisited. Physical therapy of the
cervical and thoracic spine. Clinics in Physical Therapy. Grant R (Ed) Churchill
Livingstone. New York.*

*Butler D.S. (2013) Integrating pain awareness into physiotherapy - wise action
for the future. In Gifford L.S. (Ed) Topical Issues in Pain I. Whiplash science and
management. Fear-avoidance behaviour and beliefs. CNS Press, Falmouth.*

*Butler D.S., Gifford, L.S. (1989) Adverse Mechanical Tension in the Nervous System
– Part 1, Testing for dural tension. Physiotherapy: 75, 622-629.*

*Butler D.S., Gifford, L.S. (1989) Adverse Mechanical Tension in the Nervous System
– Part 2, Examination and Treatment. Physiotherapy 75, 629-636.*

*Butler D. S., Slater H. (1994) Neural injury in the thoracic spine. A conceptual
basis to management. Physical Therapy of the Cervical and Thoracic spine. Grant
R. Churchill Livingstone. New York.*

*Elvey R., Hall T. (1997) Neural tissue evaluation and treatment. Physical Therapy
of the Shoulder (3rd Ed.) Donatelli R. (Ed) Churchill Livingstone. New York.*

Elvey R. L. (1986) Treatment of arm pain associated with abnormal brachial plexus tension. Australian Journal of Physiotherapy 32: 224-229.

Elvey R. L. (1994) The investigation of arm pain: signs of adverse responses to the physical examination of the brachial plexus and related neural tissues. Grieve's Modern Manual Therapy. J. D. Boyling and N. Palastanga. Edinburgh, Churchill Livingstone: 577-585.

Elvey R. L. (1995) Peripheral neuropathic disorders and neuromusculoskeletal pain. Moving in on Pain. Shacklock M. O. (Ed) Butterworth-Heinemann. Australia.

Elvey R. L. (1997) Physical evaluation of the peripheral nervous system in disorders of pain and dysfunction. Journal of Hand Therapy 10(2): 122-129.

Gifford L.S. (1997) Neurodynamics. Rehabilitation of Movement: Theoretical bases of clinical practice. Pitt-Brooke. London, Saunders: 159-195.

Gifford, L.S. (1993) Examining and treating signs of neural tension. In Touch: The Journal of the Organisation of Chartered Physiotherapists in Private Practice, 68: 16-24

Grieve G. P. (1981, 1988) Common Vertebral Joint Problems (1st & 2nd Eds) Churchill Livingstone. Edinburgh.

Grieve G.P. (1986, 1994) Grieve's Modern Manual Therapy. Churchill Livingstone. Edinburgh.

Harrison D.E. et al. (1997) The sacroiliac joint: a review of anatomy and biomechanics with clinical implications. Journal of Manipulative Physiol. Ther: 20(9):607-617

Maitland G. D. (1979) Negative disc exploration: positive canal signs. Australian Journal of Physiotherapy 25: 129-134.

Shacklock M.O. (1995) Neurodynamics. Physiotherapy 81(1): 9-16.

Shacklock M.O., Butler D.S., et al. (1994) The dynamic central nervous system: structure and clinical neurobiomechanics. Grieve's Modern Manual Therapy. J. D. Boyling and N. Palastanga. Edinburgh, Churchill Livingstone.

Shacklock M.O. (2005) Clinical Neurodynamics: A new system of neuromusculoskeletal treatment. Butterworth-Heinemann. London.

Section 4

EARLY AH-HA MOMENTS

Chapter 4.1

Pat Wall's chapter... Ah-ha! - Chronic Pain begins to make sense!

Chimes Of Freedom

Far between sundown's finish an' midnight's broken toll
We ducked inside the doorway, thunder crashing
As majestic bells of bolts struck shadows in the sounds
Seeming to be the chimes of freedom flashing
Flashing for the warriors whose strength is not to fight
Flashing for the refugees on the unarmed road of flight
An' for each an' every underdog soldier in the night
An' we gazed upon the chimes of freedom flashing.

Starry-eyed an' laughing as I recall when we were caught
Trapped by no track of hours for they hanged suspended
As we listened one last time an' we watched with one last look
Spellbound an' swallowed 'til the tolling ended
Tolling for the aching whose wounds cannot be nursed
For the countless confused, accused, misused, strung-out ones an' worse
An' for every hung-up person in the whole wide universe
An' we gazed upon the chimes of freedom flashing.

By Bob Dylan (first and last verse)

From the album 'Another side of Bob Dylan' (1964)

Back to the physiotherapy practice in Cornwall and back to a good many patients like 'Volvo Vivien' who've had pain for twenty minutes and want to be better yesterday. Yes, the pressure and frustrations of private practice – where you are alone. There's no one to discuss new ideas or difficult patients with, there's no one to learn from and there's plenty of pressure to get results. You need to be good at teaching yourself. Yes, but I was free. Free to do my own thing and work at my own pace in my own time.

From 1988 into the early 1990's, I basically worked the practice hard did the odd 'Maitland' lecture and a few very basic weekend 'ANT' courses. Dave had given me a few copies of his teaching slides and I cobbled together piles of ghastly overheads to supplement them. No such thing as Power- Point then. The courses had a balance of early nerve movement theory, mobilisation theory using a Maitland approach to the nervous system and plenty of hands-on practice of the new 'ANT' tests and techniques. I enjoyed teaching the physical tests and the theory but I didn't enjoy teaching the treatment approach and the techniques – because what I taught really wasn't what I did or what I believed. But back then I didn't know what I really believed. That bit was hard.

Dave was starting to teach and travel widely and I 'assisted' on a few of his courses here in the UK and occasionally in Europe too. His new book (Butler 1991) had been out for a while and was everywhere. There was a big 'ANT' buzz about and Dave's unique informative and entertaining lecturing and presenting style was in great demand.

It was while on one of these course tours in Holland that my major 'career changing' moment occurred.

Whenever we met up Dave and I always had with us a pile of books that we were reading. On this occasion Dave had some pain books and lent me one to have a look at. I can't remember what he said to me about it, probably something like, 'I think you'll find a few chapters in there of great interest Louis...'.

The book was called: 'Pain mechanisms and Management' edited by J C D Wells and C J Woolf – two eminent figures in the pain management and pain science research world. Anyway, in the book was a chapter by Patrick Wall who, along with Ronald Melzack as most of us know, is famous for the 'Gate-control theory' of pain – something we were all briefly taught as students but could see little relevance to physiotherapy apart from the fact that it told us how TENS machines work – and so we sadly, ignored it.

Pat Wall's chapter was titled 'Neuropathic pain and injured nerve: central mechanisms'.

It blew me away and led me quickly into the pain literature to find out more. It had a great many answers to all the questions I had been asking. My professional life changed very quickly from there on. Before I explain, I'd like to briefly present what I like to call 'the body chart of the unknown pain warrior.'

Figure 4.1 is a typical chronic pain patient body chart.

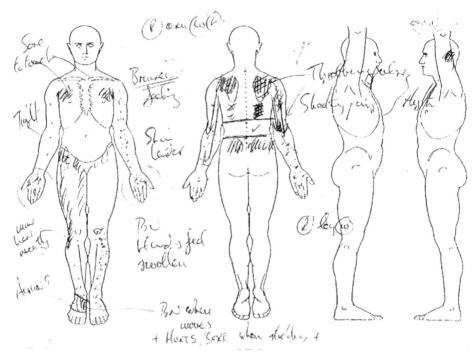

Figure 4.1 The pain of the patient who isn't described in any textbooks.

Here (figure 4.1) is the pain of the patient who isn't described in any textbooks but who is everywhere. This body chart is rather like the 'tomb of the unknown soldier' in that it is representative of all the unidentified pain sufferers who have died or will die without anyone ever acknowledging them and ever really knowing, recording or explaining their reality. *These* are the patients who have been dismissed or not taken seriously, who 'have nothing wrong with them', who have been given no explanation and no diagnosis; and as I keep saying, these are the patients who are not in the textbooks. You could say, well they are now. Well are they – where? Have medicine and the 'therapy' professions taken any notice of the pain revolution? Have educators started teaching and explaining chronic pain, showing students body charts like this one and helping them to understand what's going on? Why am I so sceptical even now? It's because the patients still come in saying: 'No one has listened to me, no one takes me seriously and no one really believes me.'

These are the patients who have had all the 'tests', there's bits of this and that – yet nothing big enough to really substantiate a 'solid' pathology or diagnosis. I've had many pain patients who come to dread the negative result of 'further tests'. 'If they could only find something then they could end this torment.' The torment of not knowing, of lack of credibility and of being in a 'cureless' state.

Look at the body chart and note the weird distribution of pain – or even the weird distribution of the areas of no pain! Pain is all over the body, it has varying qualities, mostly it is deep inside, it has vague ill-defined boundaries and if you really listen to these patients, it drifts and moves around. This body chart would be different next week, next month and next year.

All physical tests done tend to hurt – you could call it the 'everything is positive syndrome'. Standard movements of the spine and limbs hurt, all the 'tension tests' hurt, everywhere you palpate brings on pain. Nothing feels good at all. Some are almost untouchable and for those therapists locked into their favourite physical impairments, they can easily find them – I call it the 'If you look you will find' presentation. What I mean is that with these sorts of pain problems it's easy to find something minor physically 'wrong' to work on or correct, but the reality is that these issues are either non-existent, being in the eye of the enthusiastic beholder, which is rather harsh but probably true, or if they do exist are of actually of no relevance whatsoever. How on earth can a sacro-iliac up-slip account for our body chart here? No, it's not an adequate explanation, even though many would have us believe so, even the great and the good. Here's an example that sticks in my mind.

On many occasions working at Geoff Maitland's, he'd call me into his cubicle to meet whoever he was treating and show me what he had found, what he thought and what he was doing with the patient. I knew I'd soon be taking over the patient from him! Geoff worked part time, had a full list for weeks ahead and would want the patient seen within the next day or two. This time he introduced a man in his mid 40s with chronic buttock pain radiating down the both legs to the backs of his knees. The man had been off work for about a year and was 'at his wits end' with his problem. He'd been sent to Geoff by another manipulative physiotherapist in Adelaide. Geoff told me about all his difficult movements and then proceeded to ask me to palpate the fellow's back. 'I want you to do a transverse accessory from either side through L3, and tell me what you think.' I dutifully went about my task knowing I had to find some difference. I can remember thinking, 'Yup, that's solid to the left,' then going round the plinth and pushing the other way and thinking, 'Yup, that's solid to the right too.' I also remember thinking, 'I can't say that, he's after some subtle difference between the two.' 'Geoff, I think the left transverse accessory is slightly firmer than the right, if I was to draw a movement diagram of it the left graph would be steeper more quickly than the early right. 'Exactly,' Geoff enthused and that was virtually it – I would take over the patient. This was the key finding for the chronic low back patient and I would work on it 'daily' for a fortnight and we'd then review him together. I am not kidding.

That is no different from for example, a chronic neck, upper quadrant and headache problem being analysed as having a foot pronation problem on early stance phase of walking or an ilio-tibial band problem. Sadly, this type of analysis is still with us today.

So, to blame one structure, one pathology or your favourite fancy physical finding is untenable, but perhaps not quite as bad as blaming the person who has the problem.

With chronic pains like those on the body chart, small activities may hurt a little or not at all, but then later hurt a lot and the exacerbation can go on for days and days. It's rare to ever find a clear and reliable connection between activity or inactivity and the pain. Little things produce responses out of all proportion to the force used. Walking on the moon would probably hurt. Even the *thought* of some activities may cause pain to get worse.

How on earth can it all be explained? Didn't anyone want to know? Back then I felt I was completely alone. Well, there was 'ANT' – the latest fad from Australia!

These patients have often had loads and loads of treatment – all eventually floundering. Sometimes a little success is achieved early on, but almost always it all returns. They seem to lurch from therapist to specialist and back to therapist all of whom often believed that they had cured them or significantly helped in some way.

My observations from the patients' experience is that medicine just wants to get rid of them or tell them to pull themselves together, or say something nasty to them which will make them 'get-a-life' and stop pestering them for some impossible cure. Medicine, in general, tends to think of them as time-wasting head-cases who are psychologically weak in some way and unsurprisingly they are deeply frustrated by them. I can fully understand their attitude in their time pressured world with a massive lack of adequate resources to pass them on to. It is my belief that these patients are the **hardest in all of medicine to deal with** and they need something more than pushing, pulling and playing around with; they need something more than repeated trials of ineffective and often quite toxic drugs and they need more than injections and desperate attempts to help using surgical intervention.

So, they were/are, the patients with the crazy body chart. And now the seeds of an explanation – delivered by Professor Patrick Wall, hidden away in a chapter of a rather expensive and highly specialised pain science book, but an explanation of startling superiority to any tissue based proposal could ever achieve as far as I was concerned.

What was it in Pat Wall's article that so fired my interest up? It's worthwhile reading the chapter for yourself. For me, this chapter, plus a re-read of Melzack and Wall's paperback 'The Challenge of Pain' and many other articles that fed from them, all led to a marked change in my understanding and management of pain.

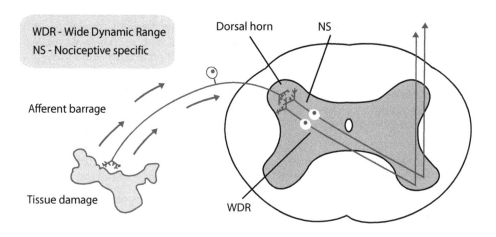

Figure 4.2 The afferent barrage from injury going to the spinal cord – very crudely illustrated...

What follows is a brief overview of what I gleaned, I've put some of the big 'ah-has' in bold!

Figure 4.2 is a very simple diagram that shows a section of the spinal cord – with its grey and white matter and the 'laminated' dorsal horn area of the grey matter highlighted. It is here where pain science first discovered that a great deal goes on when an injury in the 'periphery' (the tissues) has taken place. Please take a moment to read the footnote below.[1]

Onto this basic figure (4.2) is superimposed the very first part of a sensory pathway – that runs from injured and inflamed tissues in the periphery – into the spinal cord and then up towards the brain. A single 'pathway' in the nervous system is often described as having multiple neurones arranged in 'series' (one after another). One neurone, connecting to another then another and so on, making them 'multisynaptic'. All that's illustrated in my figure are two neurones of the initial part of the ascending pathway. Although it is usually called a nociceptor, I like to think of the first neurone in this pathway as a 'tissue monitoring or 'sampling' nerve fibre' – it has its terminal fibres spread throughout the tissue it innervates – and if anything disrupts or threatens that tissue it may fire and send impulses into the central nervous system. Its message to the central nervous system might be interpreted as...

'Look I'm hurt, just letting you know I'd like you to check me out and that I might need looking after for a while!' Or a lot more simply: 'Heeeeeeelp me!'

---

1 - *A rather lengthy footnote on 'nerves', which may sound a bit basic for some of you, but is important to clarify before going on. There's much potential for confusion!*

- *Most of us know a few nerves: like the sciatic, radial, femoral, ulnar and median. These are 'peripheral nerves' and usually form from several nerve roots. For example, the ulnar nerve derives from C8 and T1 roots and occasionally a little from C7; the sciatic nerve roots are numerous, spanning from L4 to S3. Nerve roots reach from the spinal cord to their exit from the spine just outside the intervertebral foramen. They are divided into two parts – the dorsal or sensory root and the ventral or motor root. When the two roots merge together just outside the intervertebral foramen they're often referred to as 'spinal nerves'.*

- *In between the root/spinal nerve and the nerves of the limbs are, in order from roots out, the various 'trunks', 'divisions' and 'cords' of the brachial or lumbo-sacral plexi – making the wiring diagram nicely complicated but an excellent shock absorber and disperser of longitudinal forces.*

- *Inside all the nerves, trunks, divisions, cords and roots are many hundreds of thousands of individual nerve cells. Nerve cells also get called 'nerve fibres' and 'neurones' or 'neurons'.*

- *Nerve cells have terminals at the end of their axons; cell bodies that contain the nucleus and dendrites that make contact with other neurones with which they synapse.*

- *The dorsal part of the nerve root contains 'afferent' or sensory fibres – their impulse direction is classically from the tissues into the cord and CNS. Afferent fibres include fibres from the gut which are sometimes described as 'autonomic' afferents.*

- *The ventral root contains 'efferent' or motor fibres whose impulse direction is away from the CNS towards the tissues. Motor fibres obviously go to muscles. Autonomic 'efferents' may go to smooth muscle, various glands, as well as into just about all the tissues of the body where their nerve ends secrete a variety of chemicals.*

A nociceptor is kindly, as it continually 'samples', monitors and looks after the tissues it supplies.

Nociceptors and other peripheral sensory neurones are often called 'first order neurones'. They send their impulses from the tissues into the spinal cord, usually terminating in the dorsal horn outer lamina where they form a synapse with a 'second order neurone' and so on, via a variable number of neurones and synapses up into the brain. First order neurones that are nociceptors may be either classed as 'C' fibres if they are unmyelinated, or as 'A-delta' (Aδ) fibres if they are myelinated.

In the parlance of the original 'pain gate' that Wall and Melzack described in 1966 the second order neurone was called the 'T' cell or 'transmission neurone'. But, in Wall's article, he described how in-coming afferent impulses, that had arisen as the result of tissue damage in the 'periphery', may synapse with two types of second order cell. The 'T' cell was found to be heterogeneous, meaning several different types. Here he described two types:

- an 'NS' or nociceptive specific cell

- a 'WDR' or wide dynamic range cell.

NS cells normally only respond to noxious stimuli, so if I rap my knuckle hard down on my head – nociceptor terminals in the tissues rapped will respond and send impulses into the cord – which in turn cause second order NS cells to fire and send their messages on to centres in the brain that process the threat. If I'm in a reasonably conscious state the end result will be pain that's uncomfortable enough to warn me that doing that sort of thing is not a good idea.

NS cells do not fire to light touch, normal movement, normal tissue stretching etc.

WDR cells, as the name suggests, fire off to a wide range of inputs – from gentle touch through moderate pressure, right up into the threatening and noxious range of things.

This is the usual state of affairs in the nerves that innervate the tissues of a normal uninjured non-pathological body. It is what is sometimes called the 'control' state; it's basically the normal sensitivity setting. So, tap very lightly with your knuckles on your head – and it feels quite innocuous, almost therapeutic , now gradually increase the tapping force... until you reach a point where it's not nice, it's pain, and the harder you rap the more it hurts. That's the control state.

As a quick aside, but a really important one, note that this 'control-state' setting can fluctuate since it is under the control of CNS 'central mechanisms' (see section 5). The result is that for any given input the sensation that we come to feel can be quite different. We can be more, or less sensitive to pain in different situations – which all depends on the 'context' or meaning of the input and the situation. For example, someone you're having an argument with mistakenly trips or steps on your foot as they walk round you... compared to... you're standing up to let someone pass your seat at the local football match just when there's some encouraging goal mouth action and they step on or kick your foot with exactly the same force as the previous example... 'Oh, sorry mate'... 'No worries, didn't feel a thing'... and the bloke passes by virtually unnoticed.

When there has been an injury the nervous system may shift up or down from the control state in quite dramatic fashion; either into a 'sensitised state' or to a 'desensitised state'. You would expect the first to be the case when there has been an injury, but in fact the second is often a good option where there is a lot of environmental threat about. For example, say you were crossing a busy road and you twisted your ankle – the last thing you would want at that instant in time is a lot of pain and a 'sensitised' state, much better to be 'desensitised' and be able to get across the road quickly and safely. Not the best example perhaps, but imagine you twisted your ankle while being chased by a bunch of very threatening thugs, or if you were a hunter-gatherer and you were running for your life from a neighbouring tribe. These are the situations where a powerful and reasonably prolonged desensitised state is vital for survival. Let the sensitised state and the pain that accompanies it come later when you are safe and can assess and look after the injury, as indeed it does. Think of how sore you feel after strong physical activity and contact sports like rugby, yet how at the time you were quite unaware of any injury or bruising?

If only we could shift all our chronic pain patients from the highly sensitised state to this desensitised one! Well, we could actually – if we could frighten them enough. Technically, it's called 'stress induced analgesia'.

Spend a few moments studying figure 4.3 – it's a useful one to use with patients occasionally, or one to actually get them to build up. On the left is a list of things that dull sensitivity and on the right a list of things that can enhance it.

In the modern relatively 'soft' world in which we live, we generally expect the sensitised state to follow tissue injury. Patrick Wall and others tell us what happens to the cells we are now describing when there has been an injury:

First up the tissue injury causes the local nociceptor population to produce a massive volley of impulses – the 'afferent barrage'. This barrage of electrochemical activity arrives at the dorsal horn synapse and bombards the NS and WDR cells to such an extent that their excitability state is rapidly increased. This means that they can quickly come to fire more easily and freely so that any arriving input is quickly converted to an even bigger on-going and upwardly travelling output.

So: the initial big injury input causes pain, hopefully helping us to escape or avoid further injury – at the same time as giving us a massive indicator of where the injury is located. Then, the injured area rapidly or gradually gets much more sensitive, to the extent that modest movements and gentle touching or prodding that doesn't normally hurt now does. The system becomes sensitised. For years I thought this sensitisation was all to do with activity in the tissues themselves – like inflammation, and changes in the first order neurone. I didn't for one minute think that changes might take place in the central nervous system and that these changes can go wrong—but they do— and they can sometimes be quite dramatic.

So far I have explained that the nociceptive pathway into the central nervous system is one neurone, the first order neurone, followed by a second order neurone 'in series' with the first. This one to one ratio is actually not the case at all, it helps us understand it, but it's a cartoon. It is far from this simple. For example in another of Pat Wall's writings (Wall 1994) he describes how some nociceptors, or afferent fibres, have a dendritic spread in the dorsal horn that covers many segments above

Total analgesia / no pain ←————————————————→ Extreme sensitivity / agony

SUPPRESSED STATE	NORMAL / 'CONTROL' STATE	SENSITISED STATE
Hypnosis	Fluctuates/varies depending on:	Injury
Meditation	Situation	Inflammation
Pain denial	Context	Low general health – vulnerable organisam
Fear	Intensity of stimulus	Disease
Anxiety	Attention/concentration	Tiredness
Stress, anger	Mood or emotional state	Low mood
Exercise		Anxiety/fear - related to pain or illness
Distraction		Anger and frustration
Activity		Psychological Stress
Being occupied		Physical stress
Socialising		Increased attention to body/symptoms
Having fun		Tension/spasm/altered mvt. patterns
Sex		Need
Pleasure		Time of day
Drugs		Genetic?
Optimism		
Genetic?		

Figure 4.3 Three basic states of the nervous system in relation to pain:-
Suppressed, Normal and Sensitised.

and below the incoming level (see figure 4.4). He cites the work of Arvidsson and Pfaller (1990) who reported that afferents entering the cord over upper cervical roots could send caudal branches at least as far as the lower thoracic segments! These long terminal branches have dendrites that end making contacts and synapses with second order neurones. Thus, one incoming neurone may, in some circumstances, have the ability to excite a great many second order nerve cells. Imagine if a single nociceptor in an elbow joint was stimulated by some local inflammation and this nociceptor then went on to stimulate all the thousands (possibly hundreds of thousands or even millions) of second order neurones which its dendrites came in contact with? What would the brain make of that? What chance would it have of giving all the inputs generated in these second neurones an accurate localisation? Could this help us understand the pain body chart in the above figure? I for one, certainly think it must do so.

Here are four important things:

1.   Because of the spread of the dendritic trees, one incoming sensory fibre has the potential to make contact and influence a great many second order cells. As far as the brain is concerned a great many second order cells represent a great many parts of the body – hence the potential for relatively minor inputs from small areas provoking far-reaching pains (think complex regional pain syndrome 1, for example).

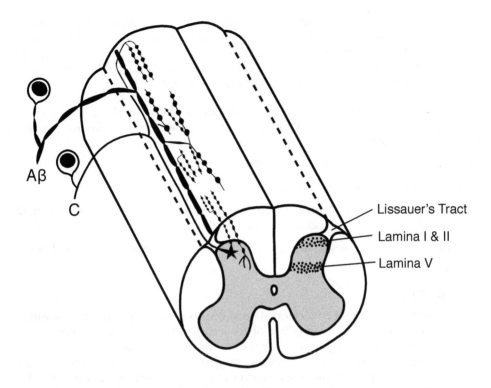

Aβ

C

Lissauer's Tract

Lamina I & II

Lamina V

Figure 4.4 Showing the massive potential of dendritic spread in the dorsal horn of first order C and Aβ fibres. Redrawn from: Fields H 1987. Pain. McGraw-Hill, New York.

2. Thankfully, it doesn't always do this because many of the contacts, or synapses, are inactive, appearing to be dormant. Thus, there are active and 'awake' synapses and 'sleeping' synapses and the amount of each varies depending on the situation.

3. On the other hand, it's known that a great many synapses would be instantly active if they were allowed to be! These 'potentially active' synapses are constantly 'held in check' by the activity of on-going inhibitory neurons – what's referred to as 'tonic' inhibitory activity, 'tonic' – meaning constant. A further consideration is that these tonic inhibitory impulse streams originate from the brain and descend in nerve tracts to the dorsal horn of the spinal cord. A great many early experiments on the dorsal horn of mice and rats looked at what happened after the spinal cord above the level being investigated was cut through. The point of this was to stop any downward 'tonic' currents interfering with what they were observing. What they found was that the dorsal horn sensitisation process (detailed in section 5) was vastly amplified, almost uncontrollably, due to this loss of inhibition. The tonic inhibitory currents can therefore be seen as a very powerful and important 'control' mechanism: the 'dimmer switches' that can prevent or allow onward and upward information

transmission. This mechanism insight made me realise that vast changes in pain intensity and pain distribution could be made very, very quickly, and – that the individual's attention could play a major part in controlling the dimmer-switch. The brain, and therefore the person, was directly attached to the dorsal horn information filtering process!

Here's a conversation that was recorded live (ahem!) between the person with the elbow pain and a little devil sitting on their shoulder, who could influence things in the brain quite easily.

'You interested in the pain from your elbow? '

'Why, yes I am, it's got me worried.'

'Right then, let's turn the controlling dimmer switch right down and that'll turn the volume right up for you to feel it better...'

'Hey, thanks, wow it's massive, and it's spreading too. I'm even more worried now...!'

'Up again then...'

'Yeah, go on ...'

4.   Individual second order dorsal horn cells receive a great many 'potential' inputs from a great many first order sensory fibres. Thus, one second order neurone may have many thousands of contacts and therefore potential synapses with other incoming neurones from far reaching tissue sources. The area that these neurones innervate determines the second order neurones 'receptive field'. As you might expect, the size of the receptive field is capable of varying, in this respect it's said to be 'dynamic' – being dependent on whether the contacting neurones have 'awake' or 'sleeping' synapses, or whether tonic inhibitory controlling currents are dulled or enhanced.

Here's an astonishing example from the work of Gillette et al (1993). These researchers showed that *individual* second order cells in the dorsal horn of spinal segments L4-5 of the cat have potential receptive fields in the back/hip/ leg. Dramatically, many *individual cells* were found responsive to stimulation from many different somatic tissues including skin, muscles, facet joint capsules, ligaments, dura, intervertebral discs and periosteum. That's one second order neurone!

As I found all this out I started to realise that it is probably quite easy for the CNS to make mistakes and go crazy. Think about Mary from chapter 2.2, if her hip really was the problem, then the CNS got it wrong telling 'her' it was her thigh and knee! Doh!

Perhaps the most remarkable thing is to wonder why more of us are **not** chronic pain sufferers!

When you start out with trying to understand pain it is best to get the groundings by describing the nervous system as a simple 'in-series' wiring diagram, but then to always remember that in reality there is a great 'in-parallel' potential too – especially when sensitised.

In Pat Wall's, 'Wells and Woolf' chapter, he mentioned that in his and others experiments, they found that **the NS cells in the dorsal horn actually change their physiological characteristics as a result of the afferent barrage – they change to take on the characteristics of WDR cells!** This means that a pathway normally only dedicated to noxious inputs can suddenly process light touch and non-noxious inputs too. Think how gentle palpation or gentle passive movements of chronic pain patients often create a massive amount of pain—could their light touch system have become linked—or even wired itself, into the pain system? Because of the nervous systems fluctuating 'in-parallel' potential, it looks as if it may well do, and most importantly, it fits with and explains, the clinical findings – the 'everything is positive' pain presentation.

Wall also described how the afferent barrage makes the WDR cells hyper-excitable and how, in some circumstances the barrage can cripple local inhibitory activity. The end result here is that every input that comes into the dorsal horn causes a huge reaction, which cannot be controlled well due to the loss of normal inhibitory controls! Further, if this situation carries on for any length of time the 'temporary' state of hyper-excitability has the potential to become 'permanent'. It seems that on-going high levels of incoming impulse activity to the dorsal horn causes the release of large quantities of neurotransmitters called 'excitatory amino acids' (glutamate and aspartate) and that they then may cause nerve cells in the vicinity to degenerate and die (known technically as excite-toxicity). Inhibitory neurones have been found to be particularly at risk and the process is called 'induced' degeneration. The term 'cripples' seems a good way to visualise it to me.

Permanent hyper-excitability! Wow!! Once pain is in the system, it can't be changed? Once inhibitory neurones are gone, they're gone forever? So all that pain treatment is a waste of time? Maybe! Back then, this thought certainly had a huge impact on me and as a result, how I managed and treated pain from there on.

What further fascinated me was the finding that **the second order neurones (the NS and WDR) in this 'induced degeneration' situation can reach such a high excitability state that they become spontaneously active. They fire without any input from the periphery arriving at all!**

This was it! Here was a situation where pain that felt like it was in the tissues, pain that felt very real, even pain that had a clear 'mechanical' behaviour – could be being generated from within the nervous system. Phantom pain without an amputation!

This meant that the pain had no value; that hurt did not mean harm; that a chronic pain patient if he or she were to choose to load their body in some way, had no more chance of harming themselves than any other person of similar fitness would. 'Useless' pain! Pain of no value whatsoever! I was astonished, all those years of taking pain seriously and getting anxious and fearful when my patients' pain flared up and got a lot worse. All those years of backing off, of feeling anxious that I might have injured them in some way and telling the patients to back off, rest, avoid the pain – I was shocked and relieved at the same time. The major affect on me was that *I was no longer scared of on-going pain*—the pain was pointless—it had no helpful meaning and yet it somehow happens. Is it a dreadful cost that stems from our being so complicated, the price we pay for being brainy?

This knowledge, combined with the realisation that massive sensitisation could lead to the potential for distant inputs from normal tissues to access the pain system as it became more 'in-parallel' bowled me over.

Here was a fantastic and quite logical explanation; that in some patients when they are injured their central nervous systems plastically change in an unhelpful way, so that instead of quietly returning to normal sensitivity and normal processing settings as tissues recover and heal, their nervous systems do just the opposite; they go on to become highly sensitised such that even the smallest of inputs become amplified in a crazy out of all proportion way and, their pain remains imprinted in their system long after healing has taken place. What a terrible state to be in – and no wonder no scan or investigative test ever shows anything to make sense of it; a pain 'imprint' and neuroplasticity are impossible to see because their presence relates to a dynamic state of a nerve circuit, to electrochemical activity and not gross anatomy. Let's not be fooled and let's not fool our patients that there's some fancy diagnostic test which visualises all this!

WOW!

At last, 'FREEDOM!'

Chapter 4.2
Ah-ha number 2...
'Secondary hyperalgesia'

The Afterlife

After I died and the makeup had dried
I went back to my place
No moon that night
but a heavenly light
Shown on my face
Still I thought it was odd
there was no sign of God
Just to usher me in
Then a voice from above
sugarcoated with love
Said 'Let us begin'

You got to fill out a form first
And then you wait in the line
You got to fill out a form first
And then you wait in the line

Paul Simon (2011) from the album: So Beautiful or So What

Kylie

… was a patient from my pain 'transition' phase – hence, in the bad old times was an 'Oh no/oh shit' patient – to the new era where she was a 'I'm not scared of your pain or you... but I don't know what to do with you, but I'm getting a better handle on it,' type patient.

Kylie has a chronic pain condition. She is 35 years old, likes food and smoking, doesn't like exercise and never will. She works as a receptionist and has a great sense of humour. Three years ago she tripped over a mat in her office and hurt her left arm and her low back. It started hurting and it never stopped. The arm pain was originally just in the shoulder joint but after about three or four weeks it spread to the arm. She had had all the x-rays, scans and tests that you would expect as well as all the various treatments and drugs you would expect. She took pain killers all the time in order to stay at work and keep functioning.

Her life and her past and present are complicated and I guess that she scores 100 on the frustration scale. She is fed up with being asked about her pain and people testing her all the time without anything active and useful being done.

The scans and x-rays revealed nothing. According to them she is normal yet she is in constant pain.

I'm about to examine her left arm, she's standing facing me and I have had a quick scan of her physical 'shape' – which looks pretty normal, pretty good. For her lifestyle she is only very slightly over-weight. She undressed quite normally, she didn't grunt or groan and there was no apparent guarding or avoiding of note. You wouldn't know she hurt so much.

'What's the pain situation right now Kylie?'

'Whole arm aches, the hand is burning and feels swollen, there are sharp shooting pains over my shoulder and I've got this feeling like someone is driving a screwdriver into the ribs just behind my shoulder blades.' She tries to reach the area with her right hand to show me.

'Give it a pain number out of ten if you can,' I ask.

'About five or six,' she smiles.

I tell her we are going to do some movements and to let me know about the pain response each time. I also tell her that I will demonstrate the movement before she has a go.

I shrug my shoulders loosely up and down.

She frowns and takes a breath.

'I'll do it,' she says.

To watch is to watch despair. Such a simple movement performed so jerkily and with such tension. The shoulder judders upwards and back, it barely goes up more than an inch. I raise my eyebrows waiting for her response.

'Eight out of ten and it's right down to my hand.'

'Can you do it again but this time, try a bit more smoothly?' I ask.

The same thing happens again, perhaps going an inch further.

'It's ten now and it's going to get worse.' She reports.

I pause and look at her. I'm not feeling sick in the guts, but I'm internally wincing – and I'm thinking 'What on earth am I going to do with you today?' I've been here so many times in my career and I desperately want this situation to change. At least I am starting to have a rational understanding of it all.

'Could you try lifting the arm up?' I demonstrate lifting my arm to about the horizontal.

She's obviously not keen but tries with more tension and now holding her breath. She manages about 40 degrees...

I then shift to seeing what neck movements are like. She flexes fully and reports: 'It's like a long ripping feeling going from the middle of the back of my head down to my shoulders.'

All her other neck movements are of good range but of similar response – at end range they produce wildly more discomfort than they normally would.

I give up with the active tests.

She lies down and I find that her reflexes are quite normal. I also do a few passive tests of the shoulder and arm; I try some rudiments of an ULTT and I also try palpating the shoulder and arm. Everything hurts, she flinches and pulls away all the time, the pain level doubles and her back and neck are now hurting too. Yet another nightmare (for me and the patient), and not an uncommon occurrence for most physiotherapists, I think you'd agree!

Kylie illustrates plenty of the features of what the pain mechanism articles are talking about and explaining with reference to neurobiological changes in the dorsal horn and beyond. There was no doubt in my mind then that these 'central change' mechanisms were a very big factor in explaining the responses and findings like Kylie's and many others, and explaining them much better than any tissue based models do. It cannot be much at all to do with the tissues, yet paradoxically, if you go looking in the tissues, there is so much hurt to be found.

Here are some of Kylie's findings that are linked to known central mechanisms:

- There is a hugely decreased pain threshold, meaning, small things that would not normally hurt at all, now hugely hurt—pain science calls this excessive sensitivity 'allodynia'—allodynia to touch, to small movements to all the physical tests. Her central nervous system takes normal non-noxious sensory inputs and processes them as pain and it all boils down to the high dorsal horn sensitivity state and beyond into the depths of CNS and brain pain processing. Nothing seems to be adequately controlling accessibility to the pain system. No harm causes lots of hurt.

- There is an increase in flexor withdrawal reflex. Following central changes motor reflexes can lose their inhibitory veil – hugely useful when an injury is raw and vulnerable but useless if it lingers for too long. At worst this is the jumpy response by the patient, the one who tenses and flinches to the slightest touch or passively performed test or movement and at times even before any physical test is begun.

- Repeated stimulation causes an increased response with each repetition. Recall that by the second repetition of shoulder shrugging Kylie was reporting that the pain had gone from 5-6 to 8 for the first attempt and 10 after the second – and even then it was still increasing afterwards. This is incredible sensitivity – almost ridiculous perhaps. No wonder such reactions get rewarded with disbelief and frustration by the medical and caring community. But, peer into the world of the dorsal horn 2nd order cells and we find that these cells when highly sensitised will, in response to repeated inputs, sequentially increase their outputs. It is now called 'wind-up like phenomena' by pain scientists, surely a term that needs no change for the patients?

- There's an increased response to something that is normally noxious. This is the definition that pain science uses for the term 'hyperalgesia'. It means that if something normally hurts a bit, now it hurts a great deal more. I think the definition and use of the word by pain science is somewhat confusing, as you will see when I discuss primary and secondary hyperalgesia shortly. For now, go along with the definition and note that for Kylie it equates with the responses given to the end range neck movements. Normal end range neck movements for most people produce a sensation of tightness, pulling or deep moderate discomfort, (extend your neck to end range to see what I mean). These are all sensations that while not necessarily labelled as noxious for most of us, do represent a message that is saying 'not much further thanks' or, 'if you do go further, be careful'. For Kylie the end range response is massive and clearly, inappropriate. Something that is normally a modest warning or slightly uncomfortable becomes highly noxious. Think how she might respond if you took her shoulder joint to end of range and gave it firm overpressure? The not nice becomes super nasty. Hyperalgesia is simply sensory amplification but commonly also includes a massive increase in the area of response too.

Note where you feel the sensation when you flex your head forwards – for me it's mainly at the base of the neck spreading slightly onto the top of the shoulders – but everyone is different. Note what Kylie had!

- There is a spread of pain and a spread of sensitivity/tenderness. This is related to not only increases in central sensitivity states, but also to a massive expansion of receptive fields in the central nervous system sensory neurones as discussed above. When pain spreads away from the area of injury, or is not even at the sight of injury the pain is 'referred pain'. Most practitioners feel quite comfortable with referred pain – especially when it falls into typical referral patterns. Patients seem to accept the idea quite readily too. For example, most would be quite comfortable about the fact that the pain of angina that comes from a distressed heart is not only felt over the left chest area, but also can spread into the left shoulder and down the arm. What they (patients and practitioners!) don't find so easy is the idea of referred tenderness and sensitivity. Tenderness is so real, surely anything that is tender has to be injured, bruised or inflamed in some way? The idea that tenderness/increased sensitivity can be referred really does take some believing. Patients (and Drs and therapists too) need an example to be convinced and even then, it's a big ask to accept such a shift.

Before giving a useful example, it's important to appreciate what the terms 'primary' and 'secondary' hyperalgesia mean. Understanding, or realising the clinical importance of, 'secondary hyperalgesia' was another massive moment for me and I'll show you why.

A great deal of work on peripheral mechanisms of nociception and early central changes that result from tissue insult or injury, has been done using skin. It's easy to see why; skin is more or less two dimensional, is accessible, is easy to injure in a very precise way in the lab, it's full of nerves that can be reached without undue damage and it's easy to test its sensitivity. When pain scientists want to make a precise injury it's often either thermal, for example produced by using a laser, or chemical, produced via an injection of chilli pepper solution (capsaicin).

Following an insult the *injured area* of skin quickly becomes sensitised to mechanical and heat/thermal stimuli, (note how sensitive to temperature a fresh cut is when you run cold water over it or get in a hot bath). This increased sensitivity is predominantly a result of local changes in the nociceptors and is called the region of 'primary hyperalgesia'. Think about it and you realise that this is an example of 'peripheral plasticity' of sensory neurones which very usefully results in the area of damage becoming sensitised. Not only that, within about five minutes or so an area surrounding the damaged zone also becomes sensitised, but this time only to mechanical stimuli, not thermal. The area is quite large and goes well beyond the area of flare that occurs with a skin injury. What we now have is an area whose tissues are *not damaged* showing enhanced sensitivity. Tissues that are not damaged but which are sensitised so that they produce soreness, discomfort and hurt when lightly stimulated, are said to be exhibiting 'secondary hyperalgesia'.

There are thus two types of tissue sensitivity or tenderness; primary, where the soreness is a reflection of tissue damage, and secondary, where the soreness is not – this type of sensitivity appears to be telling lies! The first is a true positive; the second is a false positive when considering the tissues in the light of clinical testing.

The term 'soreness' is useful when considering skin but deeper tissues can also become sore, or sensitive in the same 'primary' and 'secondary' way. Thus, there may be a great many tissues that clinicians test using pressure, movement, stretch, compression and contraction, that produce positive pain responses yet may be exhibiting secondary hyperalgesia – and therefore be quite normal. We may well be wrongly assuming tissue abnormality due to this 'false positive' factor.

Think clinically like this:

Gordon

... with an acutely injured knee from the sports field comes in to see me. (It turns out to be a simple medial ligament sprain). The pain is worse in the area of the medial knee but spreads as far up the leg as the groin and down as far as the ankle. It happened about five hours ago. Everything hurts – all the movements, all the various knee tests, and everywhere I palpate around the knee and for about twenty cms above and below it. Testing that relies on pain response is therefore fraught with difficulty if I'm looking for a culpable tissue to label. The best 'guess' as to the site of injury is down to where it is most sensitive and the site most likely to be injured given knowledge of the injuring event. To me, the main thing that's _anatomically_ worthwhile, if the pain will let me, is to test for ligamentous stability – but even this is met with a pain response and a fair degree of holding/hesitation (increased tone and flexor-withdrawal, remember!).

Here the situation contains two components relevant to the discussion: first, there is a mix of primary and secondary hyperalgesia, but one where there is a huge bias towards the secondary component, (everything physically tested produced pain – even the slump test was positive!). I hope you're reminded of Vivien in the Volvo earlier (chapter 1.2). Second, there is a significant amount of referred pain. Both can be viewed as being biologically very smart, or 'adaptive', because they're hugely protective in the vulnerable early days of an injury when the tissue regeneration and healing mechanisms are being readied and prepared to begin operations. It forces the region affected to be used with a great deal of caution and it makes the owner very vigilant and protective of it.

On the other hand is the amount of pain and spread of sensitivity here, at the very onset of an injury, a lot more than required? It's certainly more than is usual and probably more than is actually required by the tissue injury, so, yes it looks as if it is. Perhaps we should consider that a large amount of pain helps you to remember not to do that sort of daft thing again!

Normal recovery events usually lead to a rapid settling of pain and a decrease in pain and sensitivity spread as the problem starts to heal and begins to mobilize and this is what happened with Gordon. Within four to five days the marked hyperalgesia (everything positive) settled to become much more localised and thus, very much more in proportion to the extent of the referred 'spread' of pain which also contracted and diminished in intensity. It was now very much easier to do more meaningful physical testing to the joint so as to ascertain the stability and location of the tissue injury (i.e. the source of the primary hyperalgesia).

Contrast Gordon with Kylie, whose pain was very long standing, but, in a similar way to Gordon, everything you moved or touched or tested was positive in the extreme. The difference between the two is that for Kylie the healing process of the original injury must have long since moved on and settled—but the pain and sensitivity have continued and spread—instead of contracting in size and getting less. The marked unhelpful sensitivity that Kylie had and it seems that of Gordon too are extreme examples of totally unhelpful secondary hyperalgesia – one chronic and one acute.

Both are also wonderful examples of what makes clinicians confused and frightened of pain states. Again, you don't see Gordon's presentation in any sports injury or orthopaedic texts and you don't see Kylie's anywhere! The terms 'maladaptive' and 'adaptive,' are useful when considering a given pain and its presentation.

Biologically anything that is unhelpful is termed 'maladaptive', an evolutionary term, meaning of no advantage to the organism and its future. 'Adaptive' is clearly helpful.

To me Kylie and Gordon presented with maladaptive pain and sensitivity (primary and secondary hyperalgesia). See that Gordon's primary and secondary hyperalgesia was 'far more than required by the injury' – but that there was an injury. In Kylie's case, the hyperalgesia was wholly irrelevant to the tissue status since healing will have long since finished. Those tissues that were originally injured would now be healed *to the best of their ability*. If scar tissue should remain, as it most likely often does, a small amount of remaining sensitivity might be appropriate. 'Maladaptive' then, applies to any response that is unhelpful or out of proportion to what is needed. Clearly this designation can sometimes be very difficult to judge fairly, but in many chronic pain presentations it seems reasonably straight forward to see that the pain they have is way too much and lasted way too long. Their tissues, even though horrendously sensitive and reactive are probably best regarded as 'deconditioned' – not pathological, but merely weak and lacking fitness.

Let's continue.

Imagine for a moment that Kylie's pain was a bit less intense and reactive and you could perform many of the standard physiotherapy movement tests reasonably well:

When I tested her upper limb tension test of her good right arm it produced a fairly normal response – pulling discomfort in the arm, most pronounced over the anterior elbow region, plus a little drawing feeling and slight tingling in the hand. The range of each test component was also within a reasonably normal range too. However, when I then tested her 'bad' left arm the response was marked, the test range was very limited and pain increased in the whole arm, plus she got neck pain and her hand felt swollen and on fire. When I let off the scapular depression component of the test all the symptoms quickly subsided. She had a clearly positive ULTT. What's the interpretation now?

I'm asking the question because I've struggled for years with physiotherapist's interpretation of physical testing, especially when it comes to neurodynamic tests like the ULTT. Most, in my experience, tend to favour labeling this as a neurodynamic problem – and a great many would want to try and find the exact location along the nerve trunk as to where the 'ANT' impairment might reside. Because the response is so mechanically on and off the belief is that there is a simple tissue source to the problem. I disagree and would like to state that I am a neurodynamic atheist in this type of chronic pain situation and also with less chronic problems too. Even though it is so clear cut, this response, to my mind, is much more likely to be secondary hyperalgesia. The hugely positive test is merely a normal input, from normal (or relatively normal) tissues inputting into a central nervous system that is processing what should be modest hurt as massive hurt. All that has happened is that the central nervous system representation of the pain is being kick started or 'rekindled' by the sensory input derived from the test. Or, put another way, a normal modestly stressful movement is being over-amplified to produce a massive neural response resulting in massive pain. In this scenario, that's massive pain at the instant of the test and a quick abatement of the pain and hence of the associated representational activity, when the test is stopped.

For me, the bias has to be in favour of maladaptive central processing rather than tissue abnormality or pathology. All we are witnessing is the impact of a movement or test that is moderately uncomfortable anyway being amplified by a very badly over-reactive sensory processing system. If there was appropriate loss of muscle power, muscle bulk, loss of reflex and clear sensory abnormality my interpretation would be very different. I would want to investigate the nerve and its health in a lot more detail.

The key message here is that chronic pain, on-going pain, unhelpful pain, maladaptive pain, whatever you want to call it, can still behave in straight forward mechanically patterned way.

Understanding secondary hyperalgesia clinically is so important. I was thrilled to realise that when I found all those clinical tests to be positive in the chronic pain patients – palpation, passive movements, neurodynamic tests, all physical tests; that they were best interpreted as being non-pathological and therefore not an indicator of something badly wrong – a 'false positive' for the tissues under test. Again, hurt not equating with harm, but hurt equating with 'central over-amplification'. It meant that my physical examinations for these highly reactive pain states became a process whereby a patients spread of sensitivity and their pain response was being mapped and recorded. I no longer had to try agonisingly to find some 'source' of the problem in order to treat and manage the patient. For those of you who may be a little concerned about the importance of diagnosis and fear that I may be rather dismissive of it, I will discuss this further in the Graded Exposure section later.

Angina pectoris is a good and well known clinical example to use with patients in explaining the phenomenon of 'false' tenderness – secondary hyperalgesia, and also to show us that therapy applied to plainly non-pathological tissues can actually significantly alter any pains status and even the pathology itself!

Angina typically refers pain into the left side of the chest and the left arm. Often the arm becomes tender and is moved with difficulty. Patients with intermittent angina attacks have an increased number of tender points in the area in which they feel the full-blown angina pain when an attack occurs. Here then we have a situation of chest and arm pain, where the arm may be difficult to move and in which there are multiple sites of muscle tenderness. Without the knowledge of angina that we have today, one could be forgiven for concluding that the origin of the pain was somewhere in the arm, perhaps even in the arm muscles. Further, the apparent peripheral site of the disorder does contribute to the sensation. The evidence for this is that if the arm is anaesthetised with a brachial plexus block, the threshold for angina produced by activity is greatly elevated! Treatment of the arm or of the heart, both reduce the severity of the angina, even though the primary disorder is undoubtedly cardiac (see Wall, 1993).

In a way this is all rather good news. To treat pain, you don't have to know where it is coming from– because treating the site of the pain helps it! Pretty obvious really, we've all been manipulating and massaging our pain for millions of years. Animals lick their wounds too. Treat anywhere and you may well be influencing the primary source of pathology and even if not, you may be helping to relieve symptoms and producing a more pleasant life for the sufferer.

There are two final things to discuss before moving on.

Firstly, the confusion, regarding the definition of the term hyperalgesia. The International Association for the Study of Pain (the IASP), define it as an increased response to a normally noxious stimulus, yet in general usage it's taken as being simply 'enhanced sensitivity'. For example, this is exactly how it was used in our discussion above of primary and secondary hyperalgesia and is often the case in much of the literature. I've always seen a problem, in that there is an overlap with the term 'allodynia' – which indeed there is! In my day to day clinical work I think of allodynia as skin hypersensitivity; for example, the incredible pain when simply brushing the skin of those who suffer with shingles and which often occurs with complex regional pain syndromes (CRPS), the occasional nerve root problem and frequently with other neuralgias. It also occurs with patients like Kylie and Gordon – two ends of the acute to chronic spectrum that demonstrate the 'almost impossible to touch' situation.

I've often wondered why a pain term hasn't been invented to describe the increased response to movement and movement tests that physiotherapists do all the time. For now 'movement allodynia or hyperalgesia' has to suffice, and is occasionally used.

The second thing is that you may have noted that highly sensitised Kylie moved and undressed quite normally until I began the physical examination process. Then, she could hardly move and the pain reports flooded in. I am sure most observant clinicians have noted this in many of their chronic pain patients, one minute they are talking and moving their arms around freely, or they are bending to take off their shoes and socks... yet once the physical examination begins, it's as if the pain has been suddenly switched on.

Well, it could be, or the patient could be exaggerating in some way, but it may well be worth using a bit of 'evolutionary reasoning', discussed later (Graded Exposure section), to interpret this in a different way. It's all about different 'contexts', different situations and different goals. So, for now, reason like this: functional, goal orientated movements are processed by the nervous system quite differently to the stereotyped pain focused movements that clinicians request ('Where's the pain? What's happened to the pain? Think about the pain, tell me about the pain, pain, pain, pain... talk pain!'). Put yourself inside the patient's processing head when they're standing exposed in their underwear and you've just announced you're going to start the physical exam. 'Ah, it's time to concentrate on what happens when I move... OK, ready when you are...'

If you observe this type of 'one minute they're moving fine the next they can't' type response – especially in the context of long-standing pain, try to think 'maladaptive processing' rather than logging it as yet more evidence you're dealing with a 'non-organic, over-reactive, system manipulating, attention seeking, no-good-for-nothing, time-wasting malingerer!' These types of maladaptive behaviours can be very effectively managed – what you are observing is something that needs to be addressed in your management rather than criticised!

Section 4
Read what I've read

Arvidsson J., Pfaller K. (1990) Central projections of C4-C8 dorsal root ganglia in the rat studied by anterograde transport of WGA-HRP. Journal of Comparative Neurology 292: 349-362.

Gillette R. G., R. C. Kramis, et al., (1996) Characterization of spinal somatosensory neurons having receptive fields in lumbar tissues of cats. Pain 54: 85-98.

Melzack R, Wall PD. (1965) Pain mechanisms: a new theory. Science: 150(699): 971–979.

Meyer R.A. et al., (2006) Peripheral Mechanisms of Cutaneous Nociception. In McMahon S.B. and Koltzenburg M. (Eds), Wall and Melzack's Textbook of Pain (5th Edn). Churchill Livingstone. Edinburgh.

Raja S.N. et al., (1999) Peripheral Neural Mechanisms of Nociception. In: Wall P.D. and Melzack R. (Eds) Textbook of Pain (4th Edn). Churchill Livingstone. Edinburgh.

Wall P.D. (1991) Neuropathic Pain and injured nerves: central mechanisms. British Medical Bulletins: 47(3) 631-643.

Wall P. D. (1994) The control of sensory input by control of impulse propagation. In Boivie J., Hansson P. and Lindblom U. Touch, Temperature, and pain in health and disease: Mechanisms and assessments. Seattle, IASP Press. 3: 407-419.

Wall P. D. (1993) Neurophysiological mechanisms of referred pain and hyperalgesia. New Trends in Referred Pain and Hyperalgesia. L. Vecchiet, D. Albe-Fessard, U. Lindbolm and M. A. Giamberardino. Amsterdam, Elsevier.

Wall P. D. (1993) The mechanisms of fibromyalgia: a critical essay. Progress in Fibromyalgia and Myofascial Pain. Voeroy H. and Merskey H. Elsevier. Amsterdam.

Wall P.D., Melzack R. (1996) The Challenge of Pain. Penguin. London.

Woolf C.J. (1994) The dorsal horn: state-dependent sensory processing and the generation of pain. In: Wall P.D., Melzack R. (eds) Textbook of pain. (3rd Ed). Churchill Livingstone. Edinburgh.

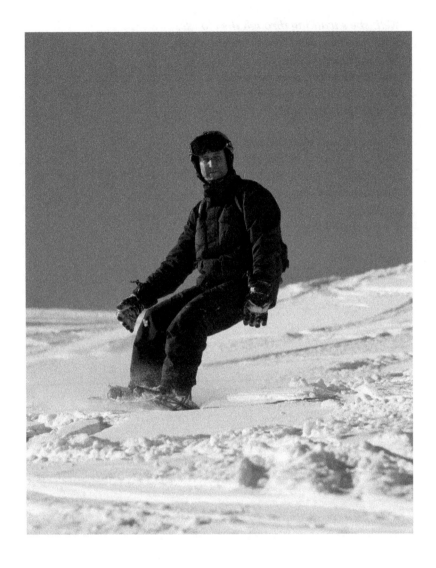

Little Wing

Well, she's walking through the clouds,
With a circus mind that's running wild,
Butterflies and Zebras,
And Moonbeams and fairy tales.
That's all she ever thinks about.
Riding with the wind.

When I'm sad, she comes to me,
With a thousand smiles she gives to me free.
It's alright, she says it's alright,
Take anything you want from me,
Anything.
Fly on little wing.

Jimi Hendrix

Section 5

THE DORSAL HORN

Chapter 5.1
The Dorsal horn tale: Coderre et al 1993

One of the keys to happiness is a bad memory.

Rita Mae Brown

After the wonderful pain 'Ah-ha' experience gifted to me from the Pat Wall chapter in the Wells and Woolf book, I quickly became engrossed in as much pain literature as I could get my hands on. I wanted to know and feel at ease with all that pain physiology offered and make more clinical sense of it. I saw that one of the first things I really needed to understand was the neurobiology of the dorsal horn plasticity changes that had been so inspiring – but it was so depressingly difficult, even though I had good physiology grounding from my zoology days. Nobody seemed capable of explaining it with any clarity – back then or now!

The golden article I grappled with over and over again for a great many hours was:

Coderre TJ, Katz J, Vaccarino AL, Melzack R (1993). Contribution of central neuroplasticity to pathological pain: review of clinical and experimental evidence. Pain 52: 259-285.

It's a fantastic article but it's difficult to understand and follow in the later sections when the neurobiology of the central 'mechanisms of pain' are explained.

Two of the authors (Joel Katz and Ron Melzack) had done a lot of work on phantom pain and in the article there was some mention of 'pain memories' in amputees. I'd like to quote a passage from the article that really registered as clinically important:

> *'A striking property of phantom limb pain is the persistence of a pain that existed in a limb prior to its amputation. This type of phantom limb pain, characterized by the persistence or recurrence of a previous pain, has the same qualities and is experienced in the same area of the limb as the pre-amputation pain. Case studies of amputees have demonstrated pain 'memories' of painful diabetic and decubitus ulcers, gangrene, corns, blisters, ingrown toe nails, cuts and deep tissue injury.' (Coderre et al 1993)*

Up to then I had always thought that phantom limb pain was just any old pain that made its presence felt in the phantom; what Melzack and Katz were saying was that the pain had incredible precision, even phantom in-growing toe nail pain! I was to later read that patients, who had years of pain and stiffness related to knee rheumatoid arthritis who then had an amputation, still continued to suffer the very same pain and stiffness in the phantom joint with the same pain behaviour. For example, in its former 'real' life, the knee was worse when the weather changed, stiff in the mornings; yet now in the present, the patient noticed that when their intact limb knee joint suffered a flare up of symptoms, so did the phantom joint! They still suffered when the weather changed and morning stiffness continued. Further, the sensations of stiffness that occurred when they 'moved' their phantom knees responded to the usual non-steroidal medications (see Haigh et al 2003). So much for a 'tissue' based explanation for this type of pain!

Thus, removing a body part that hurts or destroying its nerve supply won't necessarily rid the sufferer of the pain. Some further interesting examples: stomach ulcer pain has been reported to persist after vagotomy, or gastrectomy with removal of the ulcer. Patients have reported labour pain and menstrual cramps following total hysterectomy and rectal and haemorrhoid pain following removal of the rectum.

The Coderre article also discussed pain persisting after 'de-afferentation'. This is where a nervous system injury has taken place resulting in complete loss of any possible sensory input from the tissues. Brachial plexus avulsion injuries and spinal cord injuries are classic injuries where this occurs. Think about these injuries and for the brain it's 'as if' an amputation had taken place. The only evidence for a limb is via their eyes and the weight of the limb dragging on, or pressing against, tissues with intact sensory systems.

All this was strong evidence for the proposal that pain can have a 'central representation', (or as Mick Thacker prefers and is likely to be more correct, is 'centrally constructed') and that anyone can have 'somtatosensory' pain memory – not just amputees and the neurologically injured.

How about this example from the article:

Leriche (1947) described a patient who did not experience phantom limb pain until 6 years after amputation, when an injection into the stump instantly, and permanently, revived the pain of a former painful ulceration of the Achilles tendon.

Pain when it has been committed to a central representation cannot only be incredibly persistent but it can also be incredibly precise, in quality, in location and in intensity. No wonder it is so hard for us, for medicine and for our patients to believe that a pain in our muscles and joints might not be coming from where it is located and where it feels so real, but be generated from within our nervous system. No wonder clinicians and Drs persist with tissue based explanations: 'Your on-going buttock pain is due to a tight piriformis; or, one leg being longer than the other; or, your tight lilio-tibial band; a cranio-sacral dysfunction; an imbalance in yin and yang'... etc. ad infinitum.

The idea that pain memories might come about _without_ amputation or dramatic nerve injury and deafferentation fascinated me and I puzzled that no one else seemed to be thinking of it. This was back in the early 1990's. Could conditions like chronic low back pain, chronic RSI and whiplash have **pain** and **hypersensitivity** that is a mere memory module, something installed in the nervous system as a ghostly reminder of previous misadventures?

The exciting notion of pain existing in the central nervous system as a 'memory-like' representation prompted me to start to look into the memory literature in the hope that better explanations would come along. They did.

The next important read was this one.

'The Making of Memory – from molecules to mind' by Steven Rose.

I also read some of Eric Kandel's books and articles too. Kandel won the Nobel prize in 2000 for his work on the physiological basis of memory in neurons; as far as I'm concerned he is _the_ world authority on memory biology, the big-daddy grandfather figure! Steven Rose is a professor of biology and neurobiology at the Open University in the UK and another humble and brilliant brain/memory authority (and was a great mate of Pat Wall to boot!).

I read a great deal and felt inspired to write a letter to Pat Wall. Which, I rather nervously thought he might think was rather naïve; even so, I pointed out the similarity between the dorsal horn physiology of pain and sensitisation and the biology of short and long term memory. I expected a 'yes of course' reply but was quite surprised to receive a letter of great interest, including an invitation for me to come up to discuss pain and memory biology; he would ask Steven Rose along too!

Unfortunately Steven couldn't make it but we both had some good correspondence for a while. With Pat I had one of the professionally most memorable evenings of my life. I sidled my way into Pat's little flat, in Grays Inn Road, London. There was a blazing fire and lots of books and dust. There was a rather 'Dickensian' feeling about it all. He opened a couple of cans of beer, we smoked roll-ups and discussed the pain and memory biology and surprisingly revealed that he hadn't really linked the similarities between memory and pain. We also talked about broader issues of pain and the problems that Drs, medics, physiotherapists and others had in seeing the bigger picture that pain understanding revealed. Pat gave me the confidence to go out and start talking and teaching – even though I was a 'lowly' physiotherapist.

'You people in physiotherapy are the great observers of clinical manifestations,' he said. He urged 'us' to 'record what you observe in every detail and then hand it to the scientists to make sense of.' He urged physiotherapy to give more attention to recording and writing up their observations of the disorders treated rather than over-focusing on clinical trials of therapy. *'Those who first described angina, they hadn't a clue what caused it, but they described it with such fine unbiased detail and in a way unknown to modern medicine'* he said. He was firmly saying that we really only tend to hear and record the features that fit with what we believe and that medicine has forgotten how to listen and record without prejudice.

Pat Wall revealed that he struggled with persuading his own medical profession to understand and see the bigger picture when diagnosing and understanding the pain patients they confronted every day. 'They're all stuck in the bloody Cartesian model' he said. Meaning medicine thinks about causes being in the tissues and if it can't find an adequate cause there, it blames 'the mind' of many a poor and misunderstood patient.

The infinite possibilities for variation in pain/nociceptive activity interpretation and expression due to 'modulation' in the CNS/brain he found particularly difficult to convey to his colleagues, even though he was a masterful teacher. As I shook his hand after our meeting he said, 'Good luck,' with a wry twinkle in his eye. I knew that he was wishing me well with a task that he had struggled with all his life and that I would too.

One thing was for certain – yes, the mechanisms of memory did seem to have great similarity to those of pain.

Chapter 5.2
The Dorsal Horn –
some spinal cord basics

....'Moreover, understanding science is a hierarchical process: it is extremely difficult to understand the more advanced concepts until the basic concepts have been mastered.'

Lewis Wolpert

The dorsal horn is a small area of the spinal cord that pain science seems to know more about than anywhere else. Why? Because it's the easiest part of the central nervous system to access and experiment on! As I mentioned in the last chapter, the other area it knows a lot about is in the skin.

Cut through the spinal cord and look at the section and you see what's shown in figure 5.1. The important part for now is the upper right or left poles of the grey matter – the 'dorsal horn' area. This is the first 'junction-box' for sensory information arriving from the body. It is where first order sensory neurones meet second order transmission cells (like the WDR and NS cells discussed in the last chapter) and influence each other. It is where new connections and associations are made and terminated and it is where some of the most important first steps are made in either remembering or forgetting the pain of tissue injury or disease. The dorsal horn 'junction-box' is where millions of neurones synapse with one another. Yes, millions. Those who like numbers should know that a match-head's worth of your central nervous system contains about 1 billion potential connections and that 10,000 neurones can fit into the space of a pin head. It is incredibly complex and yet we draw simple drawings to try and understand it! The endeavour here is not to get too lost in complex molecular and neuro-biology, but to make what is known easy and relevant to physiotherapy management of pain.

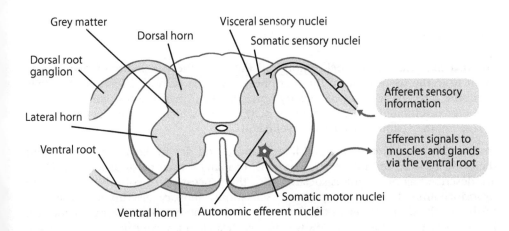

Figure 5.1 Section through spinal cord showing basic anatomical details.

Figure 5.2 is a crude rendition of the roughly 'H' shaped 'grey matter' of the spinal cord, that all physiotherapists should be vaguely familiar. The figure shows the principal 'inputs' into the three 'horns' of grey matter: the dorsal horn (DH), associated with sensory processing; the lateral horn (LH), associated with the sympathetic/autonomic system; and the ventral horn (VH) which is dedicated to somatic motor control. Note that I've also drawn two 'output' arrows from the lateral and ventral horns—they exit the cord in the 'ventral root'—which is illustrated in figure 5.1.

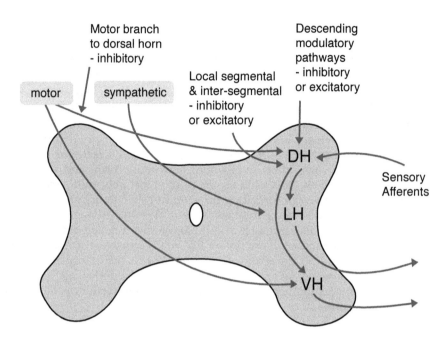

Figure 5.2 Grey matter of spinal cord - mainly to illustrate inputs to the dorsal horn

Of great importance for nociception and therefore the possibility of pain, is the input from the tissues—from the 'periphery'—via the sensory afferents. You may recall the three basic types of sensory fibre: the Aβ (A beta) fibres which are large diameter myelinated fibres; the Aδ (A delta) fibres which are smaller myelinated fibres; and the C fibres that are unmyelinated.

In the normal uninjured state, Aβ fibres send useful day to day information about the body into the central nervous system. In many formal medical texts Aβ fibres are described as not being associated with the processing of pain, but to do with proprioception, light touch, pressure sensations, sensory discrimination and so forth. It's thanks to Aβ fibres that I am aware of my body. Close your eyes and you know where your body is, you know where each segment of your body is positioned, you feel pressure on your buttocks if you're sitting and if you move you don't have to look to see where your limbs are to know what they are doing. Aβ transmitted information is constantly streaming into the central nervous system.

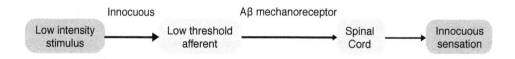

Figure 5.3 'Normal' processing of 'light touch'

Figure 5.3 illustrates normal Aβ processing and the resultant feeling 'output' from the brain– 'innocuous sensation'. What a dull uni-dimensional, boring, lab-scientist generated diagram that is! Try this, or just think about doing it. Gently rub your hand up and down on your thigh and you feel a gentle rubbing sensation. What you see is clearly what you get! Or is it? Think about what happens when the situation changes. For example, what does having your thigh rubbed in exactly the same way feel like when it's in a romantic situation? – mmmm. Or, having your thigh rubbed inappropriately by someone – yuck, or, have it happen totally unexpectedly, or even totally unexpectedly when you're feeling a little anxious.

Here then, are several different situations (the control/experimental; the luvy duvy, the yucky, the unexpected, the anxious and so forth), where Aβ fibres are firing in exactly the same way in each, yet the system is somehow changing the end result. This is modulation. It may be worth also thinking about extreme pain and its modulation. I found having the cane for misbehaving at school extremely distressing, but change the context and being whipped and caned can, for some, become extreme pleasure. Ahem... moving swiftly on!

The central nervous system 'modulates' sensory inputs to produce a wide variety of responses that are hugely dependent on the situation, or context you are in, or the situation you think you are in and this applies to pain just as much as any other input. The thigh rubbing is a good example to use when you are explaining pain and its processing/modulation to patients. I'm not sure that I have used the whipping example ever!

Modulation, as described here, adds a complex spectrum of feeling, colour, texture and meaning to the sensory information that constantly bombards the central nervous system. Modulation can also be reduced to a simple switching type mechanism for 'allowing' or 'not allowing' entry into the CNS or, more relevantly, up into consciousness. This switching is the 'pain gate' described back in the 60's by Ron Melzack and Pat Wall (1965).

Let's come back to the sensory fibres again. The other two, the Aδ and C fibres, are the 'tissue monitoring' fibres that were described and discussed a little in chapter 4. They're rather like those creepy little kids at school who were always 'telling' on you for mucking about. When something's amiss at the back of the class up goes their bloody hand... 'Sir, sir, sir... Gifford's lighting matches with Fatty Hall, Sir... Sir... Mr Chalk Sir.' Luckily this time the teacher's fed up with Creepy Jenkin and ignores him to get on with the class. 'Belt up Jenkin and listen or you'll be in detention.' Jenkins been modulated out for the time being, but if he persisted his pleas may well get investigated and modulated back in, and the end result might vary hugely depending on what mood old Chalky is in at the time. Just like nociception and pain production!

The thing about Creepy Jenkin is that he 'tells' on everything... Sir, sir, Gifford's just given me a 'V' sign. Again, just like peripheral nociceptive mechanisms, which have the capacity to report everything from hardly threatening to extreme danger; leaving it up to the central nervous system to sort out the relevant from the irrelevant, and it sometimes messes up. If you think in evolutionary terms, and we will a good deal more later, then it would appear wise to always err on the whimpier, better listen inside of things, if you have the opportunity to – just in case something is ignored at one's peril.

Injured tissues bring about dramatic changes in the local chemistry. Chemicals that are not normally present in tissue fluid are released or quickly manufactured from the damaged cells or arrive from local circulation and local immune cells. A great many of these 'damage' chemicals provide a 'help me' message and as a result draw in and trigger mechanisms that can provide it. Think of 'damage' chemicals like prostaglandins, leukotrienes, bradykinin, histamine, hydrogen ions, neuropeptides and the many interleukins for example. Many of these 'help me' messengers stimulate mechanisms local to the tissues, for example, the complex process of inflammation that sets the scene for clearing up the mess, making immediate repairs, and then initiating and organising the longer term healing process (for more detail, see sections 11-13).

These chemicals also powerfully stimulate the 'tissue monitoring' Aδ and C fibres and off they go, firing away and sending their volleys of impulses into the dorsal horn with the message singing out, 'Help me, help me, help, help, help… there's damage down here, damage down here, and you need to know, need to know…' etc. Just like Creepy Jenkin.

Now, the dorsal horn/CNS must be getting these sorts of messages from the tissues all the time (see section 11), after all, we continually knock, strain, over-stretch, over-pressurise (sit for hours and hours!) our tissues, that then need some kind of attention to be relieved or put right. If the CNS constantly accepted these incoming signals and brought them up into consciousness, my reckoning is that we just wouldn't be able to get on with life and do anything. Nociceptive 'incoming' volleys of impulses from these local tissue 'stresses' and modest injuries have to be assessed on individual merit and for the most part modulated out in some way. The dorsal horn 'assessment' may well run something like: 'I can hear you, I can hear you (*thinks*: little buggers, those tissues are quite capable of looking after themselves, there's no need to inform him up there, so I'm going to ignore them, blank them off and let him get on with what he's doing).' The nociception gets filtered or 'modulated' out – it's ignored, just like Chalky ignored Creepy Jenkin to get on with what he was focusing on.

But, Chalky was actually ignoring some quite dangerous behaviour – Gifford and Fatty Hall were lighting matches. Creepy persisted though, he went on and on and eventually Chalky investigates and finds out the full extent of the problem. Nociceptive activity has to compete with activity in the rest of the nervous system to get attention and it finds it can do this by going on and on, by shouting louder and louder, or a combination of the two. The extent to which modulation asserts its control over nociception is hugely influenced by what is going on elsewhere, in the environment, in the body and hence in the nervous system and the mind of the individual involved. It's as if there is an active competition going on for a valuable slot in the mind's busy schedule. I hope the reader is starting to think about those patients who feel the slightest pain all the time and that their system seems to have the modulation sensitivity set ridiculously high. If you are, you're 'getting it'; you're seeing that sensitivity exists on a spectrum, with super sensitivity at one end and very dull sensitivity at the other. Think soccer players v rugby players.

As will become evident, the biology of the dorsal horn reflects the need for gating and modulation.

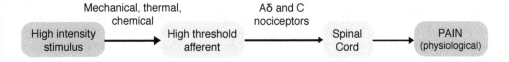

Figure 5.4 'Normal' processing of a 'high intensity' stimulus

Figure 5.4 illustrates normal nociceptive processing where the subject is in the 'control' state, i.e. doing nothing much in some pain researcher's laboratory but aware of what is going on.

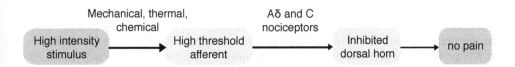

Figure 5.5 Dorsal horn 'inhibition' of 'high intensity' stimulus

Figure 5.5 illustrates the 'Chalky ignoring Creepy Jenkin' effect, i.e. inhibition! Think of the number of times you have noticed bruises on your body and cannot remember hurting yourself. Gardeners, manual workers, and rugby players for example will be particularly aware of this phenomenon. Also, anyone who has been involved in a serious accident is likely to have experienced a time of relatively little pain even though there may be evidence of significant injury. Gating can be very powerful when it needs to be.

Let us now return to and complete the discussion surrounding the contents of figure 5.2. Noteworthy, from the immediate discussion, is the presence of incoming excitatory and inhibitory connections to the dorsal horn. The wiring is such that sensory information coming in from the periphery, whether it is nociceptive or related to more benign sensation, meets up with terminals of neurones that can influence its onward passage into the CNS. These neurones are the modulators.

Thus, the dorsal horn receives input from above – from the brain. Therefore, it can be influenced by anything from simple reflex responses via the brainstem to the thinking, feeling and reasoning individual whose brain it is. I want to emphasise that conscious you and your brain activity, have an influence over what is 'let-in' and how much is let in, and therefore, over what you ultimately may feel. The reality is, it's conscious/semiconscious and unconscious – sort of all at once! I'm saying that because we rarely think to ourselves… 'Right, no pain now, don't let any in.'

Try this: if you are sitting, uncross your legs and place your feet on the floor. Think about and give all your attention to your left foot! Can you feel the pressure of the floor? Where precisely do you feel the pressure? What about temperature? Warm? Cold? Where's it warm or cold? Any tingles? Anything else? See what you can find? I hope that from this simple task it's plain to see that your attention, that I've directed, or similarly, your own interest or concern, are powerful influences on the neural activity that leads to conscious awareness. This little exercise is a good example to use with patients[1].

I want to make the point that 'gating' and modulation are going on all the time. Also, that there is a constant sensory input going on too and—if you choose to—you can wander round your body and listen to it all day long. Continuously scanning your body on the look-out for sensations and abnormalities and then thinking that something might be wrong is often referred to as somatising. We tend to somatise much more when we feel vulnerable. We may also somatise when we're bored and have nothing to do! Think about the times when you go off on a little scan round your body and note stuff. Think about that becoming a habit of attention? Think about the relevance of this to a chronic pain sufferer?

Wherever your mind focuses it causes a local lifting of inhibitions and a facilitation of excitations. Give attention to anything and you change the filtering and modulation that is going on in regions of the CNS relevant to where that attention is directed. You change the activity, you change the volume, you change the tone—this is what might be called a 'Top-Down' directed effect—the 'top' being the thinking conscious 'you'. It's very important to appreciate this in the understanding of pain and its consequences.

Modulatory activity doesn't just come from the 'you' above; it can also be generated locally, inter-segmentally and a great deal further afield too. Hence, pain in one area of the body being dulled by a whole variety of stimuli from elsewhere. When the stimulation is quite intense, remember 'pain relieves pain' – it produces what is often called 'hyperstimulation analgesia'. For example, TENS, massage, strong manipulation, ice, heat etc. The stimulation doesn't always have to be intense though.

Clearly the 'elsewhere' can be from a long way off: think about treatments like 'cranial osteopathy' that fiddles with the head and 'reflexology' that does fiddling on the feet! While it's hard to make sense of what these practitioners tell us about how it's supposed to work, the point is that if it does make a difference to someone's pain, some kind of processing change, or modulation, has occurred somewhere in the system, and this could well include the dorsal horn. Certainly the massive network of connections is sufficient enough to allow it to happen. For me, anyone who claims to have a treatment that changes pain should first-up explain it from a perspective that embraces changing processing – not changing some 'energy field', some muscle imbalance or, some minor anatomical discrepancy.

Interestingly, descending spinal cord *motor* pathways are known to send inhibitory branches to the pain processing lamina of the dorsal horn (see figure 5.2). It surely

---

1 - Apparently this is the basis of the 'Mindfulness' approach.

makes evolutionary sense that movement should inhibit pain. 'Clinical' pain is usually associated with stopping you moving or altering how you move in order to protect the wounded, weakened or healing tissues. However, in times gone by and at times today when conditions are rigorous or threatening, there are many instances where, regardless of injury or pain, one has to move to survive. Powerfully inhibiting pain to allow essential 'survival orientated' movement has therefore evolved–a nasty hook through the mouth 'ain't gonna stop that there fish on yer line from fighting its heart out to try and get away! It may well be at some cost to the individual tissues that get traumatised by the hook, but it is ultimately of overall benefit if the fish manages to get away.

I've often darkly pondered the need for some kind of therapy that makes use of this neat evolutionary aspect of pain. In my pondering I call it 'machine-gun therapy' (or MGT). Now my Philippa tells me that I just cannot recount this, it's too politically incorrect. I used to on my courses. No? NO! So I'll instead use a pack of bloodthirsty Rottweilers trained to kill anyone who isn't running except me!

Take a group of chronic pain patients to the gym and line them up against one of the walls.

'Today, we are all going to have a run round the gym. You are all going to run faster than you have ever run in your lives if I get this right.'

Pause. Everyone's looking at each other and frowning. None of them have run for years. Many are hanging on to crutches or sticks, several are trussed up in some kind of corset and most are holding their breath and grunting. I'm smiling and looking confident. I'm standing in the corner of the room next to a door.

'We're going to do a new kind of therapy, it's called 'R-W therapy' and in all the clinical trials so far it has 100% success rate for your kinds of problems.'

I pause. There's a little babble of hopeful chattering.

Slowly I open the door and bring out two of my trained Rottweilers. They're on quick release leads.

'Let me introduce 'R' and 'W'. These guys are trained to bring down and make a mess of humans who are either standing still or walking; they're happy and won't bother you if you're running. They usually go for humans one at a time and the nearest to them is the one that gets targeted.'

'The rules: I blow my whistle once and you guys start on your run. If you're not running I blow the whistle again and after that you have one more chance. After the third whistle I let R and W go and they'll go for the nearest of you who's not making an effort to run. Clear?'

 Blow the whistle.

No one moves. They don't believe this is real.

Second whistle.

'Last chance to get going!' I quip.

Third whistle, they don't budge, so I let the dogs go.

The dogs quickly down Geoff; 'R' grabs his arm and holds onto it and 'W' does the same with one of his legs.

The others are now running quite nicely and the dogs are happily standing guard over Geoff.

'Come on, you're all looking good; let's see those smiles now... look as if you're enjoying it...'

Sorry, I know it's very wicked of me, please don't be offended; it's my devilish sense of humour designed to keep a flagging class awake a little longer. The notable thing to realise and understand is that maladaptive chronic pain often stymies movement very badly, but the sufferer's anatomy, muscles, bones and joints of movement are perfectly capable of producing good movement. The emphasis of 'cause' is therefore on 'processing' not abnormality, or disease, of structure. Good chronic pain management can get some determined sufferers to be running, falling over, tumbling and doing a great many other enjoyable physical activities that they never thought would ever be possible again.

In figure 5.2 both the lateral and ventral horns are illustrated and both receive inputs from the dorsal horn. Both areas are part of 'output' or motor pathways whereby impulse traffic leaves the CNS in order to influence peripheral tissue targets. The ventral horn, via somatic motor nerves, influences movement, while the lateral horn, via pre and then post ganglionic sympathetic fibres influences more 'visceral' systems.

When thinking in terms of nociception and pain we tend to neglect its origins and purpose in favour of thinking about the sensation and its unpleasantness. Clearly, the purpose of nociception is to have some influence on other systems in order to conjure up support and help where it's needed. For example, a freshly twisted ankle requires conscious 'you' in partnership with the somatic motor system to alter muscle tone for guarding and to change patterns of movement in order to avoid undue stress while healing begins.

The sympathetic system helps, by supplying inflammatory/healing related chemicals direct to the tissues, as well as, in organising appropriate circulatory responses (see section 12). It is therefore hardly surprising that there are direct links from nociceptive processing sites to those involved in providing help where it is needed, i.e. the motor and autonomic horns of the cord. Both these 'motor' sites in the cord are of course under the influence and controlled by processing at higher levels—they are thus modulated—just like the dorsal horn. I think that it is important to appreciate this 'higher centre' involvement and influence and to link it to consciousness, at least to some degree, every time. What we are looking at here are some of the terminal pathways of the 'mind-body' network. Meaning; how we think and feel, how we focus on and how we give value to a given situation can all influence the biological processes going on in the tissues of our bodies. 'Top-Down' can be very important and has great potential to be influenced in useful ways.

There are likely many more connections, but those discussed are all that are needed to illustrate the point.

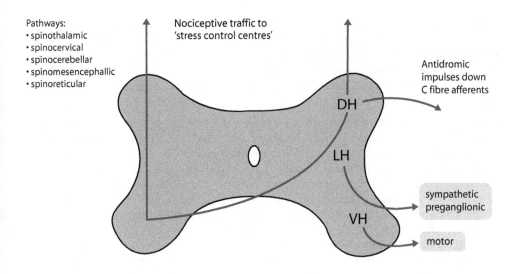

Figure 5.6 Grey matter of spinal cord—mainly to illustrate dorsal horn outputs.

Let us now have a brief look at spinal cord 'outputs'. Figure 5.6 details them.

Clearly, the dorsal horn 'outputs' to the brain. I think it's worth separating the terms nociception and pain, after all pain is often a result of nociception but it is not the only product, especially when seen from the perspective of stress biology. As I will discuss later, nociception is a response to a real physical 'threat' that has potential impact on an individual's wellbeing and survival. As we know from the stress literature, anything that is deemed threatening triggers some form of stress response whose purpose is to maintain the viability of the system. So, rather than thinking that nociception relays on up to the brain's 'pain-processing' centres, think more that it relays to threat-processing centres, of which pain-processing is just one compartment and option.

Nociceptive activity routes from the dorsal horn to the brain via a great many pathways – some that are evolutionarily old, like the tracts that are sometimes prefixed by the term 'paleo'; whereas others are evolutionarily more modern and hence are prefixed 'neo' in the older textbooks. The paleospinothalamic and the neospinothalamic are two examples of tracts taking nociceptive information to the thalamus. This terminology has been sadly dropped for a more modern anatomically descriptive one which is a shame I think. That aside, the most important thing, as I see it from an evolutionary biased perspective, relates to quick and slow pathways.

Quick pathways have very few synapses, in this way the information gets to its important destination quickly and hence can yield a quick response in turn. If you grab a plate that is very hot, you want to let go fast and you do thanks to those fast pathways. It's thanks to fast pathways that we react quickly and prevent an injury from being more damaging than it would be otherwise. Fast pathways tend to be precise in the information they relay, hence you know exactly where the pain is coming from and the type of pain too. These pathways all nicely relate to the 'sensory-discriminative' dimension of pain, i.e. where the pain is located, the quality or type of pain and its behaviour over time. It's the basic information that sets us thinking about it and working out what it means for us now and in the future. The dimension of pain that relates to our applying our thoughts and previous knowledge to pain so that we can evaluate it is often referred to as the 'cognitive dimension' of pain.

Slower pathways have more synapses and more interactions and are obviously of less importance when it comes to quick reactions and avoidance. These pathways tend to course in the more ancient tracts and run up through the deeper 'medial' parts of the brain stem; they link up with more primitive cortical and sub-cortical brain areas associated with the assessment of stress and threat and responses to it. The sites involved are all part of what's often called the 'limbic' brain and associated with emotional reactions. Pain, on the whole, links to centres that generally make you feel emotional. The three key emotions linked to pain being: fear, anxiety and anger for obvious reasons. This aspect tends to relate to the 'emotional dimension' of pain or more correctly, the 'motivational-affective' dimension. As we all know, feelings and emotions, especially strong ones, motivate us to get going and actually do something about the situation. Emotions drive behaviour. If you're whacked on the head by someone the subsequent pain plus the fear or anger that accompanies it, quickly motivate you to do something – fight or flight, get stuck in! Other situations with pain may motivate a 'do nothing-get grumpy-go to bed' type reaction.

All the systems interact and feed off each other of course and it would be naive to suggest that separate pathways in some way isolate each type of response. I would suggest the reader reviews Melzack and Walls brilliant paperback, 'The Challenge of Pain' to get the full picture from the horse's mouth.

Back to figure 5.6 and now note that the dorsal horn also outputs back down the sensory fibres! These are called 'antidromic' impulses and are defined as those that seem to go the wrong way down the axon. 'Orthodromic' impulses are 'orthodox' which is the term applied to those impulses that go in the right direction – hence go from the periphery into the CNS for sensory or afferent fibres and from the CNS out for motor and autonomic fibres and pathways. Antidromic impulses will be discussed in further detail later (section 11).

Spinal cord outputs, (figure 5.6), from the lateral horn go out into the sympathetic chain via 'preganglionic' sympathetic fibres; and from the ventral horn to somatic muscle via the peripheral nerves. Simple! The point is that nothing goes in without something coming out in response. Pain is always taught from the bottom-up, meaning starting in the tissues and describing injury and inflammation; then onto nociceptor activity and sensitisation; then spinal cord processing and finally up to the brain and... STOP. That's linear and it's daft. As we will see, I hope, pain involves circular and parallel processing with continuous input, processing and output components all the time in every patient and at all levels.

Don't let this confuse you, but if you think about it, the terms 'input' and 'output' only exist if you stop and consider one point on any given 'processing circle'. Thus, the output from the dorsal horn becomes the input at the next point you care to stop and ponder. This might be say, the brain stem, or the lateral horn of the spinal cord.

Chapter 5.3
Sex and the dorsal horn

'I am male. We males account for less than 50 percent of the population, yet we generate an incredibly disproportionate percentage of the violence.'

Robert Sapolsky

From this and the previous chapter the reader should be getting the basic idea. It's not boring, it's all about sex. Look at it this way and, daft though it may be, hopefully it will spark a little concentration in an otherwise potentially terminally dull topic.

Figure 5.7 is a cartoon, a schematic, of simple pain anatomy from the dorsal horn's perspective. The tissues get injured in some way and the nociceptors start screaming (Help, help, help, help, me, me, me, me, etc...). The afferent barrage bombards the dorsal horn and things start to happen.

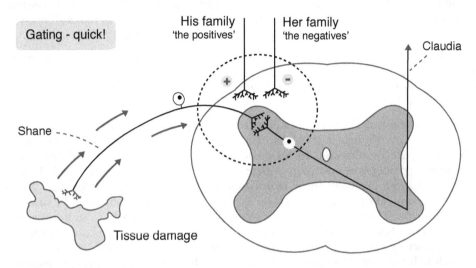

Figure 5.7 A very basic schematic of the dorsal horn

Think of the nociceptor as a virile young man, Shane, and the second cell, the transmission cell or 'T' cell as the cute female, Claudia. The little male and female signs are on the diagrams that follow. Claudia sends impulses up to the brain when she feels like it.

Shane is trying to 'get-off' with Claudia so he is showering her with all sorts of gifts (impulses and their 'neurotransmitter' consequences). Does she respond? Well, it's all down to the influence of their respective families.

As you can see the two families are present: Shane's family are all for the marriage to Claudia (she's good looking, has a good family and they've got loads of money); his family are the 'positives' – they're the 'facilitators' and they're going to do all they can to encourage the relationship. Claudia's family, on the other hand, don't think that Shane's are anywhere good enough. He's got a pretty common sounding name; he's not got a job with good prospects; he's always going out with his friends; he drives a crummy car; he doesn't live in the right area; he seems to drink too much and worst of all he smokes and farts in public. Also Shane's family, are unreliable; the brothers and sisters are claiming benefits and there is a pile of extra kids from various relationships. Claudia's family is of the opinion that the marriage is doomed to failure and they'll do anything to get in the way of it, if they can. Her family are the 'negatives', the 'inhibitors' and they want the whole thing off.

Facilitators and inhibitors are everywhere – they have local (segmental and inter-segmental inter-neurones), as well as more distant sources (e.g. descending excitatory and inhibitory neurones from the brain stem).

So, Shane's bombarding Claudia with all the stuff he thinks any girl loves while being greatly urged on by his scheming family. At the same time though, the whole thing is being wearisomely stifled by Claudia's doggedly mistrustful family unit and the natural coyness of the female species. The war is on! This is biological competition at the cellular level where the end result can be a tie up – marriage and possible permanent union; or even an all out, never-ending sexual orgy where it's all messed up, or perhaps a fleeting relationship that eventually fizzles out not to endure.

The moment to moment jostling that is going on between the family factions equates to nociceptive or pain 'gating'. Let's call the marriage on! ... Nociception gated 'in'. Let's call it off! ... Nociception gated 'out'. Pain-on, pain-off all the time (or the potential for this).

I'll discuss the normal behaviour of pain in later chapters (11.5 and Graded Exposure 3), a point now though is to realise and accept that **it is normal for all pains, whether acute or chronic, to wax and wane and come and go all the time.** Gating for nociception and pain is therefore a very active, on-going and shifting process. To me, clinically, there is no such thing as a truly consistent pain if you really listen and ask the right questions – sensory processing changes all the time. As a result, we must be very careful in our interpretations of pain behaviour in response to treatment. For example, are we just mucking about with the relative quantities of inhibitory or excitatory processing with our passive treatments? Is what we do enough to be of more than just fleeting benefit? That was certainly the case with the types of patients I saw in Geoff Maitland's practice in Adelaide.

In order to understand more straightforward chronic on-going pain as well as the related but more weird and crazy on-going pains, we need to look further and deeper into the biology of the dorsal horn, to the area enclosed by the dotted circle in the Figure 5.7. In other words we're going to look at some of the details of the synaptic and molecular biology of our 'affair' and the structural changes to the neurones that can result.

We are looking down to the level of one synapse, but the reality is more likely to be hundreds or even thousands of them. It is said that one CNS neurone on average connects with 1000 others (see Robertson 1999). Figure 5.8 helps this perspective a bit, I feel. See how one transmission cell is covered by the Triffid-like dendritic ends of terminating neurones. From our narratives perspective, the big cell in the middle is Claudia and all the fronds that surround her are the dendritic arms of Shane (and those of many other blokes who may or may not be willing to have a go too!).

As explained briefly in section 4, synapses can be in several 'activity' states. Firstly they can be asleep, or dormant; they're just there in close physical proximity to their target neurone minding their own business having no part in the general action that might be going on around them. Dormant synapses are termed 'refractory' and need to undergo a slow waking-up process to become active. Secondly, synapses can be designated as 'inactive', meaning that they are capable of being instantly active; it's

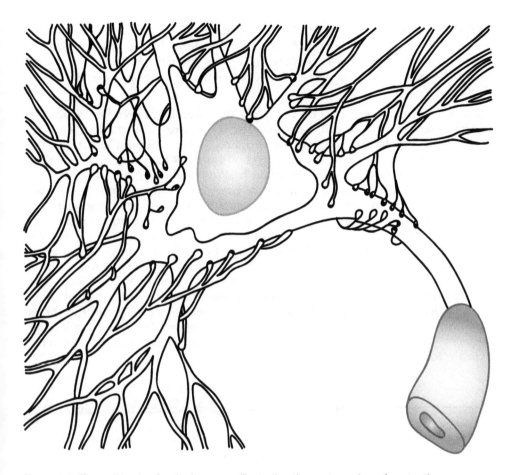

Figure 5.8 The cell body of a single neuron illustrating the vast number of contacting synapses.

just that they happen to be doing nothing at any given moment. Inactive synapses don't need to be woken-up they just need something to do. 'Active' synapses, our third state, are clearly hard at work forwarding messages and communicating with each other.   Finally, though not quite a synaptic 'state', is the formation of new synapses between cells. When one neurone makes another neurone fire, they develop a relationship and the more they keep firing together, the stronger their bonding becomes; when one fires, the other fires with ever increasing ease – unless some inhibitory process intervenes. The simple slogan 'cells that fire together wire together' is often referred to as 'Hebb's Rule' after Donald Hebb a Canadian psychologist who investigated learning back in the late 1940's. The real rule is this:

> *'When an axon of cell A is near enough to excite cell B or repeatedly and consistently takes part in firing it, some growth process or metabolic changes take place in one or both cells such that A's efficiency, as one of the cells firing B is increased.'*

Hebb didn't know what happened back then, but we do now. When neurones fire together they change structurally, forming new synapses among other things and indeed do almost literally wire together. I'll show you later, but let's now have a comfortable journey into the world of just one of the synapses between Shane and Claudia.

Figure 5.9 shows the synapse: on the left is the incoming nociceptor, Shane; on the right the transmission cell, Claudia. The seven arrows on the left represent the incoming impulse barrage from the periphery. When electrical activity like this gets to the end of a neurone it can't travel onwards. What it does do though, is to very efficiently stimulate vesicles (little bags of chemicals) that are chock full of neurotransmitters to burst open and release their contents into the synaptic cleft. The classic excitatory neurotransmitters are the amino acids, aspartate and glutamate. Out they go into the cleft and across the space to Claudia, the second cell. Does she react? Will she respond? Will she fire and send the message on? Will Shane have gained her attention? It's all down to her level of interest and this is down to the presence or not, of amino acid transmitter *receptors* and *ion channels* in the cell wall of her synapse. If she has none, or the ones she has are dormant or refractory, then she won't respond. If she has one or two, she may respond a little and if she has a great many she'll respond a great deal. *Sensitivity changes, in the first instance are all about the presence and amount of available receptors and ion channels.* As you can see in the diagram she has twelve receptors but only three of them are active.

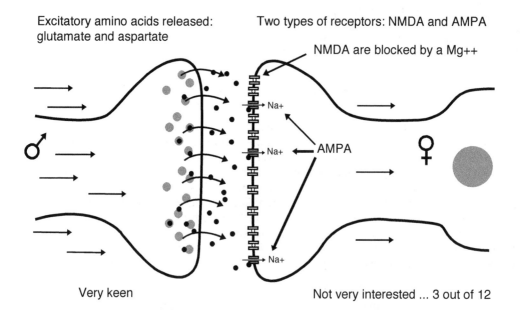

Excitatory amino acids released: glutamate and aspartate

Two types of receptors: NMDA and AMPA

NMDA are blocked by a Mg++

Na+

Na+ ← AMPA

Na+

Very keen

Not very interested ... 3 out of 12

Figure 5.9 A single synapse between two neurons, incoming barrage on the left from 'Shane' and little interest from 'Claudia' on the right.

We now need to side-track a bit to explain and feel comfortable with ion channels, receptors and neurone firing.

It's easy! Remember that in order for a neurone to fire off and an action potential to occur and travel down the axon, there is a sudden flow of sodium ions from the outside of the cell, through the axon cell wall, to the inside. Sodium ions being positively charged (Na^+), make the inside of the cell change from having a relatively negative charge (-70mV), to now having a more positive one (+50mV). This rush in of sodium ions and change in polarity is what produces the electrical current–the 'action potential' of a neurone.

Sodium ions pass through the cell wall via tiny pores called ion channels. Figure 5.10 illustrates four different kinds of ion channel. Ion channels can be opened and closed and in this way, they are said to be 'gated'. Opening an ion channel 'gate' allows chemicals like sodium ions to pass through and closing prevents the flow. What opens an ion channel then? Figure 5.10 shows four ways. The top ion channel has a chemical receptor built into it on the outside aspect of the channel. Chemicals in receptor biology are often called 'ligands'–hence this ion channel is called a 'ligand-gated' ion channel. The ligand binds onto the receptor and this then causes the ion channel to open. Weird though this may seem at first, it soon becomes fathomable when you understand that all ion channels and receptors are simply protein structures, which have a definite shape and configuration. They are physical 'structures' and hence are a part of the physical anatomy of the neurone. What is thought to happen when an ion channel opens is that it changes its shape or configuration when the ligand locks into the receptor on it. It's rather like a tiny Boa Constrictor snake that is tightly coiled around its prey, but then suddenly relaxes and releases it. The release of the prey leaves an open space (opens the gate) – in rush the sodium ions and off goes the impulse action potential down the axon. When neurotransmitter ligands like aspartate or glutamate lock into a receptor on an ion channel they 'reconfigure' it so that it opens and with a rush of ions across the membrane, current subsequently flows. No receptor/ion channels for aspartate and glutamate equals no flow and no effect. (Note, in figure 5.9 Claudia has three available channels and seven that are blocked or refractory).

Two ligand gated receptor/ion channel protein complexes are involved in the transmission of nociceptive impulse traffic and they are shown in the diagram: the AMPA (alpha amino-3-hydroxl-5-methyl-4-isoxazole!) and the NMDA (N-methyl-D-aspartate) receptor/ion channels.

Now, sometimes, receptors and ion channels are separate from one another on the cell wall. What happens here is that the neurotransmitter arrives at the receptor and locks onto it as before. This time, it produces its effect on the ion channel by triggering a series of chemical reactions *inside* the cell. These internal reactions eventually open the nearby ion channel by a process called 'phosphorylation' – a phosphate group is added to the protein of the ion channel and it is this that causes the configuration change, so that the channel opens. Crazy! But it's just the way some ligands and ion channels seem to work. Phosphorylation is illustrated in 'B' on the figure. Examples of this type of effect are seen with the neurotransmitter 'substance P' which we will discuss shortly.

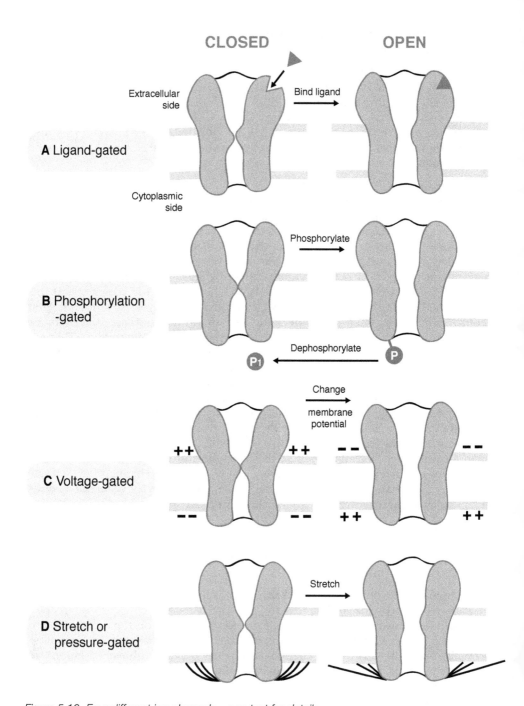

Figure 5.10 Four different ion channels – see text for details.

The third type of ion channel illustrated ('C') is a 'voltage-gated' ion channel. Simple! A given threshold voltage around the channel forces it open. It's rather like giving the coiled up Boa Constrictor an electrical jolt causing it to relax its grip! Voltage gated ion channels are found all the way along axons. Thus, once an impulse starts in one part of the neurone it will then pass on down the neurone given sufficient voltage gated channels along the way. No ion channels, no impulse propagation, but the more there are – the easier it gets.

'D' at the bottom of the figure, shows a 'stretch or pressure-gated' ion channel and is the presumed mechanism that relates to mechanosensitivity of a neuron. Think clinically, of physical movements that put physical forces on tissues and nerves, i.e. most movements do. If you bend your finger back sensory fibre nerve endings in the subcutaneous tissues and the ligamentous tissues of the joint are likely to get stretched. As the nerve is stretched the forces are transmitted to the cell wall and eventually the stretch activated ion channels get pulled open and off goes the flow of ions and then the impulse. The requirement for mechanosensitivity has to be mechanoreceptors! If there are none, or if the ones that are there are refractory, then there will be no pain with the physical tests that stress the tissues.

If you are like me in your clinical observations, you can think of plenty of sciatic pain problems that have frank loss of conduction and neuropathy, yet the SLR has no or very little sensitivity to movement, the SLR is of virtually normal range, yet the pain rages on! Those SLR's that are pain producing at 30 degrees or so, are likely to be well endowed with active mechanoreceptors/ion channels.

Back to Shane and Claudia. I hope you can now feel comfortable with what is going on here. Shane is giving Claudia everything he's got thanks to the afferent barrage and release of the glutamate and aspartate. She's only got three active AMPA receptors/ion channels and a few sodium ions are flowing into her cell, causing a modest response – she's being coy! (Her message is 'give me a ring next week if you like, I might be in'). All the other receptor/ion channels illustrated are NMDA's and these are special because they are kept in a refractory state by a magnesium ion (Mg^{++}), which blocks the channel. The Boa Constrictor is curled up round a big lump of magnesium which stops it from letting go.

But Shane keeps on firing and Claudia's AMPA channels let in a bit of Na^+–this results in the adjacent cell walls of the synapse becoming modestly electrically charged. There is now a 'voltage-differential' and which leads to a configuration change in the nearby NMDA channels, resulting in the magnesium ions popping out. Our Boa Constrictor is basically given a bit of a shock and it uncoils enough to let the magnesium ions make their escape.

This is all shown in figure 5.11. As you can see there are 3 open and working AMPA channels plus three more NMDA channels that have been activated. Claudia's interest has doubled; she's got six out of the ten channels available and a stronger current is now flowing. Things are looking up for Shane right now. The trouble is that Claudia's family can mess things up, or, Shane might run out of steam.

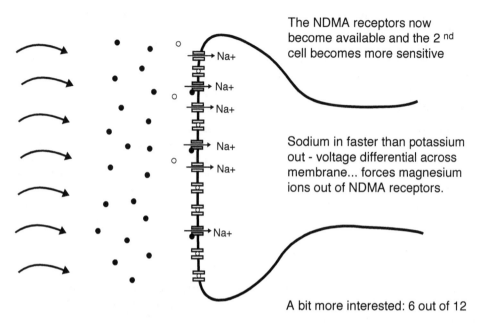

The NDMA receptors now become available and the 2 nd cell becomes more sensitive

Na+
Na+
Na+

Na+
Na+

Sodium in faster than potassium out - voltage differential across membrane... forces magnesium ions out of NDMA receptors.

Na+

A bit more interested: 6 out of 12

Figure 5.11 A slight increase in excitability. The AMPA receptors (dark) allow sodium ions through. The subsequent increase in membrane voltage forces Mg++ ions out of a few of the NMDA receptors (light) – which in turn allows more sodium ions in and an increase in responsiveness.

This is shown in the next figure, (5.12). Mg^{++} can go back into NMDA channels, they thus have the capability of being able to revert to being refractory. This happens when there is an increase in 'inhibitory' neurotransmitters in the vicinity ('2' in figure 5.12) or if the amount of excitatory neurotransmitters decreases ('1' in 5.12). In other words, Claudia's family (what on earth does she see in him?), are heavily intervening by releasing their inhibitory transmitters into the area. Examples of these are: the endogenous opioids (dynorphin and enkephlin), glycine and GABA (which stands for gamma amino butyric acid–the drug gabapentin is synthetic GABA). They work in two ways, first by clamping down on Shane's release of excitatory amino acids and second dampening down the excitability of Claudia's synaptic cell membrane. In this way, Claudia's family are quite intrusive in that they don't just have a go at her, they take it up with him too. They thus have both 'pre' and 'post'-synaptic effects. Clearly there would be little effect if Shane and Claudia were devoid of any inhibitory neurotransmitter receptors i.e. dynorphin, enkephalin, GABA and glycine receptors.

So, at this early stage the sensitivity of the dorsal horn second cell is dependent on:

1.   The amount of incoming activity. So, if the situation in the tissues improves and the nociceptive barrage diminishes, so too will the sensitivity situation centrally.

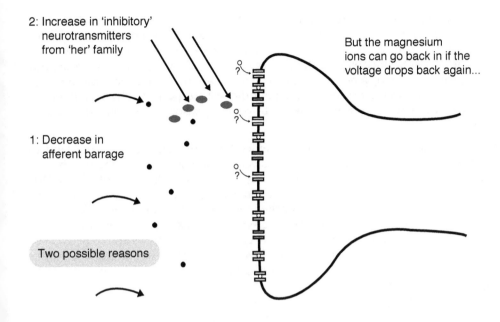

2: Increase in 'inhibitory'
neurotransmitters
from 'her' family

But the magnesium
ions can go back in if the
voltage drops back again...

1: Decrease in
afferent barrage

Two possible reasons

Figure 5.12 Loss of excitability/inhibition – the presence of inhibitory neurotransmitters dampening the effects of the excitatory neurotransmitters (glutamate and aspartate) and the decrease in excitatory barrage.

2. The amount of inhibitory activity going on there. In fact, inhibitory activity is going on all the time, to prevent any activity getting too out of hand. This continuous activity is termed 'tonic' activity, meaning ongoing. Intermittent inhibitory bursts of activity also occur and are termed 'phasic'. Shane has quite a wall of inhibition to penetrate.

    (And, if you are still with me, can you relate what's going on here to the brain and the environment and hence the needs of the individual? For example, Claudia's family will be really 'upping' their game if Shane's massive-incoming-nociceptive-afferent-barrage-trying-to-create-pain is competing with the individual's ability to save their own skin in a life-threatening situation. Think the absolute opposite too – the supersensitive individual who may be finding the whole pain experience a total and utter 'disaster-darling').

3. The amount and availability of the various receptors and ion channels related to the excitatory and inhibitory neurotransmitters.

What has so far been described, relates to simple 'gating' of nociceptive information – that allows it to wax and wane as conditions elsewhere in the organism or environment dictate. But, this doesn't explain clinical pain states and on-going chronic pain states to any satisfactory degree. There is more to it.

So far, Claudia and Shane are merely holding hands very loosely and only from time to time. Their attachment is easy to break at this stage. But Shane has more ammo. He doesn't just let rip with excitatory amino acids (glutamate and aspartate), he also releases 'substance P' into the synaptic cleft. Substance P is a neuropeptide (i.e. a protein made by a neuron), that is well known for its presence and influence on inflammation in the tissues – remember the flare response? Substance P, among many other functions, powerfully helps to produce vasodilation and extravasation in the tissues.

The bigger blobs in figure 5.13 are substance P and the dark squares on Claudia's cell wall are substance P receptors (they haven't suddenly appeared they were there all the time, I just didn't illustrate them). They're actually called neurokinin, or 'NK-1' receptors and are the type that have no ion channel attached to them. Receptors that have no ion channel directly attached, are called 'metabotropic' receptors, if you're interested. You are interested? Well then, you also need to know that when a receptor is attached to an ion channel, like NMDA's and AMPA's are, they're called 'iontotropic' receptors. Neuroscientists love to make things complicated, but it's neat to learn the basics! Hopefully, it'll make reading complicated pain mechanism papers easier for you.

Let's continue with increasing sensitivity ...

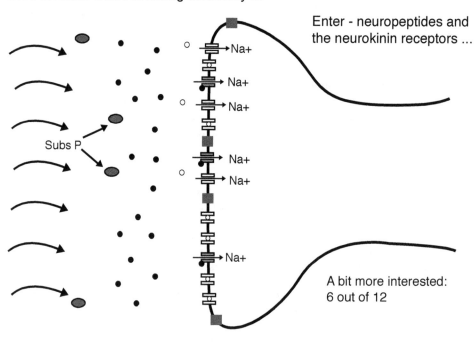

Enter - neuropeptides and the neurokinin receptors ...

A bit more interested: 6 out of 12

Subs P

Na+

Figure 5.13 The arrival of substance P and the start of a longer term excitatory state. The substance P or 'NK-1' receptors are the dark squares. See text.

Right, so now we have lots of substance P going across the synapse and Claudia's got the wherewithal to deal with them. Figure 5.14 shows the substance P neuropeptide snugly binding to the NK-1 receptors. What now? Well, it's extremely complicated, but basically when substance P combines with the NK-1 receptor it causes a re-configuration of the receptor protein component that's inside the cell, which in turn triggers a series of chemical reactions within the neuron. Stick to this: Claudia's getting a tingling feeling inside her and Shane's starting to make a real cool move here.

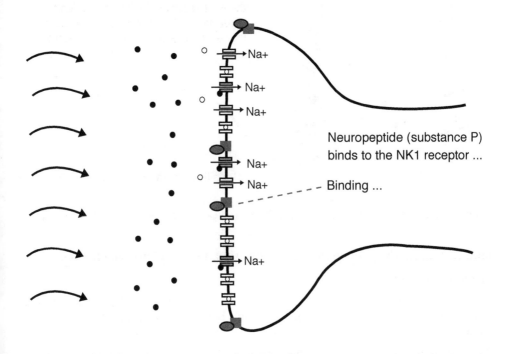

Neuropeptide (substance P) binds to the NK1 receptor ...

Binding ...

Figure 5.14 Showing substance P binding to the NK receptors

What do these reactions end up doing to Claudia then? They make her release calcium ions (Ca^{++}) from intracellular stores, which has a very positive/excitatory effect on sodium ion channels but also wickedly dampens down and inhibits the GABA, glycine and endorphin receptors that *her* family are so dependent on! Shane's really freeing her up nicely and he's smashed the enemy lines too!

Further, yet another set of calcium ion initiated chemical reactions within the cell causes, the NMDA 'Boa Constrictor' to relax and release its Mg^{++}, as well as increasing ion-channel 'opening time' of all excitatory receptor-ion-channels (i.e. AMPA's) too. The ejection of the Mg^{++} is shown in figure 5.15.

Thanks to Shane's 'substance P' gambit, he's now got her into a state that every time he sends a signal to her (incoming afferent barrage), she responds progressively

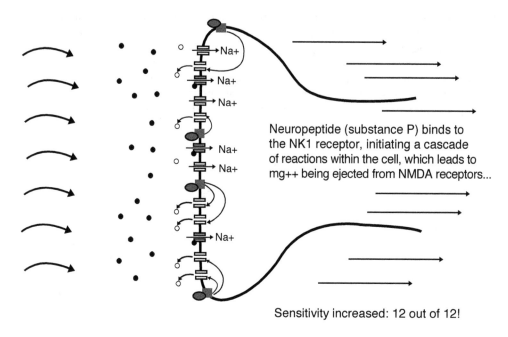

Neuropeptide (substance P) binds to the NK1 receptor, initiating a cascade of reactions within the cell, which leads to mg++ being ejected from NMDA receptors...

Sensitivity increased: 12 out of 12!

Figure 5.15 Internal cascade of reactions leading to ejection of Mg⁺⁺ ions from NMDA receptors.

more each time. The pain literature calls this situation 'wind-up like phenomenon'!

A patient example:

Keith has come in with a shoulder problem; he's had it ages and he's elaborated at length about the pain and what a bad time he's having. You start to do the physical examination...

'Right Keith, let's see what your movements are like – any pain in it right now?'

'Nagging in here, down here and over this bit here too'

'Can you lift it forwards and up? How's that?'

'Not bad, Lou, bit of a twinge under here.'

'Now try out to the side, good, doesn't look bad range wise.'

'Nasty under here and over the back now, Lou...'

'So pain resting compared to just now?'

'Doubled and spread a bit too.'

'Let's just finish the movements to get the full picture. Try behind your back like this. Yup, good range again, your shoulder mechanics look pretty good.'

'Hmmm, big deal, bloody throbbing and pumping now.'

He looks grey, he sits down with a thump – water, ah, right, better lie down a minute.

'This happens all the time, it moves fine, but just builds up and up and up.'

And so on. We all know it and it's maddening to deal with. Couldn't explain it in the old days, but can now! Yes! Manip physios call it 'irritable' – too right, but that didn't tell you why or what the reaction meant. Think about it, four or five movements and the pain more than doubles – to the point of feeling faint. There's no way that tissues, anatomy or even inflammation can do that as quickly. But nerves can. Considerations here are two fold, one, via central wind-up mechanisms, two, via peripheral nerve related mechanisms. I will discuss Marshall Devor's work at length in the Nerve Root section of the book. For now, it's enough to note that mild mechanical stimulation of injured peripheral nerve fibres can create massive impulse activity, sufficient to cause this type of reaction.

Everybody's probably now going, 'So how do you treat it then...?' And the answer is that it's not easy, but understanding that there's a central mechanism or a peripheral neurogenic mechanism going on, makes it a great deal easier to fathom and explain than in the old days. For now, see this type of reaction as highly maladaptive; it's very unhelpful and it is way out of proportion to any damage done. For treatment, the key is pain treatment and management alongside a desensitising approach. The use of effective anti-inflammatories/pain killers may be essential. Just as small mechanical stimuli can cause a massive reaction, so too small amounts of inflammation.

So why have this wind-up; why does it occur?

If you apply a hot probe to the skin, one that is hot enough to create a slight reddening or minor burn – it's uncomfortable. If you repeat it again to exactly the same spot with the probe at exactly the same temperature, you hurt it again but this time it's slightly more painful. Keep repeating and every time you repeat, the exact same stimulus causes a progressively more intense response – the pain 'winds-up' and often leaves an 'after-pain' too.

This example is clearly a wise response, repeated minor injury on injury equates to a bigger injury and the tissue is in danger of serious injury – if this activity continues. So, the reaction is adaptive; it's useful and stops us doing too much to one tissue and repeatedly injuring ourselves. The maladaptive response, like Keith's above, or like some peripheral nerve injury related pains, that produce incrementally more pain with repeated light touch, when there is no, or very little, evidence of injury or abnormality, indicates that the processing system itself is responsible for the problem. If I press 'K' on this computer just once and this comes up: kkkkkkkkkkkkkkkkkkkkkkkkkkkkkkkkkkkkkkkkkkkkkkkkkkkkkkkkkkkkkkkkkkkkkkkk...... then given that the keyboard is fine (think the tissue), the problem must reside with the processing in the computer itself (i.e. in the nervous system or in the nerve fibres going from the tissues to the nervous system).

Let's return to the Shane and Claudia romance.

Claudia is now twelve out of twelve in our figures (5.15). In the laboratory, this state of affairs doesn't take long to happen. Think of the repeated heat stimulus above; it could just as easily be a repeated mechanical stimulus – (try jabbing yourself repeatedly in the same spot with a sharp needle!). We are talking a relatively few seconds. No wonder we don't repeatedly perform a movement that has just caused us pain.

Shane and Claudia are now making out with abandon but things could still get a lot worse. The synapse is now well oiled and setting up the potential for a strong, possibly permanent union. If only Claudia's family could help.

Perhaps you are starting to work out why many pain-killers can be ineffective? Yes, the inhibitory receptors are blocked and no available inhibitory receptors, equals no-chance of controlling the situation. The key is ultimately Shane quelling his incoming afferent barrage activity, for example, rest the tissues, or inhibit the inflammation and hence keep the nociceptive nerve endings in the injured tissues as calm possible. While increased 'nociceptive' activity at the dorsal horn level is the result of Shane's excessive activity and his effect on Claudia, it ultimately comes to side with Claudia's family because the pain that the brain ultimately produces brings about a change in behaviour that does its best to keep the tissues calm. Resting and looking after the part that hurts is likely to be the best way to stem the nociceptive flow early on in the injury and recovery process, but significant endorphin release in the tissues may be a big, but under-rated and little researched possibility too. If you think about it, a lot of pain is such a rotten experience that it makes you not feel like doing anything – you basically feel crap! I deal with the 'sickness response' in the Vulnerable Organism chapter later (chapter GE 2.3).

Back to the nitty-gritty; down in the synapse...

Claudia's now highly charged and responding impressively. Shane has nearly got her! Calcium ions are the key to their more permanent union, and now they don't just get released from internal stores, they enter freely from outside the cell via calcium ion channels and NMDA channels too. Figure 5.16 shows the calcium ions entering via the NMDA channels and figure 5.17 shows calcium ions being released from intracellular stores.

Claudia's excitability now starts to spread beyond Shane's lonely connection to her. Sleeping synapses with other neurones become activated and hence, start to come into the picture – recall that she could well have around 1000 potential connections to other neurons, whose individual receptive fields may be far and wide. These connections include normally silent ones like those with $A\beta$ sensory fibre branches – with the result that when they become activated, they can start to excite her too. This is turning into a bit of an orgy!

Pain science tells us that if you experimentally stimulate a nociceptive C fibre to produce a very high intensity burst of activity for about 10-20 seconds, it will not only enhance the sensitivity of the individual Shane-Claudia synapse, but also of other synapses on Claudia that are nothing to do with it and don't normally have any effect on her at all. This can happen within seconds of the burst of activity. So, put aside the notion that 'central mechanisms' are only relevant in chronic pain, they're there in acute pain too, almost from the word go. They're fine if they are useful but they're a big problem if they are not.

We could call the $A\beta$ fibre 'Cedric' perhaps. A bit upper class, not interested in mucky nociception, just there to send on regular missives about comfortable and

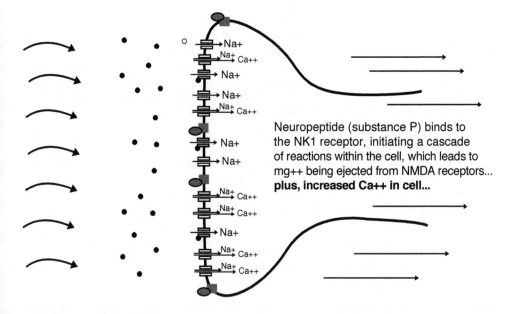

Neuropeptide (substance P) binds to the NK1 receptor, initiating a cascade of reactions within the cell, which leads to mg++ being ejected from NMDA receptors... **plus, increased Ca++ in cell...**

Figure 5.16 More established excitability state and the influx of Ca++ ions.

Further internal cascades (messenger systems) lead to release of more ca++ from intracellular stores

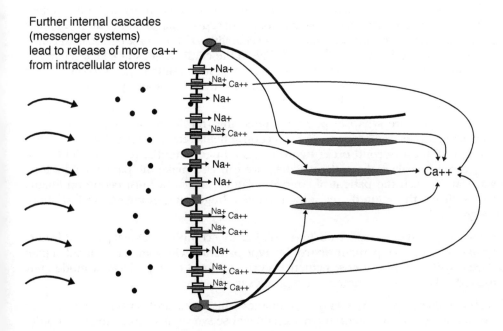

Figure 5.17 Further cascades of intracellular reactions via various 'messenger systems' leading to further build up of Ca++ ions.

pleasant things via other synapses and much quicker pathways (dorsal columns). The Cedrics of the world are normally well behaved but when times are ripe for them, they actually rather like to be part of a full on proper orgy–hence a few tentacles out to 'alert' Claudia. So, Shane's sensitising of Claudia isn't just about his synapses with her (so called 'homosynaptic' sensitisation)—he also ends up finding that many other synapses of hers start getting going with other fellows too (hence, heterosynaptic sensitisation) – including all the crafty Cedrics!

This neatly explains primary and secondary hyperalgesia. As we saw in the previous section (section 4) primary hyperalgesia is all about the sensitisation of nociceptors in the damaged tissues, so that when you move the injured part, or put pressure on it or touch it in some way, it produces pain – it's the 'true positive' for the tissues under test. They hurt, they're injured – period. Secondary hyperalgesia is all about non-damaged tissues sending messages into the CNS and causing pain. Testing produces a false positive. They hurt – they're not injured. This is 'Cedric' pain; pain that is mediated via Aβ fibres that normally only report non-noxious stuff like proprioception and light touch. So, the reason they can get wired into the pain pathways is just because old Cedric has a few of his little tentacles giving Claudia a gentle touch up and when she gives the OK, they're both happy.

Pain science tells us that this orgy situation not only occurs very rapidly, but also outlives the stimulus by many hours. Thus, stop Shane from performing and Claudia carries on partying regardless. Also, even if Shane settles down a bit and sends in relatively low levels of activity, still the sensitivity remains high and causes it to persist even longer than a few hours. Peripheral nerve injury and the resultant 'ectopic impulse' trains (chapter Nerve Root 1) of activity that arise and then bombard the dorsal horn, are found to maintain excitability for very long periods, so called 'prolonged central sensitisation'. Just like in the clinic, it doesn't take a second to make someone a lot worse and then it's well nigh impossible to get it to calm down again. You know, you've stirred someone up, and everyone's seen patients who have been badly stirred up by other clinicians.

The effect of more synapses being recruited into the 'orgy' also has the effect of increasing the second order neurons' receptive fields. Remember in the last section (4), one of these second order neurons has a huge potential receptive field. Not only can we easily make patients worse, we can also make the pain spread a long way too. So can the patient of course! Claudia, instead of just taking on Shane, whose 'from' the injured area, now recruits a huge gang of guys from just about everywhere!

At the worst end of the spectrum here, think of the 'complex regional pain syndrome' (causalgia/reflex sympathetic dystrophy) type patient—whose massive spread of pain started with a minor almost pathetic injury—a bump on the elbow, a moderately twisted ankle, a minor surgery are typical examples.

We see similar responses, but not so dramatic as this, day in and day out in clinical pain treatment and management: the neck pain whose symptoms spread to the shoulder blade and shoulder joint; the hip pain that spreads down the leg into the knee and later seems to start in the opposite leg. We now have a scientifically viable mechanism and explanation to validate these presentations and it's most likely all to do, or mainly to do, with processing changes. As an aside, it's worth noting that processing changes are highly likely to be responsible for the vagueness and inaccuracy of dermatomal and myotomal boundaries. Clinically, as far as my case load of patients over the years is concerned, the dermatomal referral patterns illustrated in neurological, orthopaedic and musculoskeletal textbooks are a complete myth.

The big question is why does it happen in some patients but not in others? I'll come back to this soon, because it's a question to which I've always wanted the answer.

Pause. A bit more here. Claudia gets so excitable, she wants more than Shane. Those Ca^{++} also trigger chemical reactions leading to the production of nitric oxide (NO), a gas. She releases the NO back into the synaptic cleft, which diffuses back to Shane (and others too!) and tries to get him stirred into even more action. NO is a 'presynaptic' excitatory chemical and is thought to work by promoting the release of excitatory neurotransmitters from the vesicles that contain them. (I see NO as acting like a pheromone, a bit of a scent that encourages increased arousal and sexy behaviour!).

Let's just recap a little. So far the central sensitisation can be put down to:

High activity of nociceptors (Shane)–hence lots of excitatory neurotransmitters: i.e. the excitatory amino acids glutamate and aspartate which act on AMPA and NMDA receptor-ion channels and neuropeptides – substance P was mentioned, but others include calcitonin gene related peptide (CGRP). Substance P acts on the NK-1 receptor and initiates **multiple cascades of chemical reactions** inside the second cell (Claudia), which…

Block or greatly inhibit receptors for inhibitory neurotransmitters that reside on the second neuron, effectively preventing inhibition from working – the term used by pain science is 'disinhibition'. Hence this blocking of inhibitory ligand receptors can stop the effects of dampening and inhibitory currents (Claudia's family), whose effects are mediated normally by the endorphins (enkephalin and dynorphin); GABA and glycine.

An increase in the efficiency and effectiveness of active excitatory receptors and linked ion channels as well as **making inactive or refractory ones become active**. E.g. unplugging the Mg^{++} block in the NMDA receptor.

The activation of previously dormant or silent synapses that the second order neuron has with other sensory fibres–hence Aβ fibres now accessing nociceptor/pain processing pathways.

The second order neuron to **release NO,** which diffuses back and then encourages the **pre-synaptic neuron to release excitatory neurotransmitters in even greater quantities**.

But it goes even further; the internal chemical reactions and cascades of reactions that have been mentioned can also lead to the switching on of genes – hence production of proteins, the synthesis of new cell 'components' and possible physical changes to the cell too.

I hope that you can remember 'protein synthesis' from school/college biology? The important thing to understand is that the structure of the cell and a large percentage of its chemical constituents are manufactured within the cell itself. Proteins give structure to the cell, for example, the 'cytoskeleton' and the cell wall contain proteins. A neuron cell wall also contains ion channels and receptors, all of which are protein-based structures. Neurotransmitters are proteins. Non-protein products are manufactured in the cell too and the reactions to produce these require enzymes to bring them about. Enzymes are of course proteins and different enzymes are required for different reactions.

Proteins are made up of massively long strings of amino acids, remember the twenty amino acids which are put together in specific sequences for specific proteins. The sequence of amino acids for a specific protein is determined by a specific gene and it's the gene that needs switching on, in order to produce the required protein.

Let's think of further ways that Claudia can get excited or be excited:

1. Make more ion channels and receptors and install them in the cell wall. Yup, this is what can and does happen given gene activation specific to those elements.

2. Grow more and make new synapses and connections; instead of Shane and Claudia just holding hands, they're now totally embraced with huge surface areas of contact. For this, there's good evidence from the science of memory and that concerned with 'long-term-potentiation' (LTP) – terms that are now being used with more and more frequency in the pain literature. Memory will be discussed shortly. The point is that sensitisation equates with the growth and formation of new synapses–the cell structure actually changes.

3. Up regulate the level of neurotransmitter production. Yup, that happens too...

For these things to happen, the appropriate proteins and protein complexes have to be synthesised. This means that specific genes have to be switched on relative to the desired protein product. For example, the gene that codes for substance P might be engaged and activated in the nociceptor (Shane), or a gene for the NMDA receptor in Claudia. When genes are switched on, messenger RNA has to be assembled adjacent to that gene (on the DNA... in the chromosome... in the nucleus) and released with the specific protein's code contained within its base sequence. This is then used as a template to organise the collection and slotting together of the appropriate amino acids in the correct sequence. To do this, RNA has to leave the nucleus and enter the cytoplasm of the nerve cell. Recall that it's 'transfer RNA' (tRNA) that is responsible for roaming around and picking up each individual amino acid from the cytoplasm and then bringing it to the appropriate 'slot' on the RNA, for the protein to be formed.

To understand pain and hypersensitivity, as well as the suppression and treatment of pain, it seems we have to have an appreciation of gene activation, or gene 'expression' as it is referred to in the literature. I would quite confidently suggest that any successful pain treatment is likely to be manipulating gene activity and hence: cell structure, cell physiology and cell function. One thought is that switching genes on and off and hence altering sensitivity states throughout the nervous system, is likely to be a far more potent mechanism to explain therapeutic interventions that relieve pain than anything that may, or may not, be happening in the tissues. As Mick Thacker points out, we might like to view ourselves as rather subtle, but very competent genetic engineers. While tissue changes must of course have an influence, for much of the time they just plod slowly on: living, metabolising, healing, adapting, strengthening and weakening in response to their unique but changing situation and the ageing process. The really big deal for me is that for pain expression, it all ultimately boils down to 'changes in processing', which I'll discuss more of later. For now, an important thought is to realise that changes in processing can be brought about from within the organism. Hence any changes in the way and extent to which a patient copes, thinks, deals with, moves, exercises, works, functions, gives attention to, worries about their pain and the situation it brings, may have huge implications on the way it is processed and perceived.

Why do some individuals suffer more than others? How can two people who sustain the same injury go on to have quite different outcomes? Why might one of these individuals go on to have a chronic pain problem while the other recovers well?

Here are some possible mechanisms:

1. ***Some people have more efficient pain inhibitory systems.*** We all know of people who have recovered remarkably quickly from what appears to be quite substantial injury. They soon get going again and they report little pain and show little pain behaviour. A great many of my patients over the years have turned out to be like this – all they've wanted from me was to know whether it was safe to get going or not. Should they get active or should they rest? They're easily managed and usually do very well. Others are the exact opposite – minor injuries equates with major pain and major functional problems. At the time of writing, I am treating two patients with twisted ankles. One has quite marked swelling, but has good stability and good balance. At three weeks he's starting to run again. The other patient is at six weeks. There's virtually no swelling; he's still hobbling and I can hardly touch the lateral ligament area or perform any end range modest stretches due to the sharp and intense pain. This guy has only just started to try going up on tip-toes. Clearly all of us are endowed with an 'anti-pain' system and it is my belief that like any other 'trait' we might care to observe, there is likely to be a spectrum, or continuum, from one extreme, for example, a very poor pain control system where individuals hurt at the slightest strain or stress, to the other –where the individual has a very powerful pain inhibitory system. Quite often these individuals don't report hurt until quite extreme forces are used, or, more commonly, they are capable of tolerating a great deal of pain. Are these individuals differently endowed with pain inhibitory systems and networks? Do they have a correspondingly different quota of inhibitory neurones, neurotransmitters and receptors? Are their brains wired differently? They must be. Their systems' efficiency or lack of is like all those other traits and nuances of

an individual, down to the unique effects of environment acting on an individual's given genetic blueprint.

2. ***The response of a given individual to the pain may be a big factor.*** How we respond psychologically to the 'pain situation' must have an impact on the processing that occurs. For example, if we show concern and give a great deal of attention to the problem and the pain, surely the end result will be a lifting of inhibitions, just like I showed earlier when we focused on the left foot and thought about different sensations and feelings. With pain, if you focus on it, get anxious about it, give it attention, get angry with it, all you are doing is shifting the nervous systems' processing to favour the perception and amplification of pain and in so doing lifting inhibitions. In large part it's individual 'you' doing it—'you' and the situation and context of what's happened to you—are what's allowing Shane and his family to get a grip and prevent Claudia's family from doing their 'inhibitory' work. In animal studies it has been shown that where descending inhibitory currents from the brain are prevented from reaching the dorsal horn (by cutting the spinal cord!), there is a dramatic increase in the level of plastic change that occurs there. Cutting the descending inhibition frees the shackles of inhibition and the 'orgy' scenario forges ahead unhindered. Continuous inappropriate attention and preoccupation with pain may have similar effects. No wonder a great deal of research into the development of chronic pain focuses on the negative early effects of issues like: beliefs and attributions, distress, what the patient has been told is wrong, their emotional state, the influence of work and family and so forth. A large part of these 'Top-Down', or, individual, brain to cord effects are likely to directly link to these neuroplastic imbalances of excitation/inhibition in the CNS and that are now thought to be such an important part of maladaptive pain states. I would press every clinician to think beyond, or in-parallel, to the biology and physiology here; it is all mere minutiae unless linked and considered in relation to, the person who suffers – the context of their problem and the way they are reacting to it. All nervous systems just do not react in the same way, we are all different.

3. ***The responses of injured peripheral nerves, is known to vary between one individual and the next.*** This is all to do with the known on-going and high levels of afferent barrages from injured and abnormal peripheral nerve fibres and will be discussed in the nerve root chapters later on (NR 1).

4. ***Different people heal at different rates.*** Dealt with in the healing and natural history chapters (13-15).

5. ***Some people may have deficiencies in peripheral control mechanisms.*** E.g. in the control they have over the amount of inflammation that is allowed to occur in a given situation. This is discussed in the healing and natural history chapters (13-15).

6. ***The patient being in a 'vulnerable' state.*** Dealt with in the 'Vulnerable Organism' chapter (GE 2.3).

That's it, that's sex and the dorsal horn. I hope I've managed to maintain your attention? Thank you!

Section 5
Read what I've read

Coderre, T.J., Katz J. et al., (1993) Contribution of central neuroplasticity to pathological pain: review of clinical and experimental evidence. Pain 52: 259-285.

Haigh R., McCabe C. et al., (2003) Joint stiffness in a phantom limb: evidence of central nervous system involvement in rheumatoid arthritis. Rheumatology 42: 888-892.

Kandel E.R., Hawkins D.H. (1993) The biological basis of learning and individuality. Mind and Brain. W H Freeman and Company. New York.

Kandel E.R., Schwartz JH et al., (1995) Essentials of neural science and behavior. Prentice Hall. London.

Kandel E.R. (2006) In Search of Memory. The Emergence of a New Science of Mind. WW Norton and Company. New York.

Melzack R., Wall P.D. (1965) Pain mechanisms: a new theory. Science 150 (3699): 971–979.

Melzack R., Wall P.D. (1996) The Challenge of Pain. Penguin. London.

Ridley M. (2003) The Red Queen. Sex and the Evolution of Human Nature. Perennial. London.

Robertson I. (1999) Mind Sculpture: Your Brains Untapped Potential. Bantam Press. London.

Rose S. (1992) The making of memory: From molecules to mind. Bantam Press. London.

Section 6

MEMORY BIOLOGY

Chapter 6.1
Circuits in the brain –
pain as a 'memory' circuit

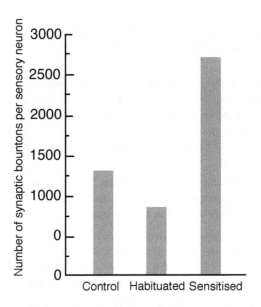

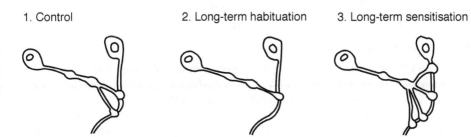

1. Control 2. Long-term habituation 3. Long-term sensitisation

Figure 6.1 Shows the physical increasing of synaptic boutons with learning or sensitising and the actual decrease in them with forgetting/habituating or 'getting used to it.' The bar graph gives the actual figures the lower three drawings illustrate the loss/growth of synaptic boutons relative to a 'control' state. Figure redrawn from unknown source – possibly from one of Eric Kandel's early papers or chapters.

The memory analogy

I've already mentioned Donald Hebb with his famous (and very useful) rule: 'cells that fire together wire together' and Eric Kandel, the world expert on memory, who won a Nobel Prize for his work in 2000. He was the one who showed that what Hebb hypothesized, back in the 1940's, actually occurred and he showed it first in a lowly invertebrate called 'Aplysia' – the sea slug[1]. What's special about Aplysia is that

1 - *Google or Wikipedia, 'Aplysia' to see what this creature looks like. Learn a bit more by watching this short vid: http://www.dailymotion.com/video/xjhxzw_memory-research-aplysia-californica-memorable-snail_school*

it has enormous neurons, so big in fact that they are clearly visible under a standard light microscope. Kandel saw that when Aplysia was given a simple learning task, the neurones involved increased the number of synaptic 'boutons' at their synapses (figure 6.1).

Boutons can be considered to be where neurones communicate with each other – the more boutons or synapses, the more communication! One of the conclusions was that when 'cells fire together and wire together', they anatomically change by physically making more/ stronger connections. As well as a complex biochemical process, learning ultimately has a physical impact at the cellular level.

I also mentioned my liking of Stephen Rose's book 'The Making of Memory'. His investigations of learning in chicks further backs up the Hebbian principle of memory, by revealing that synaptic growth and reconstruction leads to new patterns of connectivity between neurons, which are subsequently preserved over time.

These guys were the leading lights in memory biology for me, but I often prefer scientists who write more for the general public rather than for students of their own discipline; simply because they have a much neater way of putting things down and often do so in the context of the human condition and day to day life.

Ian Robertson, a professor of psychology at Trinity College Dublin, who is one of the world's leading researchers on brain rehabilitation, is just one of a few who is brilliantly gifted in the way he is able to explain things . His book 'Mind Sculpture – your brain's untapped potential' is a real gem.

Here's a quote from page 8:

> *'Everything which makes up 'you' – memories and hopes, pain and pleasure, morals and malevolence – is embroidered in a trembling web of 100 billion brain cells. On average, each cell is connected 1,000 times with other neurones, making a total of 100,000 billion connections. There are more cell meeting-points in a human brain than there are stars in our galaxy.'*

What a wonderful way of expressing the potential connectivity in the brain and thus its potential to form new pathways and new memories.

In the memory literature it is often said that if you were to start counting the number of potential connections in the human brain at the rate of one connection every second, it would take you thirty million years to complete the task! Or this: that there are more potential connections in one human brain than there are leaves in the Brazilian rain forest! Figure 6.2 may help a little, but even here the figure is far from reality.

The main point is that there is a lot of room for recording stuff in our brains – from the way to get home from the office, to the recognition of a deadly poisonous mushroom. Our knowledge, our beliefs, our ideas... are all somehow, marvellously contained in our brains and central nervous systems.

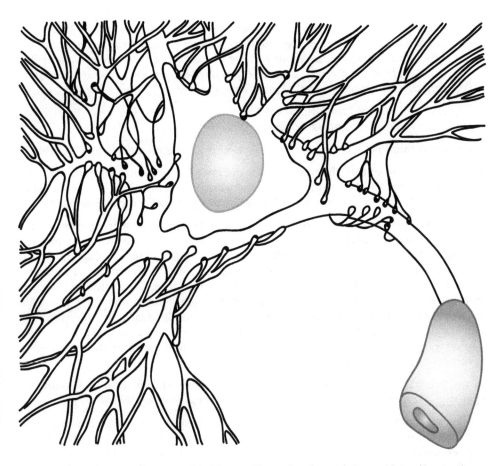

Figure 6.2 Cell body and axon of a CNS neuron illustrating the massive number of contacting axon terminals and the huge number of potential synapses there can be. I like this illustration because it helps the reader see the incredible complexity of the nervous system. In my lectures this figure was accompanied by this:- Consider that 30,000 neurons can fit into the space the size of a pin head or that a large match head's worth of your brain contains about 1 billion connections! Redrawn from Stevens CF 1988 The Neuron. In: Llinas RR (Ed). The biology of the Brain: From Neurons to Networks. Readings from Scientific American Magazine. Freeman and Company, New York. 1-19

Stephen Rose makes it clear as to how phenomenally amazing our brains are for remembering:

> 'Most of us worry that we have a poor memory, that we forget names, faces, vital appointments. Yet the scale and extent of what any one of us can remember are prodigious. Imagine sitting down and looking at a photograph for a few seconds. Then another, then another, then another... Suppose that a week later I show you the photographs again, each accompanied by a new, different one, and ask you to say which you had seen before. How many photographs do you think you could identify

*correctly before your memory ran out or you became confused? When
I asked my colleagues in the lab, their guesses ranged from twenty to
fifty. Yet when the experiment is done in reality most people can identify
accurately at least ten thousand different photographs without showing
any signs of 'running out' of memory capacity.*

*(Rose S 1992 The making of memory:
From molecules to mind. London, Bantam Press: p 2)*

It seems that there is plenty of room in our brains for the memories of a lifetime.

The main purpose of this chapter is to put the case for pain (and all the associated feelings, thoughts and behaviours that occur alongside), as having the potential to put down a CNS/brain memory circuit, just like any piece of information might.

The idea that phantom limb pains have a major component of their pain source within the neurones and circuitry of the central nervous system was first mooted by Ronald Melzack and Joel Katz back in the early 1990's. The language used was of 'somatosensory pain memories' and of pain 'imprints'. The focus was only on phantom limb pain and my feeling then was that the proposal could just as easily apply to any ongoing pain, or any maladaptive pain. Since that time the 'pain memory' notion has gained considerable support in the research literature, but sadly had little impact at the clinical level. As I've recounted elsewhere, it was nice to bring this notion to Pat Wall all those years ago and find him to quite warm and to be very receptive to the idea.

Let me present three fine cases which beautifully illustrate this notion of pain as a memory. The first two are from the work of Lenz et al (1994, 1995, 1997).

The first example involves a 69 year-old woman who was undergoing an operation to implant a deep brain-stimulating electrode for treatment of chronic leg and perineal pain secondary to arachnoiditis. Arachnoiditis is inflammation of the arachnoid, the middle lining of the dural sac, that surrounds the spinal cord and which has often been blamed as a culprit for chronic back and leg pain, following spinal interventions – like epidurals and surgery. Her past history also involved nine years of exertional angina that had been treated via angioplasty and had been stabilised. At the time of the implant operation she reported having not had an angina episode for two months. During the electrode implant operation specific sites in the thalamus were identified and stimulated. In one area, the awake patient reported feeling angina of exactly the same location and quality as she normally experienced during an attack. Further, the researchers were able to turn the angina pain on and off using the stimulator. The angina could even be reproduced in the presence of nitro-glycerin, a vasodilatory drug, normally self administered by the patient to relieve the angina. The authors pointed out that performing the exact same stimulation techniques in the same areas of other patients, but who did not have a history of angina, failed to reproduce any symptoms.

In another patient, thalamic electrical stimulation evoked intense pain in the perineal /genital region. On stimulation at one thalamic site, the patient responded that she 'thought she was having a baby.' At a second site, the stimulation reproduced pain experienced during sexual intercourse. As in the example above, intense pain experiences of the past had left their mark.

For years, the general view was that electrical stimulation of the brain did not produce pain. However, until the 1990's all brain stimulation experiments had been done on healthy asymptomatic subjects. From studies like these it was becoming clear that individuals, with a history of significant pain, may well have pain memories embedded in their nervous systems that have the potential to be rekindled.

My belief is that all new pains, of whatever origin, are bound to be making some kind of new circuit. Of course, the more significant (e.g. emotionally) and intense the pain, the stronger and more significant, or deeply embedded, will be the circuit that's produced to represent it.

The next example relates to phantom pain and was described by Hill and colleagues in 1996 (Hill et al. 1996). The female patient had had a below-knee amputation because of recurrent infection of a leg wound over a two year period. During this time she had suffered much pain following infection, multiple surgeries and damage to her popliteal nerve. The most distressing pain experienced was evoked by the treatment procedure carried out on the open drainage site on the calf, which had to be cleaned and repacked twice daily. During this time the patient was very distressed, not only by the pain, but also by the prospect of having to have the wounds dressed regularly. In order to manage the procedure, as comfortable as possible, she was administered diazepam and morphine prior to the treatment. For additional pain relief, a mixture of nitrous oxide and oxygen was also self-administered during the procedure. When even this did not alleviate her pain the decision was made to amputate.

Subsequent to the amputation, she experienced phantom limb pain of two kinds: that which was on-going, experienced only in the distal parts of the phantom limb and infrequent episodes and that which remarkably resembled some of the pre-amputation pains associated with the open drainage site. Triggers to this second pain were recorded by the researchers and varied from more physical antecedents, like a stump abscess problem after receiving a new prostheses and during a flu virus; to more cognitive/emotional ones, such as following a discussion of her pre-amputation experience with a friend and while watching a television drama, which showed an individual with a leg injury being given nitrous oxide and oxygen to relieve pain.

Thus, it seems that many tissue traumas or impairments that cause pain, can go on to leave some form of pain memory or pain circuit in the CNS. And that these pain circuits can be triggered or activated by neural processing that has its origins both in the body, as a result of some kind of physical stimulus (i.e. 'bottom-up'); as well as from in the brain/mind, via neural processing that emerges from thoughts and feelings ('top-down'), or more likely, a combination of the two working in tandem.

In order to simplify a very complex biology one way of looking at the brain and central nervous system is as a vast mass of neurons, a proportion of which are idly waiting to do something and thus have the potential to form new interconnections – hence new circuits. Figure 6.3 crudely represents a series of neurones some of which, the darkened ones, have already 'fired together and wired together'. It also illustrates the vast numbers of neurones that are idle and waiting to be used. Clearly if the brain has the capacity to hold more information in memory there must be provision for it. It seems that this is provided by this excess of idle neurones and idle connections that together have the potential to produce novel circuits. Idle neurons, becoming wired together and active, equate to new pathways and new memories! Of course a circuit or pathway only makes itself known to consciousness when it is active and when consciousness is receptive to that circuit. All of us may well have a massive library of pain circuits that are neatly referenced away in the dormant shelves of our memory library. Or, that *are* actively working away, but being 'gated-out' or ignored by consciousness.

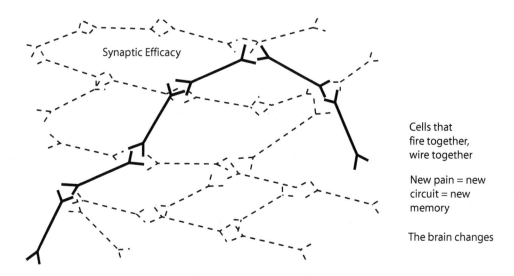

Synaptic Efficacy

Cells that fire together, wire together

New pain = new circuit = new memory

The brain changes

Figure 6.3 A very crude but quite adequate illustration of a 'new circuit' formed amongst otherwise 'idle' neurons. A new circuit represents a new memory.

I like the example of tinnitus, especially as I now have it. For me, it's a constant high pitched tone in both ears that's unvarying. When I become aware of it, it always makes me think how loud and how annoying it is, yet moments later I can be totally unaware of it. Tinnitus like this is a great example of how pain, or any symptom or bodily feeling, can be constant yet still be ignored by the brain. Or in the terms used by Wall and Melzack, my tinnitus can be 'gated' out. Because the tinnitus is always there if I go and 'look' for it, I assume that the tinnitus circuit is always firing. Or maybe the... 'when I go and look for it' thought actually turns the circuit on? Many other tinnitus sufferers report that theirs will often disappear altogether, even if they 'go and look' for it mentally, here then presumably, the circuit must be capable of refraining from firing.

The way neurons wire together to produce a memory is embraced in the biology that we dealt with in the last section, the Shane and Claudia scenario, but probably not to such a disruptive endpoint. Certainly, the biology of memory and the biology of long term pain, as viewed from the cellular level has a great many similarities and this is being recognised more and more by pain science. The literature calls the strong association of two neurones such that they fire well together – 'long term potentiation' or LTP. It also uses terms like memory 'imprint' and memory 'engram' to denote the physical thing that is memory. The reality is more likely to be an ever changing mass of inter-relations that ultimately maintains a specific 'pattern' of firing and connectivity. The end result is that important memories can be maintained throughout our lives in the face of a very changeable – minute to minute, hour to hour and day to day, neuronal anatomy and physiology. The stability of some memories over time is remarkable.

As you can see, to make it easy to explain to my physiotherapy and medical colleagues, as well as to patients, I like to think of any particular 'memory' as an individual physical circuit of some kind. When it is active and firing and able to tap into consciousness, it is then 'given to us' – 'it's recalled' and we become aware of the 'fact' – whatever it may be. This is easily illustrated: think of your telephone number! Think of your mother's and father's first names... Simple cues divert your attention to the question, your brain makes sense of it and then goes and finds the answer... the circuit switches on... ah yes, Jean and Vernon! Think of clinical questions like; 'Where is your pain right now?' And, 'How's that pain in your back?' As triggers to switching on pain circuits and maybe keeping them running! Or, if they are already switched on, like my tinnitus, to making the pathways to consciousness more efficient! Dwelling on symptoms may not be a good idea when you start thinking about pain from a neurobiological perspective.

The memory analogy is useful for understanding chronic pain and in order to see this I'm going to take a brief excursion into manic depression and epilepsy!

In the early 1990's I became interested in stress and the biology of stress (more of which later). This led me into literature on mood, anxiety and depression and I luckily came across a book called 'Listening to Prozac' by an American psychiatry professor called Peter Kramer. Chapter 5 on stress fascinated me. Here, Kramer starts off describing and explaining the 'gravest' of mood disorders: 'rapid cycling'...

> 'There are people in whom mood seems to have lost its attachment to psychological stimulus whatsoever, in whom affect has become utterly dissociated from their experience of the everyday world.
>
> These people may shift back and forth from deep depression to startling euphoria or to extreme irritability, sometimes in a matter of days or even hours. The radical swings may occur in response to very slight provocation, such as a minor disturbance of sleep. Or the cycling may be entirely autonomous – that is, the shift from mania to depression or vice versa may occur out of the blue, or even at fixed time intervals.'

I hope you can see the similarities to chronic pain with its accentuated and often greatly amplified, waxing and waning, with often little or no provocation? Just like chronic pain here is a condition that not only has a 'mind of its own', but is also sensitive to the tiniest provocation.

Kramer went on to describe the work of Robert Post, who devoted his life to understanding manic depression, or as it is now called 'Bipolar Disorder'. Robert Post did something that I think needs doing far more in many areas of medicine. He plotted and recorded the natural history of the depression/euphoria/mania disorder that so fascinated him.

Kramer summarises his findings:

> '*Sufferers would typically experience a single episode, usually of depression, in early life. Three to five years later, they might have a second episode. Two years later, an outbreak of depression would blend into subsequent mania. The later recurrences would typically include all the symptoms of earlier episodes, plus additional symptoms. The general pattern was a decrease in the interval between episodes and an increase in the severity and complexity of the episodes, until finally rapid cycling set in.*'

Robert Post noted that initial episodes and early subsequent episodes were mostly preceded by some form of psycho-social trauma. But, as time went on they would start with ever smaller stimuli until eventually, they became independent of any obvious stimuli. There was also a decreasing interval between episodes and each episode would last longer and longer.

The similarities to the development and characteristics of sensitisation and chronic pain, particularly chronic back pain, seemed to me excitingly obvious.

If you are like me, you will have listened to many chronic pain histories that started off with some kind of trauma and a consequent pain episode that eventually settled; but in the months and years that followed episodes came and went with ever increasing regularity, with more intense symptoms, and often coming for no apparent reason, until they eventually became a permanent but highly fluctuating feature.

Post was determined to study the problem and for this he needed an animal model of a condition with similar characteristics – one where repeated stimuli led to a rapidly increasing sensitisation.

The condition that attracted Post's attention was the 'kindling' of seizures that occurred in epilepsy. Probably more by luck than rational scientific reasoning and judgement (and that beautiful word – serendipity) researchers back in the 1960's had managed to create an animal model of epilepsy.

Experiments were done on rats and monkeys who had had an electrode implanted in their brains and were then subjected to a modest electrical current.

> '*If you pass a small amount of current, at first nothing observable will happen. After a series of intermittent small stimuli, the animal will have a limited seizure. If after an interval you again stimulate the sensitized site, less electricity will be required. With enough intermittent stimulation, the animal will exhibit more widespread seizures: first it will start to make*

chewing motions of its jaw and then nod its head, very soon one forepaw
will go in and out of spasm, then both forepaws, and so on. In time the
animal will start to seize spontaneously, with no stimulus at all. Eventually,
the interval between these seizures will decrease, with spontaneous seizures
occurring in ever more rapid succession and with greater symptomatic
complexity.'

To Post this was just like what he was seeing in the life charts of his bi-polar disorder patients. The process 'kindled' – just like a fire, starting off with a mere match to light it and then gradually getting greater and greater with no added stimulus needed and finally raging out of control.

Post reasoned that drugs to control seizures in epileptic patients should work on his bi-polar patients. He experimented with the anticonvulsant drug Tegretol and had marked success. Here then was a drug that worked on two quite different disorders, but where the process in common was 'kindling'. Researchers have gone on to show that when 'kindling' occurs, it is underpinned by a re-wiring of the brain. Repeated stimuli can sometimes lead to dramatic and very unhelpful changes in wiring, just like the Shane and Claudia scenario of the last section.

Importantly, kindling and the concomitant rewiring can be of 'physical' trauma origin, as in the introduced electrical current in the epileptic rat model, or of psychological trauma origin – as in those with mood disorder. Also, the rewiring is known to occur well before symptoms become evident.

Let's now look at the analogies that this seems to have with the development of chronic back pain:

- sufferers, like all of us, often undergo a variety of physical stresses and strains throughout their life (we are therefore all likely to 'kindle' a great many things)

- chronic pain histories usually start off with some kind of strain; trauma, inflammation, 'wear and tear' or overuse and a pain episode that eventually settles – though often not completely. (We have to also acknowledge that some individuals have problems that appear to start spontaneously and this needs some consideration.)

- the patient may remain good for quite a long time before another incident – which is often relatively minor; precipitates another episode that is similar in symptoms but may be more intense, spread out a bit, be more difficult to manage and last quite a lot longer

- the pattern continues with shorter and shorter gaps in between longer and longer episodes; pain often spreads, which in the worst cases can include large parts of the body

- in the worst cases the problem becomes more or less constant and in large part, has a mind of its own; patients find it difficult to be clear about exacerbating factors; their focus is generally on physical factors and as a result can end up avoiding just about all physical stressors that they believe may precipitate the flare-ups

• in some cases, just like bipolar disorder, there can be a rapid waxing and waning of symptoms; think of patients who one moment are hardly able to move yet moments later on or the next day their movements suddenly return

Pain coming and going like this cannot be explained in terms of tissue changes as tissues simply cannot change back and forth so rapidly – but processing can! Thus symptom fluctuations can be beautifully explained when changes in 'circuit-activity' or, what I like to call, 'changes in processing' are considered. Changes in processing can be the on/off activity of the circuit itself, or, as I believe for my tinnitus, the circuit continues playing but the inhibitory 'gating' process intervenes to prevent it impacting consciousness when my attention is elsewhere.

So, when we learn something, cells fire together and wire together and a new circuit forms as a result. The circuit has incoming and outgoing connections of course, incoming so that it can be started, outgoing, so that it can have some effect.

What's your telephone number? What's the name of the street you live in? What's your best friend's name... are all 'cues' that shift your attention to the areas of the brain most likely to contain the information. 'Cues', via input pathways, trigger brain circuits that end up supplying you with the answer – via output pathways to consciousness.

As I discussed, cues are essential for pain too. Here, it can help to think either 'top-down', for example, when the Dr or physio asks 'Where's your pain right now?' and the patient promptly focuses on it, or 'bottom-up', where some physical stress is put on sensitised tissues. Hence, if you've sprained your ankle a day or two previously, simply knock it somehow, or do an awkward movement and promptly pain appears. The 'cue' for the circuit here is physical and very straight-forward to clinically understand. That the aching pain is more of a burden at night time can be viewed as more 'top-down', in that it relates to what might be called 'lack of interference'. This is when the consciousness part brain has little to do and therefore easily allows in the constant aching ankle pain circuit which derived from the injured ankle and the on-going inflammatory chemicals driving it.

Chapter 6.2
'Jenny' – 'circuits that fire together wire together'

Jenny has had RSI in both arms for five years. She can no longer work. She reports that every time she uses a computer she ends up making her pain ten times worse and it stays worse for days. Fine, it therefore has a simple physical cue like the sprained ankle above? Wait a minute though, listen more carefully to her story – she can type fine for thirty minutes, the pain does build up, but it's not until two or three hours later that the pain gets really worse. Explain that! … Enquire more, listen again. It turns out that when she first started having the problem, she would find her shoulders and neck would get achy after typing for several hours without resting. A bit of rest and movement away from the typing and things would soon settle. Just like what might happen to you and I perhaps? Gradually over time, the pain came on more and more quickly with the typing and took longer and longer to settle. It also spread into her arms, eventually affecting her hands. For several years the pain linked reasonably directly to the physical input she did but gradually it got more and more sensitised. Eventually, she had to stop work as the pain became constant and, like most constant pains, it varied a great deal. Stopping activity no longer relieved the pain. It waxed and waned in a pretty unpredictable way regardless of what she did – which was hard to fathom at first. Like most people with pain in the muscles and joints of their limbs she tried to find a physical reason for the waxing and waning. On several occasions when the pain was bad she noted that she had been using the home computer a few hours previously. She admitted that the amount of typing and keyboard work was often a few minutes – but she'd note it, she'd made the link in her mind. She also started noting other physical activities that did the same thing – doing the washing up, vacuuming and ironing and so on. While quite often she found the actual tasks not particularly aggravating at the time, but she came to fear them because she 'knew' that they would make her worse later.

Jenny's pain could now be cued in by the 'expectation', or fear/concern that it would hurt several hours after computer activity or any other physical activity, like her household chores. Expectation/fear/concern circuits link with the pain circuits, so that when one fires the other is highly likely to follow at some point. It is simple conditioning, in that when one thing follows another often enough an association between the two occurs, even when the link is outwardly pretty weak. Hence, Pavlov's dogs were quickly trained to salivate when a bell rang or a light came on. Recall that the training period involved a bell and then the presentation of food. Obviously, when dogs see food they salivate in preparation for eating and digestion, a simple and vital reflex common to all of us and most of the higher orders of animals too. Pavlov kept repeating the process and soon found that just ringing the bell would produce the salivation. The dogs had learned that the bell meant food was coming. It reminds me of the school dinner bell! In the dog, the circuit that the bell switches on, becomes linked with the one relating to food and then the one that produces the saliva.

In Jenny, one circuit fires, the 'fear/expectation of pain circuit' and becomes linked or 'wired' to the other – the pain circuit.

In the dogs, if you keep ringing the bell without presenting the food the salivation, gets less and less until it stops occurring. The dog 'unlearns' the association because the rule that food followed the bell no longer holds true. In Jenny, as in all chronic pain patients, if activity can be done that doesn't produce the pain, the same disconnection can occur, but it usually requires many successful trials to be successful. The problem is that just like in the dog if the two things do occur together again, even after long periods of time, the association is very quickly rekindled.

Issues relating to this will be discussed further later on.

But is it possible to cue something in with such a long delay? And is it actually consistent? Or could it be a little to do with this? Thanks here to Stuart Sutherland for his fantastic book: 'Irrationality – The Enemy within'.[1]

Humans tend to only gather the information and facts that fit with their personal set of hypotheses, theories and beliefs and at the same time they tend to dismiss or ignore anything that doesn't fit. We're very good at finding 'facts' that confirm our beliefs and very bad at finding evidence that might 'disconfirm' them. Sutherland goes on... 'To establish that a rule is likely to be true one must try to prove it false, but this is just what people don't do.'

As an aside, this is very much a feature of Drs, physiotherapists, manual therapists, 'alternative practitioners' and so forth, who often tend to operate within hard-held beliefs in various models and paradigms of the presentations they see and the treatments they offer for them. They keep finding facts that confirm their theories and ignore those that don't fit with them and thus make their favourite diagnosis.

So, Jenny noticed that once or twice when her pain was bad that she'd been on the computer a while before and then blamed the computer for aggravating the pain. It quite often fitted so the rule/belief stuck. Fine, but did she notice the times when she did a bit of computing and it made no difference? Or the times when she did computing or household chores and the pain was actually better? According to Sutherland we may even go as far as denying the existence or relevance of contradictory evidence.

I want to make the point here that this sort of human reasoning and behaviour is not 'bad' behaviour or reasoning – it's normal, humans *normally* do this. We all do! We work hard to keep our belief systems intact and consistent – it's just that some people are far more stubborn at shifting out of them than others!

(The good thing is that now you're aware of this you can be on the lookout for it in your own reasoning and thinking!)

Linking a specific activity to a pain, especially when there is a delay in onset of symptoms, is fraught with difficulty. Linking to the computer might be fine a few times but when it's worse with no computer use what do you then put it down to? Yes, link it to anything else you might have been doing 2-3 hours before... ironing, housework, shopping etc... The list is never ending.

I hope the reader is now seeing that Jenny's pain has a 'bi-polar' behaviour; it waxes and wanes alot, but in reality it has a bit of a 'mind of its own' as well as a large chunk that is highly likely to relate to situation or context. She understandably just

---

1   *Sutherland, S. (1992). Irrationality, The Enemy within. London. Penguin books.*

happened to link it to the most obvious thing in relation to the original cause and behaviour of the pain. I hope you're also thinking of those patients who link their pain to changes in the weather!

After explaining the nature of chronic pain; I wanted to help Jenny to see that linking her pain to physical activity all the time, was stopping her doing more and more. And that this was a big factor in growing inactivity, disability and unfitness issues. She made an activity diary and she made a pain diary for two weeks. What it clearly showed was that pain increases and flare ups were just as likely to occur 2-3 hours after resting as they were after any form of 'home' activity. The diary showed that the pain had a mind of its own and this 'disconfirmation' of her beliefs hugely helped Jenny to take on board pain explanations related to 'pain circuits' and 'faulty processing', rather than those relating to abnormal or damaged structure. The diary also occasionally showed that when Jenny had done quite a lot of physical activity, she was later no worse and once or twice a lot better. Jenny freed her mind of the links and from then on started to work on getting fitter with far less fear.

'Cells that fire apart depart' or more practically for us: 'Circuits that fire apart depart'...

Important factors in the making of pain memories...

I tend to consider the following factors that may be of significance, individually or combined, in forming a circuit for a pain 'memory' that has the *potential* to cause chronic pain:

1. High levels of on-going acute pain that the patient doesn't cope well with. Here, there is likely to be a very high intensity afferent barrage from nociceptors and/or damaged peripheral nerves. Think about it – anything that is intense and prolonged is likely to be remembered. High intensity 'nociceptive signals' are highly likely to 'get in' and command a high place in conscious awareness – if given the slightest chance . My thought is that afferent barrages from damaged nerves are particularly culpable. This is discussed in more detail in the nerve root section of the book.

2. Raised attention to pain that is accompanied by a high degree of worry or anxiety about it. If you keep focusing, dwelling on or thinking about something, you soon get it into your head and – you soon learn it! You also tend to amplify anything you give full attention to. I can easily do this with my tinnitus for example. Committing anything to memory involves; attention, interest, repetition and practice and this type of behaviour is common in patients who have musculoskeletal pain. Adding emotion to anything will also help to preserve it in memory; since strong emotions enhance memory mechanisms, especially the negative emotions like fear, worry, anxiety and anger. As I will discuss later, it makes sense in

evolutionary terms that anything that is threatening to us, should be remembered. (Knowledge of how we escaped a threat may be also vital for future survival). While having a vivid memory of a situation that caused pain is very helpful; having a continual annoying pain 'memory-tune' playing all the time is a far different matter and is surely not helpful at all.

'Lifted pain inhibition due to undue attention/concern/fear/anxiety' summarises the thrust of what I'm getting at here: in the language of the last chapter, 'Claudia's family' are brutally silenced by the intense interest in the situation!

3. A poor, weakened, inhibited or otherwise impaired pain inhibitory system. This contrasts with the previous 'lifting of pain inhibition' in that rather than being an effect related to mental state, this is a situation where the pain inhibitory system is weak and inefficient, regardless of conscious factors like attention. The ability of the brain and CNS to turn pain off is hugely variable from one human to the next, as well as within the same human from moment to moment, hour to hour, day to day and so on over a lifetime. My stance is that if we observe any system, function or capability in a human it will always turn out that some of us are much better at some things than others. For example, some people are naturally talented musically, some people can be good musicians but have to practice hard and others are simply not talented at all. There is always a simple spectrum, or continuum; which at one end has incredible virtuosity, the average ability in the middle and at the other end virtually zero talent at all. Observe any system, function, ability, characteristic, sense etc. and you will find a spectrum of capability within it, both between different individuals as well as in the same individual, observed over time. I believe our pain inhibitory systems and our pain enhancement systems are subject to this variability too; having both a natural, or inherited/genes component combined with the influence of environmental factors, that ultimately leads to an individuals' current and unique sensitivity 'setting' capability.

At the time of writing there seems to be good emerging evidence that chronic pain sufferers have significant degenerative changes of grey matter in areas of the brain known to be linked to 'anti-nociception', 'pain modulation' and analgesia. Arne May's article[1], 'Chronic pain may change the structure of the brain' is a particularly informative review of the state of the art in this area. Recent research highlights quite extensive structural changes and suggests that they may well be maladaptive in nature. Arne uses the term 'structural maladaptive plasticity' which I rather like. He also asks the question as to whether the structural changes in the 'pain matrix' of the brain *precede* or *succeed* the clinical 'chronification' process. My hunch is that there is almost bound to be a bit of both, but there will be large variations between individuals. As he proposes at the end of the article, it would be very interesting to see if structural changes actually normalise with adequate treatment or when recovery occurs. He also wonders as to whether plying a healthy brain with

1 - Arne May, 2008 Chronic pain may change the structure of the brain'. Pain 137:7-15

nociceptive input over several days would produce similar structural changes or whether it would merely produce a healthy response. For example, anti-nociceptive areas may actually increase in size as the person and their brain combat and then adapt to the ongoing situation.

I've always thought that good pain inhibition, like good football skills, is in quite a large part the result of plenty of good practice – especially when you're young! Hence lots of outside play, falling over, grazes and bumps, falling into stinging nettles and out of trees and even the occasionally fisty-cuffs with your mates... All are likely to give a bit of practice to your pain 'off' systems. Other environmental factors may include how you were brought up to react to pain, how those around you, especially your parents and siblings, reacted to pain and so forth. Our behaviours and our reactions just as our pain feelings and responses are surely moulded and manipulated by our early experiences. Luckily, the wonderful plasticity of the human brain allows clinicians to think in terms of rewiring pain control related components to some degree.

The notion that chronic pain sufferers pain controlling systems could benefit from prolonged and persistent hardening up may be borne out by the claims of some behavioural programmes like the 'school for bravery' approach that has been documented (Williams, 1989).

Section 6
Read what I've read

Greenfield S. (2002) The Private Life of the Brain. Penguin. London.

Hebb D.O. (1980) Essays on Mind. Psychology Press. Hove.

Hebb D.O. (2005) The Organization of Behavior: A Neuropsychological Theory. Psychology Press. Hove.

Hill A., C. A. Niven, et al., (1996) Pain memories in phantom limbs: a case study. Pain 66: 381-384.

Kandel E.R., Hawkins D.H. (1993) The biological basis of learning and individuality. Mind and Brain. W H Freeman and Company. New York.

Kandel E.R., Schwartz JH et al., (1995) Essentials of neural science and behavior. Prentice Hall. London.

Kandel E.R. (2006) In Search of Memory. The Emergence of a New Science of Mind. WW Norton and Company. New York.

Katz J., Melzack R. (1990) Pain "memories" in phantom limbs: review and clinical observations. Pain 43:319 –336.

Lenz, F. A., R. H. Gracely, et al. (1994). "The sensation of angina can be evoked by stimulation of the human thalamus." Pain 59: 119-125.

Kramer P.D. (1997) Listening to Prozac: A Psychiatrist Explores Antidepressant Drugs and the Remaking of the Self: Revised Edition. Penguin. London.

Lenz F. A., R. H. Gracely, et al. (1995) Stimulation in the human somatosensory thalamus can reproduce both the affective and sensory dimensions of previously experienced pain. Nature Medicine 1(9): 910-913.

Lenz F. A., R. H. Gracely, et al. (1997) The sensory-limbic model of pain memory. Pain Forum 6(1): 22-31.

May A. (2008) Chronic pain may change the structure of the brain. Pain 137:7-15.

Post R. M. (1990) Sensitization and kindling perspectives for the course of affective illness: Toward a new treatment with the anticonvulsant carbamazepine. Pharmacopsychiatry 23: 3-17.

Post R. M. and J. C. Ballenger (1984). Neurobiology of mood disorders. Williams & Wilkins. Baltimore.

Post R. M., D. R. Rubinow, et al. (1986) Conditioning and sensitisation in the longitudinal course of affective illness. British Journal of Psychiatry 149: 191-201.

Robertson I. (2010) Mind Sculpture: Your Brain's Untapped Potential. Bantam. London.

Rose S. (1992) The making of memory: From molecules to mind. Bantam Press. London.

Williams J. (1989) Illness Behaviour to Wellness Behaviour: The 'School for Bravery' Approach. Physiotherapy 75(1):2-7.

Section 7

THE PLACEBO 1

Chapter 7.1
The Placebo 1: insults, pseudo-science and stigma!

Key articles and chapters that strongly influenced me ....

Wall, P. D. (1992). "The Placebo effect: an unpopular topic." <u>*Pain*</u> *51: 1-3.*

Wall, P. D. (1994). The placebo and the placebo response. <u>*Textbook of Pain*</u>*. P. D. Wall and R. Melzack. Edinburgh, Churchill Livingstone: 1297-1307.*

If I was a university lecturer teaching a 'pain module' to medics and physiotherapists I would more than likely start my lectures on pain by talking about the placebo. Why? Because it's fascinating and it forces you to be involved with the brain and the notion of 'top-down' right from the get-go.

My goal is to get you interested in it, feel comfortable with it and then help you to get to grips with how to deal with it clinically. I also want you to realise that it's a massive part of medicine, or any form of helping people and that it's real, biological and not evidence of 'imagination'.

Here we go...

You may or may not have heard and be surprised by quotes that run something like this: *'Surgery has the most potent placebo effect that can be exercised in medicine'*... and... *'The history of medicine is the history of the placebo'*... and then probably ignored them or maybe even scoffed at them. Since the placebo phenomenon started to be described and understood a great many clinicians, including those in mainstream medicine, the alternative therapies and those, like physiotherapy who are 'allied to medicine', were of the firm belief that 'their' treatments and interventions were rational, proven, scientific, 'real' and had little or nothing to do with it? Admitting to the placebo effect as a potent and major part of 'therapy' would be like admitting to hoodwinking the patient and that the treatment offered was no better than 'snake-oil'. The admission of fraud!

Perhaps you haven't heard those quotes but as a therapist you've been told by Drs and consultants that your ministrations were little more than a placebo? I have many times and it's clearly meant as an insult and a comment that points to physiotherapy as being a waste of resources that could better used elsewhere. My reply would often be three-pronged, and with or without barbs... Here is my trident...

1. I'd use the quote above about surgery being THE most potent placebo and that this makes it a worryingly dangerous form of medicine – see the placebo surgery examples later to back this up.

2. That physiotherapy is mostly about 'rehabilitation' – meaning shifting a patient from a position of relative disability into recovery and back to functioning and fitness.

3. Part of that positive and very practical process embraces the placebo as much as it can.

Alternative medicine[1] is given a hard time and a great many physiotherapists use it. Manual therapy included.

Ben Goldacre's book 'Bad Science[2]' is well worth reading. He makes the point that

---

1 - *A variety of therapeutic or preventive health care practices, such as homeopathy, naturopathy, chiropractic, and herbal medicine, that do not follow generally accepted medical methods and may not have a scientific explanation for their effectiveness. It's another name for complimentary medicine.*
2 - *Goldacre B. 2008 Bad Science. Forth Estate, London.*

inventors of therapies or therapy gurus and their acolytes go to extreme lengths to give their therapy a physiological, anatomical, biomechanical, pathological and scientific **sounding** basis. In today's culture, if something sounds 'sciency' – it must be credible! The other thing that's persuasive and very common is when the treatment has a founding-father figure who's designated 'Dr' or 'Professor'. That many of these characters have quite bogus qualifications has been discussed by Ben Goldacre. The example I found was of John Upledger, the founder of cranial osteopathy, described on one website[1] as 'a medical surgeon', when in fact he's not a medical surgeon at all; he's an osteopathic physician whose done research into 'cranio-sacral' theories. Reviews of his studies reveal that they are of insufficient quality to provide conclusive proof for the effectiveness of cranio-sacral therapy and the existence of cranial bone movement[2] – yet the juggernaut enthusiastically rolls on.

Alternative medicine therapists (funnily, just like surgeons) find the suggestion that the outcomes they reportedly achieve are mostly, or even partly, due to 'psychological' elements, or the 'placebo' effect, totally unacceptable and often go to great lengths to vilify the research and the researchers who dare make such suggestions. Dr Edzard Ernst, the recently retired highly informed Professor of Complimentary medicine from the University of Exeter, comes to mind as a particularly strong critic. His meticulous research of these therapies has drawn much ire from the therapists whose methods it investigates and has earned him the title 'the scourge of alternative medicine[3]'. All he did was set up very carefully controlled double-blind trials and reported on the outcomes.

On a positive note, in an article in the British Journal of General Practice, Ernst published a useful list of treatments that 'demonstrably generate *more good than harm*'. Cop these: St John's Wort for depression; hawthorn for congestive heart failure; guar gum for diabetes; acupuncture for nausea and osteoarthritis, aromatherapy as a palliative treatment for cancer; hypnosis for labour pain; and massage, music therapy and relaxation therapy for anxiety and insomnia.[2] At the other extreme Ernst, jointly with Simon Singh[4] – he's the rather brilliant science writer best known for his longstanding libel lawsuit[5] with the British Chiropractic Association (BCA) over his criticism of the claims of their therapy which were published in the Guardian newspaper – have criticised homeopathy and alternative medicine in the strongest terms. For example when asked what they thought about the future of alternative medicine they replied:

---

1 - *www.healthandgoodness.com/Therapies/what_is_cranial_osteopathy.php*
2 - *Green C et al. 1999) A systematic review of craniosacral therapy: biological plausibility, assessment reliability and clinical effectiveness. Complement Ther Med 7 (4): 201–7*
3 - *See Edzard Ernst page on Wikipedia*
4 - *Singh S, Ernst E 2008 Trick or Treatment: The undeniable facts about alternative medicine. Bantam Press, London.*
5 - *Singh won and as a result of this a campaign to change the libel laws in this country was successfully launched. On 25 April 2013 the Defamation Act 2013 became law. It ensures 'a fair balance is struck between the right to freedom of expression and the protection of reputation.' Under the new law plaintiffs (i.e. here, the BCA) must show they suffer serious harm before the court will accept the case.*

'For us, there is no such thing as alternative medicine. There is either medicine that is effective or not, medicine that is safe or not. So-called alternative therapies need to be assessed and then classified as good medicines or bogus medicines. Hopefully, in the future, the good medicines will be embraced within conventional medicine and the bogus medicines will be abandoned.'

Cool, but it you are solely a 'technique' practitioner or therapist – feel threatened, rightly, unless you're offering something from the list above!

What always amuses me is that while a great many 'practitioners' take umbrage at criticism of their particular therapy they are often really happy to hear that other competing therapies, medicines and interventions are well dowsed with placebo elements. Yes you are. If you love your manual therapy you love to trash electrotherapy; if you're a physician you love to trash surgeons and vice versa. My bug-bear is towards the pseudo-scientific diagnoses, explanations and accompanying flim-flam that some physiotherapists, chiropractors, osteopaths and other 'alternative' health practitioners pedal to the seemingly gullible public. I'm not one for a 'mission' in life, but my holler from the 'pulpit of logic and reasoning' to all these practitioners and clinicians would go something like this...

'If only you could all twig that you are all, ultimately, doing the same thing – **playing with processing,** yet because you don't see that, you're wasting a huge opportunity to help a great deal more and sell a great deal less.'

Sadly Ernst, as a result of his apostasy (he was trained in many branches of alternative medicine), was forced/persuaded to retire from Exeter university after a long-running spat with the university and the Prince of Wales, who is well known for being highly supportive of complementary medicine. Well, I guess we can feel comforted that at least he didn't get executed, as heretics of the Church and Crown did not so long ago.

I'd now like to discuss two perspectives of 'all alternative' approaches; the first is quasi supportive because of the importance of the 'placebo' mechanism and the second is not because it focuses on what is being diagnosed and peddled.

With regards to the first: now, it's all well and good to state, as Ernst and Singh did, that there's either 'good medicine which is effective medicine' and 'bad which isn't', **when medicine has a lot to offer the things that people complain about**. The problem with this attitude is that there are a great many ailments and problems that bother humans for which medicine has nothing useful to offer or is only of limited help with.

I think most people who break their leg or have a nasty accident, or get a nasty looking and smelling discharge, would much rather go to the local A&E department, than visit their physio, homeopath, chiropractor or cranio-sacral therapist? A plaster cast or a pin and plate are a far better remedy than a bottle of liquid essence of nothing at all, or someone holding your head for half an hour or even a session out front with the charismatic healer who's just come to town in his private helicopter. On the other hand, if you've got problems with migraines or fatigue or skin problems or aches and pains, or hair falling out... then A&E isn't where you want to go and it's quite unusual to find the average Dr to be that interested. So, who's willing to take this incurable-by-medicine stuff on? Yes, you, me and all the other therapists too and we're all in it together.

Every clinician who has listened to their patients for long enough will have heard how such-and-such a therapy cured the thirty years of migraines, psoriasis, eczema and chronic fatigue problem in two goes. While criticised by researchers and medicine as a dubious billion dollar industry (rather like medicine is, but with a little less 'dubious' ahem!) alternative therapies exist, and always will exist, as long as medicine remains only useful to a narrow band of illnesses, injuries and complaints.

So, what's good about the 'alternative' therapy is that for some people, with the right therapist in the right context – improvements can be achieved. And that improvement is achieved by the sufferers own biology getting its act together and it only gets its act together because the therapist-patient interaction provides the 'trigger'. Well, it's more than that, it's a bit of everything; a smorgasbord of therapist; the warm, cosy treatment parlour; the fragrance, the smile; the being on time; the smile, the nods, the smile; the affirmation, the care, the smile; the listening; the therapy session; the chat; the advice; the quiet time and the smile and touch... and the smorgasbord is called 'the placebo'. Some kind of 'perceived treatment' is a major requirement for the trigger to take effect.

The next few chapters will explain it how I would like to have it explained if I was training now and how I would like it explained to all practitioners if I was all powerful – from Drs and surgeons to manual therapist, osteopaths, chiropractors and all those other alternative therapies or therapies that have 'no proven physiological effect,' (but you wait and see). What medicine has to realise is that the placebo isn't just in pills made of chalk, it's also a major part of the pills and interventions that actually do do something too, as you will see shortly.

Now to my second much more critical perspective on alternative medicine – it's as I've already stated, it's brimming with pseudo-science, or to put it more basically brimming-with-bullshit. Please read Ben Goldacre, Edzard Ernst and Simon Singh to explore the pseudo-scientific flim-flam that all the alternative therapy paradigms are based on and which is passed on to patients. It's no longer good enough to say 'but it works' and reel off the most improbable mechanisms by way of explanation. If it works as the proponents say it does then a far better and more rational science is ready and waiting. Steve Robson and I offered our contribution from a neuroscience and pain science perspective for manual therapy in 2006 in our chapter: 'Manual Therapy in the 21st Century,[1] and Max Zusman, a very widely read and thoughtful physiotherapist and lecturer from Curtin University in Perth Australia, has made a significant contribution to the manual therapy 'mechanism of action' debate over the last 15 years or so. Max has not held back being critical.

A quick summary of a few things from the discussion above:

- the placebo is earning a great number of therapists a great deal of money
  – so is medicine

---

1 - Robson S, Gifford L 2006 (2013) Manual Therapy in the 21st Century. In: Gifford LS (Ed) Topical Issues in Pain 5. CNS Press, Falmouth.

- a great many therapists are working with paradigms that are rationally and scientifically redundant

  (so are parts of medicine, but they're working on it much better than the alternatives; as you'll see, surgery is getting a bit of a pasting)

- alternative therapy isn't going to go away unless medicine has better interventions for the things that it isn't good at helping – that is unlikely

- understanding the placebo is essential to making headway with the mechanisms of all alternative therapies. This should lead to more effective interventions and management strategies. (Physiotherapy is well placed to bag them, but is sadly unlikely too)

- it's my humble opinion that wise folk like Singh, Ernst and Goldacre (and Richard Dawkins too, I've heard him criticise alternative therapies and talk about placebo... badly!) don't fully understand the placebo in the context of the bigger picture.

  As an aside, trying to kill-off alternative medicine from 'humanity' is almost as nuts as trying to think that getting rid of religion is possible. From this perspective, those who are vocal haven't really listened to the unshakeable devotion of true believers and I'm talking about the religious as well as the alternative therapists and their acolytes. Deluded to the eyes of logic and reason? Maybe! But 'shiftable'! Pointless! From our profession's point of view, the only way to stop 'alternative' infiltration and indoctrination of our minds and brains, is better early education – get something decent in there first, to prevent the intellectual 'drift' to the 'other-side!'

What about looking from the patient perspective?

For a patient to learn that they have responded to a placebo is discomforting, possibly even a bit insulting too – we all hate to think that we could have responded 'psychologically' and as a result of having responded to a placebo it really means that, 'Oh, there was nothing wrong with me in the first place!' Or, 'What I had wrong with me wasn't real at all. I must have been making the whole symptom and illness scenario up! Arghh... I've been found out, so bloody embarrassing... '

For those who felt that their symptoms were real it may cause them to question their own sanity or, get angry that their honesty had been challenged! 'Do you know, I took this pill for 3 weeks and my fabrication and dishonesty about it all was completely cured. How could they do that to me?'

Though rather tongue-in-cheek, will it ever be like this I wonder...?

(When you read the following paragraphs and conversation in your mind substitute the word 'placebo' with the term 'processing change'.)

Patient to the on duty 'placebo dispensary' nurse at the surgery:

'Hi, my GP, Dr Mild, says that I've got a condition that medicine has nothing of any real value which will help, so he's referring me to you for some placebo treatment. I have a placebo prescription from him, I wonder if you can help?'

'Right, let's see now, your placebo screening profile says that you'll respond better to a swallowing type of placebo treatment rather than a touchy-feely one, so I'd suggest the one where we mix a 'pathogen' with water and dilute it so much all trace of it disappears leaving only the memory of a healing force in the bottle... I'd recommend it; it cured my Susan of her allergies.... They say the more it's diluted the stronger it gets – weird if you ask me. The other option the Dr suggested I discuss with you is the 'chalk pill' which helped the last patient's eczema settle in two days They were thrilled that they've now got a really non-toxic and cheap remedy that can be used anytime there's a flare up.'

'Dr says 'weird' works for my condition so I'd like to give the 'nothing-but-water-and-a-memory-of-the-pathogen' one a go if I may!'

And this may lead to this kind of thing from the patient as they greet you... 'Hi, good to meet you Louis, I'm pleased to say the placebo (*processing change*) treatment you do has been sanctioned by my Dr!' ('Yes, and because of that, it's got funding under the new 'any qualified provider' scheme, so we're both going to be happy!')

A note on the term 'processing change' or 'processing problem'. Currently (2013 ish!), the term 'functional symptoms' has become quite fashionable to allocate a vague mechanism and to explain the nature of chronic pain and many chronic illnesses where no clear evidence for a reasonable 'pathology' exists in medical terms. Complaints that include widespread pain, fatigue, low energy and a vast raft of similar 'chronic-illness' or stress-associated symptoms and the like – that are linked to aberrant or abnormal functioning of the systems involved, are typical of those being termed 'functional'. For example, the nociceptive processing system or the immune systems 'function' is below par – even pathological... It's a 'quickie' term that misses out the human being who owns the problem, but I prefer the term 'processing problem' because of its clinical utility in my explanations with patients (explanations are dealt with in later chapters).

A great many therapists believe they are doing a lot of good and a great many patients revere their therapists as almost God-like. I've spent my life waiting to witness the 'I walked in doubled up and I walked out cured patient,' and have come to the conclusion that they don't really exist. I've noticed this sort of thing though:

Patient X...

'I had this hip pain, this amazing therapist from Australia who works on the Royals saw me walking down the corridor and instantly diagnosed a leg length problem and a pelvic imbalance... there and then he had me on the floor and stood on me... amazing!'

'Sounds like it really helped?'

'Yes, fantastic...'

'How long ago was that..?'

'In the summer, about six months ago, he even invited me to Australia for more treatment...'

'OK, well I'm pleased about that, let's get back to hearing a bit more about this hip pain... you said you had really stopped walking outside because of it just now... '

In other words, good therapist performers can make it all amazing but when the dust settles the same old thing grumbles on and the therapist carries on as if the patient was cured – especially if the patient doesn't come back again.

For me this fellow's OA hip was becoming symptomatic and was stiff and had significantly less range than his good one. I didn't beat about the bush with fancy promises of cure, but because he required it I got his Dr to organise an x-ray and a good surgeon's opinion...

'It's got obvious wear and tear fella... suggest you steer clear of me for as long as you can... Louis will show you what you need to do.'

I showed him how his movements had become limited and he got going with a good programme to get his hip moving better and stronger... alongside a graded increase in his activity levels. Five years on he's still managing fine and is not considering going to Australia or the surgeon (yet!). For interest this guy was only managing walking round his house when I saw him, he'd completely given up dog walking and would use the car even for the shortest of journeys. Within six months of first seeing him he was walking the dog daily for up to an hour and often walked for over two hours. The pain didn't go, but like all degenerative joint problems, it had good and bad phases which he understood and could cope and deal with.

This is everyday work for me, and note the celebrity styled 'Australian' king of therapy could just as easily have been any other therapist from up or down the road. I've also spent a lot of my professional life sorting out the flim-flam that people have been peddled and infected with; also, the unreal expectations engendered by therapists who haven't a clue about joint problems and their natural history. Once sorted, and it can sometimes take a lot of hard work and convincing (the surgeon was useful for Mr X as you saw), it's a case of getting them to accept the situation and get going. It's the 'guff' that they're told and the unrealistic promises that really get me.

That 'top-down' is involved has to somehow be swallowed and it can be. That a great many pain related disorders involve and are best seen as a 'processing' problem rather than frank or even minor pathology, or some 'alternative' diagnosis, has to be swallowed too. That the way a person thinks, feels and reacts to their problem has a massive influence on 'processing' has also to be swallowed... and this is massively different from the simplistic idea that 'psychology' means amplifying or making something up.

Changing processing is at the heart of what it's all about and to dismiss the potential of 'top-down' effects helping is to dismiss a massive part of the input and interaction needed to help successful outcomes.

Take the dog-walking 'hip' fellow, Mr X above, who was nearly hoodwinked by the guile, charm and confidence of a slick operator, what on earth got him to change his processing when with me? Simple, the surgeon listening and examining him, showing him the x-rays and the wear and tear and then smartly saying 'I'm always here, I can replace your hip, but it'll go for a long time yet if you act wisely... ' and then positively passing him onto me with the blessing and need for 'action' (if only these kind of words were promoted in their training!). I discussed the nature of wear and tear and how function and healthy exercise can carry on despite it. I used the pictures I have of past patients severely arthritic feet – to show him examples of people with marked joint changes, but who have remained active. My favourite are the feet which belong to 'the lady who walks the cliffs'. She came to me with back pain and I asked about her feet when she had undressed, 'Oh, don't look at them, they're awful' she said... 'But, do you know... they've never really bothered me!'

My 'hip' patient was amazed at this and it made him realise – having already seen the relatively mild OA of his hip, that he should be able to walk the cliffs too. We instigated an exercise and the graded dog walking programme. As time went on, he presented himself with the proof that his hip could do it and the more positive and reassured he became the better he functioned. Reassurance and then practicing and proving were among the most important factors that contrived to change his processing!

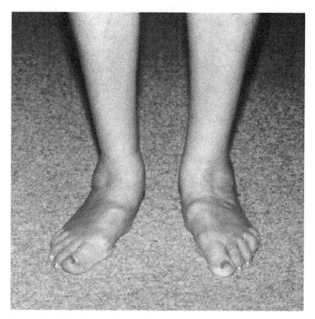

Figure 7.1 The lady who walks the cliffs

At the present time aberrant 'processing' isn't testable or visually detectable and one wonders if it ever will be. The prospect of pain practitioners one day having brain scanners to try and detect 'functional problems' or associated scan-visible changes in the central nervous system and link them to the clinical problems they face is a worrying and controversial development to me and my friend and colleague, Mick

Thacker. For one thing, fMRI scans do not reveal quite the detail that a great deal of medicine and the general public think they do, and the other is that it yet again removes the human being with the problem from the equation. The utility of scans will be discussed in section 19.

That aside, I think we now have good enough clinical skills and knowledge based reasoning to be sure that maladaptive processing is present and that it's a major issue for these 'untreatable' symptom based presentations that are so difficult to help.

For me, understanding the placebo 'properly' is central to understanding pain states and how best they can be managed. Understanding 'processing' properly is also central to understanding pain states and how best they can be managed. The placebo clearly changes processing and we need to understand, acknowledge and use it, as I did with Mr X above. It requires quite a shift from standard thinking and reasoning and a significant rejection of all the pseudo-scientific based treatments that are around. As I've discussed and illustrated with my rather facetious tone at times, the poor old 'placebo' reeks of prejudiced thinking when in actual fact it is probably the most fundamental and important process for all practitioners who deal with pain related disorders to understand and come to terms with. It 'proves' the importance of 'top-down'.

To me it would be far better to use the terms 'top-down' and 'processing change' and dump the word 'placebo' from therapy mechanism analysis. Why? Because in clinical terms placebo is too loaded with emotion. For example, it emanates from the clinicians whose methods are being challenged and labeled as placebo – they feel insulted, angry and maybe a tad embarrassed and also from other clinicians who observe and read about the therapy under scrutiny that has been given the 'largely placebo' label, and they experience mirth. Either of which are exactly what you are likely to feel as the next few chapters roll on. So, on with some classic placebo examples that had a huge effect on my thinking and reasoning when I first read about them. If they don't make you think, I've no idea what will! So, enjoy, it's fascinating!

Chapter 7.2

The Placebo 1: classic examples...

Surgery is a placebo!

There are two really good examples of trials that show how surgery has a powerful placebo element. A great deal of thanks to Pat Wall, the first one is taken from his chapter in the 1994 edition of the Textbook of Pain.

Heart surgery

This example comes from a trial done in the late 1950's on a heart operation developed in the late 1930's by a surgeon named Feischi. He reasoned that if he could improve the blood flow to the heart and the myocardial area, he would be able to relieve the symptoms of angina pectoris. It seems rather ludicrous now, but the operation involved tying off, or 'ligating' the internal mammary artery in the left pectoral area of the chest. There was no sawing through the sternum and ripping open the chest wall with massive retractors to expose the heart as in today's heart surgery–just mildly cutting the skin in the pectoral area and dissecting down to reveal the artery! The rationale for the operation was that if the internal mammary arteries were ligated, the blood in these arteries, being dammed up, would find alternative routes by sprouting new channels through nearby heart muscle, thereby improving the circulation to the heart. (Can you see the similarities here to the pseudo-scientific explanations of the cranial osteopaths, chiropractors and others given in 7.1 earlier?).

The operation was carried out on quite large numbers of patients, to the great satisfaction of many. The problem was that pathologists of the day couldn't find any of the supposed new blood vessels when they dissected the hearts of those who later died. The operation came under suspicion. Two groups of surgeons and cardiologists decided to test the rationale by carrying out sham operations on 9 members of a group of 17 who had proven angina (Cobb et al 1959 and Dimond et al 1958). Here the surgeons incised the skin, identified and exposed the arteries and then sewed the patients straight back up again. The other 8 patients had the same procedure plus the full ligation that the surgeons had been performing for all those years. The patients and their physicians did not know who had the 'true' operation and who had the 'sham'. The results...? The majority of both groups of patients greatly improved in the amount of reported pain, in their walking distance, in their consumption of vasodilating drugs and some in the shape of their electrocardiogram (ECG). The improvement in both groups was maintained over a 6 month period of observation.

Brilliant!

So, here was an operation that involved very little cutting and hacking and seemed to work well on two levels. First, at a *'subjective'* level, on the **pain** of angina and the **amount of exercise** tolerated before **pain**, and second, on the *physically/ objectively* measured ECG! Yet the operation did nothing directly to the heart, and as a result it was then relegated to the 'no-better-than-a-placebo' bin of interventions. It was rejected as a rational approach to angina. I imagine that it was ridiculed and sniggered at by the 'medical establishment' and those with other competing methods. So, an intervention that *'does nothing'* is binned...

Take note though, this operation—labeled as a placebo—did work; *it did something beneficial to the physical working of the heart for some patients, it changed their ECG for goodness sake! ... and most importantly it did something to the symptoms and way of life of the patients too. All it takes is a treatment procedure done in good faith,* and the belief and commitment of the patient and the surgeon. Merely cutting the skin, a modest bit of dissecting and the tying of a blood vessel! Think about it. How safe is that compared to a full-on modern-day operation on the heart? 'Ah, but it's not done something directly to the heart, its 'non-specific,' it's all a con, it's a rip off, it must be rejected and let's have a laugh at poor old Feischi...' may have been the response of the establishment. It almost seems a shame that this procedure got 'found-out'!

I'd like to emphasise that 'non-specific' equates to changes in processing (pain) and, as far as we can see in some people, to some significant changes in physiology/ pathology of the heart.

'Placebo' can equate to a positive physical or at least a physiological outcome. A major requirement for placebo to work is the *act of treatment* and a person with a brain that connects to its body (include the surgeons, carers and the patients!).

The big lesson here though is that doing an operation, even though it did nothing directly to the heart, caused a change for the better in the condition and functioning of the heart. Doesn't this mean that the same changes might be produced without having to resort to a high-tech surgical procedure? Couldn't there have been some way for the patient to have brought these things about for themselves? Well, er, as it so happens, yes!

A German researcher called Rhiner Hambrecht (2004) did an interesting piece of research comparing stent surgery with exercise over a period of a year. He took 100 cardiac patients and assigned half the group to surgery, where narrowed cardiac blood vessels were cleared of their plaques and a stent balloon put in place to keep them patent, while the other half, who were not operated on, were prescribed 20 minutes on an exercise bike per day and a one hour aerobics class once a week. After one year 88% of the exercise group, were 'event-free'. But only 70% of those who were operated on were!

I hope you find this sort of thing as interesting and as empowering as I do!

What's important is it seems there are a whole host of problems which, given the chance and the right opportunity, that, up to a point, the body is able to improve/ mend/cure/overcome on its own. This may require a medical intervention to trigger the 'improvement', as in the ligation operation, or, as here, a well supervised exercise programme.

What also needs to be acknowledged is that the 'trigger'—the treatment, surgery, injection, pill or 'therapy'—is likely to be accompanied by some kind of change in the patients thinking and relationship to their problem and this in turn may influence their behaviour, which for the heart includes exercising more. 'My heart is fixed. I can use it now... in fact I've been given a second chance. I'm going to look after myself far better than I did... ' Or this: 'I've got my new hip now so it must be better.' So regardless of having the leg almost sawn right off and put back again to put the new hip in–the patient gaily gets up and starts to walk.

On the other hand the patient could just as easily go: 'It's all fixed now so I can carry on with my slobby existence without any fear, pass the burger and me beer can you luv', let's watch 'telly... '

It's good to appreciate that intervention, therapy, care, information, guidance... may all be classed as 'triggers' towards better self care and well-being, and hence the removal of destructive and degrading processes and the instigation of those more geared to healing, 'anabolic' and recovery processes.

Knee Surgery!

Let's now go to a much more recent example and to a surgery that is a little more familiar to physiotherapy – arthroscopic debridement and lavage of the knee, performed on those suffering pain and disablement from osteoarthritis.

I think it is worth going into this study with some detail because it is instructive and revealing (see Moseley & O'Malley 2002).

The authors start by stating that arthroscopic surgery for the pain of arthritic knees is commonly performed when medical (drug) therapy fails and note that, in the USA 650,000 such operations at a cost of $5000 each are performed yearly. Success of the operation is widely reported (just like alternative therapists successes eh?) and in uncontrolled studies 50% report relief from pain.

How the operation works or is supposed to help OA is 'unclear'. My thoughts from a tissue biological perspective (i.e. thinking purely about the effect on the knee) is that the 'lavage' or 'washing-out' procedure would produce a dramatic, but only temporary change, in the rather fantastic balance of electrolytes, immune cells, ligand and hormone balance, fluid concentration and so forth, of the synovial fluid. It'll dramatically mess with the natural osmotic balance of the fluid in the knee, the synovium and other adjacent tissues. Quiet a physiological threat/shock really?

So, a quite logical line of reasoning might run, any abnormal state like this is actually a threat to the health of the knee and should result in *increased* pain followed by some sort of positive biological response to bring physiological stability back to normal. I guess that the new state achieved could somehow be better than before the 'lavage' but it is hard to see how this would happen and how it would last for very long.

Another perspective, and the one that's usually pedaled to patients, is that 'debris' and inflammation will be washed out. Well, perhaps, but I think smart 'biology' would tend to 'react' to this traumatic procedure and create quite a physiological disturbance! I bet no one has done any research into the physiological effect of a couple of holes being made into a knee joint? This could be done on rats or mice with good controls. I wouldn't be surprised if the rate of joint degeneration didn't speed up! Hope I'm wrong, but my research colleague Mick Thacker reckons this is 'spot on'.

I'd also like to see some research that has actually investigated and measured 'debris' in OA joints, and, if there is debris – whether the amount actually correlates with the symptoms suffered?

Could the wash-out somehow re-set and hence down-grade the level of the on-going local inflammatory response? If indeed there was one to start with?

It's a pretty simple question, but, is there a correlation between pain and the level of inflammatory markers in the synovium? Has this research been done? I've never found any.

If there was a relevant inflammatory response and it did downgrade persistently after the procedure I'd strongly err towards a significant 'central' inhibitory effect influencing the inflammation over a peripheral mechanism (see chapter 11.2).   In other words, I'm connecting the tissue 'activity' to the central nervous system and the brain and person therein! To understand this you need an appreciation of the nervous systems role in controlling and modulating actual chemical conditions and events in the tissues (sections 11-15).

From a local pain mechanism perspective, could the changed environment around the nociceptive population actually re-set its thresholds to *lower* levels of sensitivity, (even though the intervention may have created a more aggressive physiological environment?). Maybe it could, but as I intimated just now, you really can't isolate the tissues like this, anything that happens in the periphery gets 'found-out' centrally, via the reporting sensory system. This includes the nociceptors, because they're tissue monitoring devices which constantly feed information about tissue status into the central sensory and body monitoring systems. In it all goes and of course, it gets mixed in with plenty of 'top-down' stuff from consciousness. So, central mechanisms from cord to brain and self/brain back down need to be considered too... until eventually we are left with a nice multi-factorial and multi-level mish-mash of an explanation. That's really, so wise, and so fascinating, yet so unpalatable to medicine and the public's determination to keep things in the structure and hard anatomy (and a little physiology) where the patient feels the pain. Re-setting the nervous system in the operated OA knee is all about taking it from a painful default habit, to a less painful default habit and this, I would hypothesise is far more a centrally generated 'processing' change, than anything done to the tissues.   It's somewhat ironic, that in order to achieve this something has to be done to the tissues, in the patients (and the surgeons) frame of reference. Don't forget though, that if you change the processing centrally you'll also change the tissue environment too... so, damage a tissue in the right context – and it should improve!

Now, back to the 'debridement' part of knee arthroscopy operation...

Debridement involves trimming cartilage inside the joint to tidy up anything messy – although surgeons tend to use terms like 'smoothing-out' of any roughened edges, 'removal' of worn cartilage... which they call 'chrondroplasty'. Seems fair enough, it makes a bit of sense and a reasonable thing to do, if you're thinking like a mechanic does. It's important to recall that the cartilage is generally devoid of any nerve endings–

unless it's the very outer layers of the menisci, though I have a feeling that areas of degenerate cartilage and nearby osteochondral junction may well be innervated (e.g. Suri S et al 2007), which means that chondroplasty has the potential to cause more pain simply by dint of it causing an injury situation adjacent to sensitised nociceptors. But mechanically, surely having a smooth menisci has got to be good for the slide and glide and general happiness of the articular cartilage and sub-chondral bone? (Losing that horrid 'clunking' is also good for the patient's brain and the way the knees 'processed' by it/them...).

As the paper's authors point out, there are surgeons who are supporters of one or the other operations as well as those who opt for a combination of the two – yet little evidence for the operation successfully curing or arresting knee OA. The study was partly designed to see if either of the operations had an advantage over the other.

Now, the study...

All the patients had diagnosed OA of the knee with an NRS pain level of 4 or more out of 10. Patients were told and had to understand a statement that read: 'On entering the study I realise that I may receive only placebo surgery. I further realise that this means that I will not have surgery on my knee joint. This placebo surgery will not benefit my knee arthritis.'

(Hmm... an interesting way of 'prepping' the brain before the operation!). If it was me and my knee I'd be high on the 'hope it works/want it to work/can't believe they'd to nothing to me' brain trip. In the light of heart operations can you imagine this scenario 'You've got angina of the heart and we want you to understand the following statement.'

'On entering the study I realise that I may receive placebo surgery. I further realise that the placebo operation won't do anything to my heart and will not be beneficial to it.' How'd you feel! How'd you process that! (But we know that even the placebo operation does do something... remember the changes in the ECGs above?) The important thing is its good 'science' to be negative and with this part of the research it's what the surgeons actually want – a poor outcome/worse outcome with a placebo operation than the 'real' thing. So the statement is biasing their research in the direction desired perhaps! On the other hand if the 'placebo' patients do well, that'll give it (processing change) quite a nifty leg-up!

Anyway, 180 participants agreed to take part and another 144 who were asked declined–presumably they all wanted the real thing[1]!

The participants were divided into 3 groups, relating to three grades of OA, grade 1 being the mildest and grade 3 being the most severe.

Patients were assigned to one of three options for surgery:

1. Debridement only (Number=59)

2. Lavage (N=61)

3. Placebo procedure (N=60)

---

1 - *Woops, suggests a selection bias of those happy to risk have 'nothing'!! Are they 'normal?'*

For treatment options 1 and 2 there was a standard anaesthetic with endotrachial intubation. For the placebo group patients were given a short acting intravenous tranquiliser plus an opioid to make them totally buzzed-out. No tracheal tube was used.

The same orthopaedic surgeon did all the procedures.

The lavage involved 10 litres of fluid being flushed through the joint. No instruments were used except where there was an obvious bucket-handle cartilage tear–when the torn portion was removed and the remaining meniscus smoothed.

The debridement involved a lavage of 10 litres, shaving of the rough articular cartilage, removal of loose debris, trimming of torn or degenerate cartilage and smoothing of remaining cartilage. There was no removal of bony spurs but any spurs from the tibial spine area that blocked full extension were removed.

Because the placebo group were to have a different anaesthetic regime and therefore may not have amnesia the surgeon did a simulated arthroscopic debridement operation..!

So the placebo op went ahead, the knee was prepped and draped, three, 1cm incisions were made in the skin; the surgeon asked for instruments and manipulated the knee just as if arthroscopy was being performed. Saline was splashed about to simulate the sounds of lavage, yet no instruments entered the knee. The patient spent the same time in the theatre as for the true operation and also spent a night in hospital after the procedure.

The nurses who cared for all the groups after surgery were unaware of which group the patients had been assigned. The good thing about this design was that the external evidence of an operation was there to be seen in all the groups – even the placebo group. The patient can see something's been done and so can the carers, meaning that the carers in particular won't change their attitudes to the patients in the placebo condition.

The post-op regime was the same for all the patients–same walking aids, same graded exercises and same analgesia.

The use of analgesia after surgery was monitored for the 2 year follow up period, and was *found to be similar in all groups*.

The post-operative outcomes were assessed by personnel unaware of the group assignments and the operating surgeon was not involved post-operatively. (All good stuff!).

Data was collected at 2 and 6 weeks; then, 3, 6, 12, 18 and 24 months post operatively. At each follow up the patients were asked to guess which procedure they had had, patients in the placebo group were no more likely than patients in the other two groups to guess that they'd undergone a placebo procedure (which is quite amazing, or is testament to how doped-up they managed to make the placebo group!). For example, at 2 weeks, 13.8% of patients in the placebo group guessed correctly that they'd undergone the placebo procedure. But, 13.2% of patients in lavage and debridement groups guessed they had undergone the placebo procedure!

Patients were assessed on: pain scale; function – walking, bending, a 10 item physical function scale; 30 metre timed walk test and timed stair climbing.

Findings, to quote...

'At no point did either of the intervention groups have a greater pain relief than the placebo group.'

'Furthermore, at no time point did either arthroscopic intervention group have significantly greater improvement in function than the placebo group.'

'Indeed, objectively measured walking and stair climbing were poorer in the debridement group than in the placebo group at 2 weeks and at one year, and showed a trend to worse function at 2 years.' (Remember my thoughts earlier about the possibility that an intervention into a joint could trigger an acceleration of the degenerative processes?).

I want to put exclamation marks at the ends of these statements. This is simply BRILLIANT because it's such a wonderful reflection of the extent of what changing processing is capable.

This is important too...

That BOTTOM-UP is just as essential (even if it does nothing special at the tissue level) as TOP-DOWN. Yes, somewhere in our body is a recovery system and a pain-off system, whose physiological efficiency can be modulated by a combination of interventional trickery and the way we feel, think and believe. Couldn't this be seen as a most wonderful and empowering thing – that inside you, you have an apparatus that will help you to a better place? The fascinating thing is how you access it and switch it on – for many in this modern age we live in, it's via 'fix' surgery like this – but it could just as easily be a pseudo-science-cranial-sacral-tickle-up-the-Khyber too? A great deal of my career has revolved around getting the patients I've seen to learn how to enhance their own recovery and get control of their pain-on and pain-off systems. Much of the practical aspects in the Graded Exposure sections and chapters deal with and discuss how I've gone about this.

If you can change the way a patient thinks about their problem, you can change the way it's processed and hence alter its often well-trodden route to consciousness. If you can back up an initial change of processing by going on to prove that their problem works better than it did and can do a good deal more, then you should really reinforce the positive things. In other words, get the patient using it, moving it and functioning and fitter with it and you're away!

The tragedy of the cranio-sacral/reflexology/manipulation/muscle imbalance approaches is that they are one dimensional. See it as 'playing with processing' rather than playing with it, improving it then maintain it via rehabilitation with graded movement and confident functional restoration.

If your therapist only does a 'treatment' to you and misses out the 'get it moving'/ rehab/graded recovery/functional recovery process–then it's my opinion that your therapist is a complete waste of time. My determination is to try and get therapists to recognise that they're not doing this well enough or with enough emphasis.

This research was good in that it included multiple components... the operation... the first attempt at changing processing... and then the follow up procedures... which contained measurement, feedback, goal setting for activity and function, exercises, and so forth... all of which back up the initial processing change and reinforce its shift towards a new and improved default setting.

The research authors go on to look at explanations for why the operations improve patients, noting that statements like:

'Fluid flushed through the knee cleanses the knee of painful debris and inflammatory enzymes' and 'Removal of cartilage flaps, torn fragments, hypertrophied synovium and loose debris ...'

... are *'**unlikely explanations**'*. The authors attribute improvement to 'Natural history of the condition or some independent effect of the placebo... '

(Yeah, it's changed the processing?)

Their conclusion?

'If the efficacy of arthroscopic lavage or debridement in patients with OA of the knee is no greater than placebo surgery, billions of dollars spent on such procedures annually might be put to better use. This study has shown the great potential for a placebo effect with surgery...'

So even though it really does do something (indirectly), it doesn't really do anything (directly), so we'll dump it! (And sadly snigger at the surgeons who keep doing it and lambast them for wasting so much money...)

'Surgery is the most powerful placebo known to man' (sorry couldn't resist a repeat dig here). Start again: three things when doing surgery for pain related to musculoskeletal 'problems'...

Firstly, surgery for pain conditions may work best if you make sure you do enough to make it obvious to the patient that something's been done – that's a good wound in the skin, maybe a bit of bruising and swelling too.

Secondly, open up and go in but try not to do too much, or even better try not to do anything at all, resist the temptation, because the more hacking you do the worse the result (Chang et al 2005).

Thirdly, if you do go right in and you see the cause of the patient's clicking sound it's probably worth removing it so that the joint doesn't click again – if it's still clicking when the patient starts using it he won't be impressed and you'll then become a bit of a 'nocebo' sadly.

I still happily send some patients for these types of operation – they're the ones who need 'something done' to fix their problem and can't see how they're going to get better until then. Fine, don't get mad with them, accept that's the way they are and send them to a good orthopaedic surgeon with lots of positive vibes about the operation and the surgeon's outcomes.

I love this type of investigation because it is so revealing, and I would love it if someone would do the same with joint replacement – along the same lines as this, or the ligation of the mammary artery protocol described first. How cool would it be if merely the production of a big scar down the lateral side of the hip combined with a bit of appropriate 'explanation' from the consultant, could lead to a whole new relationship with your OA hip problem! Plus the vital use-it, get fitter, enjoy-it functional programme to back it up...

What's the problem? Yes, you have to lie to the patient. Here's the surgeon seeing the patient two days after the 'no-op'...

'How's your new hip going Mr J? You know it sure was bad when we got right in there and dug it out, but you've now got the latest and best replacement that money can buy... that there joint we put in would last a mountain goat 200 years.'

Then show him someone else's x-ray so he can see the new hip nicely situated. Smile, look confident and pleased say something like...

'Mr J, you're amazing and you'll continue to be amazing... I'll be in tomorrow to see how your going... you keep on walking now... bye... '

Note that this knee operation research was published in 2002, at time of writing–it's 2013 now, does anyone see the decrease in use of these types of knee operation? Ah, commercial factors, surgeons egos, countering research–there's a story! But I'm glad they're still going on, it's just a pity the patients don't get properly referred for good quality rehab afterwards.

Clinician and Patient combined...

To emphasise and repeat... a big point is, that improvement and physiological changes in the tissues are highly likely to occur if the patient set-up is right and the procedure runs well, but, **it nearly always requires a procedure to be done to set the improvement in motion**. Something has to be done or appear to be done and something has to change or appear to change. Research into interventions – which run a 'no treatment' group as well as the double blind placebo control groups, nearly always show that the intervention and the placebo groups are better than the no treatment condition. I want to emphasise that even a placebo is perceived as 'doing something' or 'having something done'.

So there's this neat thing that what's done doesn't always have to be anything really dramatic to the tissues–so long as the procedure is meaningful in the eyes of the *clinician*, and in the eyes of the *patient*. It all works better if it makes sense to both of them. Some humans are very good at knowing when they are being tricked/conned, and let's be honest a great many others are gullible and trusting and would believe anything. When you're in pain or not at all well though, you're much more vulnerable – you're in a situation where you want help and therefore want to believe...

It's not 'conning'; it's changing processing. If you're a clinician and you're burnt out and don't believe anything you do anymore works, boy, your results will suffer. When I lost faith in 'McKenzie' examination and treatment, it stopped working in a big way, in fact I made a great many of my patients a lot worse and it made me review the whole system's credibility.

One big moral of the placebo story is to work hard with your patients so they understand the intervention and get them on side. 'Sell' your therapy and rehabilitation the best you can! It's bloody hard work though...!

To illustrate the importance of **clinician** and **patient** 'belief' it's worth briefly summarising the quite well known research that was done into the effects of ultrasound on the pain, trismus (spasm) and swelling following wisdom tooth extraction. This now famous study was done by Hashish et al in 1988[1].

So, the group was interested in finding out the best 'dose' and 'intensity' of ultrasound that was required for helping the post operative symptoms. In order to do this they included groups using various ultrasound intensities and included one where the ultrasound machine was actually not emitting any output at all. The findings were fascinating in that they revealed that it made no difference as to what setting was used–all produced improvements in pain and measurable swelling (a good example of doing something, even though it might be a placebo, is better than doing nothing?). Further, and of even greater interest perhaps, was the finding that it didn't matter whether the ultrasound was emitting ultrasound or not (the researchers had doctored the machine a little!), provided that **the *therapist* and *patient*** believed that the machine was working. So long as the machine looks switched on (green lights etc.!) and the therapist and patient believe it to be working, no ultrasound is just as good as ultrasound of whatever the dose or intensity!

So, do we throw away all our ultrasound machines? Should surgeons stop doing arthroscopic lavage and debridement? We don't seem to have changed at all, 1988 is a long time ago and so is 2002 now! Why are we ignoring the results and carrying on, like faithful disciples clutching onto beliefs that defy truth, reality and logic? Answer, because we're humans!

I carry on using ultrasound and anything else 'machine' or otherwise, from time to time–it's just an 'input' that's done in the context of everything else going on in the 'treatment' and management process. It's no different from a placebo debridement or lavage operation if thought of in terms of an input with the potential, along with everything else going on, to change 'processing'.

So how do you sell ultrasound to your patients then Louis? ...

How about this... 'Ultrasound creates a very fine vibration effect that's picked up by the tissues and nerves it's going through. The nerves pick up the stimulation and relay a message into your spinal cord and brain and what comes back out is a 'control' message to nerves that produce inflammation and a control message to nerves that relay 'pain' – it basically dampens down the nerves controlling pain and inflammation, and stimulates those that help make healing more efficient. If we could go into your tissues after the ultrasound we'd find that the nociceptors (the nerves that may produce pain) there were a bit less sensitised and that there

1 - Hashish, I., C. Feinman, et al. (1988). "Reduction of post operative pain and swelling by ultrasound: a placebo effect." Pain 83: 303-311.

were more anti-pain and anti-inflammatory chemicals – you may have heard of 'endorphins' for example. This is just one tool, along with the exercises and the other things we've been doing that moves the recovery process on... it's part of the process but sometimes it really helps to trigger a much more positive response...' For many patients all that might be a bit too verbose and complicated. It's usually enough to go, 'Ultrasound has two main effects; the first is that it stimulates the release of endorphins (explain if needed) and the second is that it helps the body control the amount of inflammation going on. It simply helps to calm things down a bit...'

At this point I am feeling edgy about the mention of 'natural history' as an explanation for improvement by the authors of the knee surgery study. Fine, OA symptoms do wax and wane, but it appears that the 'surgery' triggered a wane for a great many of the operated-on here? The triggering of the wane needs investigating... What happens? What are the components? I'll leave my thoughts on this to later.

The placebo – the great testament to the incredible power of 'top-down' effects and of processing changes; especially when it is linked, associated or triggered by a 'bottom-up' treatment or intervention procedure, done by a skilled practitioner and when it makes sense to both parties.

For all those involved in pain treatment and management—the placebo cannot be ignored—you have to acknowledge it, embrace it and try and use it as much as you can, or, you will be guilty of peddling a unidimensional view of something that is patently multidimensional and multifactorial. A fairly recent term that has been cropping up in the pain literature is 'iatroplacebogenesis' – meaning to enhance the placebo effect as much as possible!

We should always acknowledge that if a tissue is alive, it is attached to a brain and a person with that brain. In turn we need to further acknowledge that the person's thoughts, beliefs, attributions, and emotions can, via the brain and outgoing pathways influence the way those tissues are processed (see the Mature Organism Model section 10).

My argument is with the pseudo-scientific explanations and the rip-off costs; that's you and your surgery, you and your energies and manipulations and force balancing and what-not...

As discussed in the last chapter, my gripe is not with the fact that anything, any form of treatment, —however bizarre it may seem—if done in the right context, can sometimes be of help. My gripe is with the unidimensional thinking that the treatment does the job on the tissues it's directed at, and that because of this thinking, the clinicians see no need for anything else to be done. For example, surgeons are notoriously bad at referring their post-op patients for rehabilitation; just like those who merely perform a treatment to a patient and again don't provide a pathway to get the patient back to 'Thoughtless-Fearless-Movement.' Sadly, Geoff Maitland and the very passive approach he taught and believed in epitomized this. I'm hoping that the reader will see what I'm getting at when I discuss and explain my 'Shopping Basket' approach later on (GE section 4).

There will never be a 'one-treatment-suits-all' situation. This means that having a good variety of treatments in your armoury has to be a lot better than being a one 'modality' therapist. A major skill may be in choosing the right thing for the right patient... and not continuing to apply the same thing over and over again when it is clearly having little beneficial effect.

But the big skill is how you present your whacky treatment in a way that fits and has a rational ring to it... how you 'sell' it – now that's a skill! Or another is getting a good result by cleverly by-passing all the laying on of hands treatments in the first place.

More later on.

Section 7
Read what I've read

Chang R.W. et al (2005) A randomized, controlled trial of arthroscopic surgery versus closed-needle joint lavage for patients with osteoarthritis of the knee. Arthritis & Rheumatism: 36(3) 289–296.

Cherkin D.C., Deyo R.A., Wheeler K, Ciol M.A. (1994) Physician variation in diagnostic testing for low back pain. Who you see is what you get. Arthritis Rheum.:37(1):15-22.

Cobb L.A. et al (1959) An Evaluation of Internal-Mammary-Artery Ligation by a Double-Blind Technic. N Engl J Med: 260:1115-1118.

Dimond E.G. et al., (1958) Evaluation of internal mammary ligation and sham procedure in angina pectoris. Circulation: 18:712-713.

Ernst E. (2008) Healing, Hype or Harm?: A Critical Analysis of Complementary or Alternative Medicine. Imprint Academic. UK.

Ernst E. (2007) Complementary Therapies for Pain Management: An Evidence-Based Approach. Mosby. London.

Goldacre B. (2009) Bad Science. Harper Perennial. London.

Hambrecht R, et.al., (2004) Percutaneous coronary angioplasty compared with exercise training in patients with stable coronary artery disease: a randomized trial. Circulation: 109(11):1371-1378.

Hashish I., Feinman C., et al., (1988). Reduction of post operative pain and swelling by ultrasond: a placebo effect. Pain 83: 303-311.

Moseley, B., K. O'Malley, et al. (2002). "A controlled trial of arthroscopic surgery for osteoarthritis of the knee." New England Journal of Medicine 347(2): 81-88.

Singh S., Ernst E. (2009)Trick or Treatment?: Alternative Medicine on Trial. Corgi. London.

Suri S et al 2007 Neurovascular invasion at the osteochondral junction and in osteophytes in osteoarthritis. Ann Rheum Dis. 66(11):1423-1428.

Section 8

THE PLACEBO, NOCEBO AND PAIN-ON AND PAIN-OFF SYSTEMS

Chapter 8.1
More Placebo!

This second placebo section explores it a bit more. Why?

1. Because it's very instructive about how we as therapists should be and act!

2. Because it gets you interested in the brain and how badly our brains sometimes interpret what is going on within us and around us.

3. Because it may just make you realise that all we are trying to do is to 'trick' the processing into a better, or more adaptive, state somehow.

There are many more examples of how the mind influences the body and its physiology. An important consideration is that, while the placebo is seen to be an 'inert' medication, 'normal' medications with 'proven' physiological benefits also have their potency influenced by top-down effects. The message is that whatever treatment you do to a patient, it needs to be 'sold' to them. For example, a great many people these days want to understand what the treatment is; how it works and also be given some indication of how effective it can be; others just do what they're told and don't ask any questions. Maybe they should though; and maybe the Dr or clinician should do their best to help them understand the treatment whether they want to or not?

An important point is to appreciate how delicate the situation clinicians and patients can be in. Clinicians can enhance their treatments via their interaction with the patient just as easily as they can stall it all, making it less effective, or not effective at all or even make things a good deal worse.

Every clinician has had patients who have been to other practitioners and been made worse, sometimes a great deal worse. Do something dramatic, like a strong manipulation or even a simple acupuncture needle and regardless of what happens to the tissues – you can run the risk of making that patient's symptoms a great deal worse. Even medication that is proven to help a condition can, in the wrong context or 'atmosphere', be surprisingly detrimental.

'Roger the foot' has just popped into my head. He came into see me with 'agony' in the ball of his right foot. He'd been given the diagnosis of 'Morton's metatarsalgia' and referred to the local physiotherapy department where a 'young physio' gave him acupuncture. That was three months before I saw him. Since then he'd virtually stopped all activity and been unable to walk far or normally. He was very angry with the physio and he was very angry with his pain...

'Tell me what happened, Roger...?'

'Well, I reckon that department is so overloaded that they haven't got time to do a good job. I was seen about forty five minutes late and I had chats with others who'd been going for a while... one bloke said, 'In you go, lie down, needles in and they disappear... writing up, seeing the next one... One day they left me flat on my stomach with needles in my back and my legs for half an hour... could hardly get off the couch... I asked to be seen by one of the others and it's been a bit better.'

'So I'm sitting there thinking, I hope I don't get the dreaded 'needler' physio... but I damn well did and to be honest with you when I saw her getting the needles out and going to put them in my foot ... I was bricking it... From the moment that needle went in the pain went shooting through my foot, it was like someone had put a match to the inside of the big toe joint... I nearly fainted.'

I'll tell you what happened to Roger at the end of the chapter.

The following examples[1] help to illustrate the power of 'top-down' in treatment and also reveal a few more thoughts on the proposed mechanisms of the placebo and nocebo.

In trials investigating treatments for gastric ulcers, comparing placebo with a drug called Cimetidine, it has been found that a placebo can reduce the size of the ulcer by an average of 46%. But note that the range of improvement, hence the different individual response is huge, the spread being from as little as 10% to a massive 91%. It would be interesting to know what and how the patients were told about the medication, or what they thought about the medication in this study. I always wonder if the poor/excellent results relate to a particular clinician involved in the research. Does the dull, monotonous, young, inexperienced looking Dr have such good results as the mature, knowledgeable and communicative Dr? I bet they don't. Of course, it may well relate to the individual patient too and factors like their beliefs, relative hopes and fears, or how easy to 'con' they are? Or more correctly, how easy it is to change or trick their processing. So an ingredient for a good result is that both parties hit it off and communicate well. The issue of placebo non-responders will be discussed later.

If patients are told that a broncho**dilator** will cause **constriction** rather than relaxation of the bronchi, the effectiveness can be halved! What a great illustration of how powerful the beliefs of the patient are in influencing the potency of an active drug!

Here's a hypothetical Dr-patient setting...

'Dr, you've suggested this medication for my problem, it's some kind of steroid isn't it, tell me if you had my condition would you take it?'

The Dr uncrosses his legs and leans forward frowning a bit. 'Look, the last time I took tablets like that I nearly passed out and was really nauseous for about twenty four hours and they didn't really help even then.'

Or, more likely... Dr, leaning forward and looking quite cross... 'Look, that's not for me to say, those tablets are recommended for the condition that I've diagnosed and they can help you, if you don't want to take them that's up to you...'

Ouch!

Patient walks out thinking... 'He hasn't a clue what's wrong with me, he didn't even examine me... '

---

1 - For detailed references see Lawes 2013

Suggestion to asthmatic patients can induce or prevent bronchospasm caused by the inhalation of distilled water! In other words do not underestimate the power that a Dr or someone who is held in high regard, can have on the outcome of a therapy. There is cause for worry here if detrimental or 'nocebo' effects are taken into consideration. All therapists know of a great many patients who were devastated by the words and actions of a highly regarded specialist or clinician and as a result their condition worsened considerably.

'Hey Dr, your attitude to me made the procedure/drug etc work against me, I'm going to sue you for noceboing me, you ******!'

'Hey Doc, next time, be nice and take time eh?'

Opioids like Buprenorphine are well known for producing respiratory depression. If patients are repeatedly exposed to the drug, they become conditioned to it. Thus, on a fourth or fifth administration, if the patient is given an inert 'placebo' Buprenorphine-like tablet the same effect as if the active drug was given will be observed i.e. measurable respiratory depression. What's fascinating is that this effect can be prevented if the subject is given another drug called Naloxone prior to the placebo. Naloxone curtails the activity of opioids by blocking opioid receptors, indicating that in this instance, the conditioning effect (the placebo effect) is produced via an opioid mediated neural pathway.

Thanks be to Naloxone! Its history in the 'proof' that the placebo has a credible biological mechanism, goes back to Levine's work in the late 1970's (Levine et al 1978).

Compliance with a given medication has been shown to have life or death consequences. Compliance, if you think about it, relates not only to an individual's self-discipline, but also to their relative belief in a given treatment or medication. If you don't 'believe' in a given drug treatment (or anything else prescribed–like exercise) you are hardly going to take it or do it with much enthusiasm or care and quite often you're likely not to even bother.

Some now quite old trials have been done on a drug for coronary artery disease called Clofibrate. This drug, like statins, is said to reduce cholesterol and triglyceride levels and hence protect against future cardiac episodes. Of interest is that the drug was withdrawn in 2002 due to its adverse effects. However, before 2002, researchers compared the death rate of a group taking Clofibrate with a group on a placebo and found the rate to be virtually identical in both.

The death rate was 21% for the placebo group and 20% for those taking the active drug (i.e. identical!). Interestingly it was noted that those who adhered to the placebo regime had a lower mortality (15%) compared with those who did not comply (28%). So, if you're given a drug which in medical terms is 'useless' (i.e. a placebo, which obviously isn't useless), but don't take it regularly and don't really believe it's going to help you – you're twice as likely to die as those who do believe in a 'useless' drug and who take it regularly... er, so long as no one tells you it is 'useless'! Right, so the 'useless' drug is not useless so long as you think it's useful and you take it as directed. Correct!

Amazing it certainly is, belief keeps you alive! In our practice we like to keep patients aware that 'BO' or 'belief and optimism' in what they are doing to help themselves, for example in their exercise programme, in their recovery, in the fundamental strength of their tissues, in their nervous systems ability to change and re-process and in a positive outcome, really helps... hugely and I often use the above example to prove it to them!

Here's another: the one year mortality of compliant patients receiving 'useless' treatment (sorry, useful placebo!) in the Beta blocker heart attack trial (1984) was 3% – compared to a mortality of 7% in non-compliant patients. As the mortality of patients receiving the active treatment was similar in relation to compliance the clinical message is clear – that adherence is a better predictor of outcome than the type of treatment received! It makes you wonder what a 'real' and 'active' treatment really is? Clinically, as I've already strongly stated – therapists and Drs must 'sell' or 'make believable' what they suggest in treatment and patients, in turn, need to believe in and comply with what they have been told to do. Clinicians have to make an effort to be believable. Note the importance (or not!) of things like: a white coat and a stethoscope, reading glasses on the end of the nose, a polka-dot dickie-bow, a good reputation... long impressive letters after your name... a high recommendation from a satisfied patient... taking time to listen... caring... etc... Different things for different people!

Seven percent is over double 3%! Just comply and you double your benefit!

A little aside so a bigger picture can be taken on board. This may be a bit of a generalisation, but folks who are non-compliant or poorly compliant are usually also pretty much in-the-dumps, low-in- spirit and down on themselves and those around them. They can't be bothered, especially if some kind of effort, like exercise is involved! Low in spirit and low in mood equates to poor self care and self worth. This adds low-in-spirit/bad health behaviour factors into the equation and is a well known accomplice to poor outcome.

Expert clinicians are good at things like: being supportive, encouraging, cheering-up, goal-setting... and nicely pressing the patient to take part and be responsible for their own health outcomes. The needy and low-in-spirit often require a great deal more time and effort. Sadly, this is often at a premium.

Let's now look at some very clever research. One of the key researchers here is Fabrizio Benedetti (2009, 2011), an Italian professor of physiology and neuroscience from the University of Turin. What a brain this guy has and what fantastic writing and research he's been involved in. He obviously loves the study of the placebo response. Read his books if you can.

If you delve into the placebo literature, you'll usually find that the underlying 'mechanisms' of its positive effects involve, EXPECTATION... 'They told me it was a strong pain killer, that's good...' CONDITIONING OR LEARNING... 'Last time I had this treatment it worked really well...' and REDUCED ANXIETY... 'Thank God something's been done at last, I'm desperate...'

Cunning placebo researchers like to screw up a potentially good result by thinking hard about what they tell the subject before the procedure.

As we've seen in the last chapter, the best kind of research is a double blind one with a 'no treatment' group so natural history can be observed. What you need then are three groups: two treatment groups, an 'active' treatment group who get the real deal; a placebo group who get the 'inert' intervention; and a third group who are, the give-nothing-just-observe contingent. None of the clinicians who deal with the subjects or patients knows which of the two 'treatment' groups a subject has been assigned to and hence are 'blind'. Only the researchers can know this and even then they only work out who's been given what after the trial results come in.

The instruction to those in the two treatment groups usually goes something like this, 'You are taking part in the trial of a new pain killing drug. You have been assigned to either a group having the new drug or a group having an inactive drug called a placebo. It's impossible for me to tell you the group you are in and you have a 50/50 chance of being in either of those groups.'

What goes through the patient's head I leave to your imagination...?

What they often do during the trial is ask the subject whether they feel they've been given the real drug or the placebo. And of course when subjects believe they've been given the placebo the effect is less, even so, there's frequently still a better result than those in the control group. So, belief and expectation may be low but the little act of taking something believed to be 'useless' may stimulate the recovery/ analgesic pathways to some degree.

When researchers want to see the influence of 'expectation' on their results, they still have the two groups but this time, tell the patient something like:

'You are taking part in a trial and you will be given a powerful new pain killing drug,' with no mention of a 'placebo' group at all. So there are still two groups but the belief of all of the participants is that they're having a real drug and they're expecting it to be good. I must say I sit here and think, 'Yes,' but some may be thinking... 'Powerful pain killing drug – that must have a whole pile of nasty side-effects...'

Now take a cohort of folks who are hospitalised for either wisdom teeth extraction operations, or, those who have had a 'VAT' procedure and do a trial. 'VAT' stands for 'video-assisted thoracoscopy' and involves an incision of about 1 cm in the chest wall and the insertion of an optical probe so the surgeon can see what's going on inside and maybe remove some tissue for later analysis.

It's good to do trials in hospitals, because the conditions the subjects are in can be manipulated and controlled more easily. It also seems that wisdom tooth extraction and VAT have a fairly predictable pain natural history.

Back in 1995, Fabrizio's research group wanted to test the analgesic properties of a drug called Proglumide and they used it on these post-surgical patients – again three groups, active, placebo and nothing. All double blind and patients told 50-50 they could be receiving an inactive placebo. Result? Proglumide was twice as good a pain killer as the placebo and the placebo was far better than no treatment. Conclusion. Proglumide is a good pain killer that acts by dampening down the pain pathways. It's a top 'bottom-up' drug therefore!

The clever bit is that they re-ran the trial but this time used a hidden infusion machine. The patient obviously has a line inserted into a vein in the wrist – a common post-op situation. The bit of kit is computer controlled so the drug can be administered without anyone being around the patient and totally unknown to them. Basically it cuts out the 'psychosocial contamination' component completely! Drug administration is therefore 'hidden'.

When a nurse or Dr gives a drug or an injection the patient is said to be having an 'open administration'. Obviously the patient is aware something is being done to them and the brain responds... mostly, it probably leads the patient to expect some relief.

Now, in the 'hidden' form of the trial Proglumide does no better than no treatment! It makes no difference at all, WOW! Proglumide in the open trial was shown to be over twice as potent as the open 'placebo'. Hide it and... Nothing... How on earth does that work?

I'll come back to the answer in a moment. Let's take a little trip and look at some other 'hidden' drug experiments on painkillers. As we all know, morphine is a very strong painkiller, being the 'gold standard' from which all other analgesic medication is compared. It constitutes between 8-14% of the dry weight of opium and works by mimicking endogenous opioids which have their effect via opiate receptors found in the CNS, the peripheral nervous system, the immune system, the gut and elsewhere in the body too. Most drug researchers are thinking CNS only though.

If you didn't know, 'endogenous' means produced by the body and it's important to understand that our bodies and just about all of the rest of the animal kingdom too – are capable of producing a natural supply of opioids and have a variety of opioid receptors. This was only discovered[1] in the early 1970's, even though opium and narcotics have been around for a very long time. It seems quite straightforward logic that if a chemical has an effect on us then we must have receptors for it or ones that it can work on... and if a body contains opioid receptors it stands to reason that it also produces its own opioids.

Right, so they gave these post-op patients between 6-8mg of 'hidden' morphine and compared this to an 'open' injection of saline where they told the patient they were getting a strong painkiller. The result. Identical pain relief in both! In other words an injection of saline accompanied by words like, 'This is a strong pain killer and will soon help ease your pain considerably' – is as strong as 6-8mg of morphine! That is amazing, I think. So if you then give the patient 6-8mg of morphine out in the open with all the 'This will help' banter, you will further advance the potency of the drug.

There's always a brain and a human being attached to every intervention and it has power over that intervention's ultimate effect! Psycho-social morphine – now we're 'smokin'' dudes!

Most of those hippies back in the 60's were all high on OXO cubes. Well, I'm pretty sure I was!

---

1 - e.g. Pert CB, Snyder SH (1973) Opiate receptor: demonstration in nervous tissue Science 179 (4077): 1011–4

'Hey Louis, your joint smells like my Mum's chicken stock...' 'Yeah well, I bought the premium stuff from the guy... who... was... right... here... a minute ago. Ah bollocks...!'

Big Point... Whenever the brain perceives that something is being done it messes and tinkers with the response of that something–could be in the direction you want it to go, but it might not be!

Comparisons of other analgesic drugs in the open and hidden conditions produced similar results. For example, an approximately 20% higher dose of the painkillers under scrutiny were needed if given 'hidden', to produce the same pain relief as when done 'open' – that was for drugs like Tramadol, Ketorolac, Buprenorphine and Metamizole. They further noted that when given as an 'open' injection the speed of onset of relief was far quicker.

Another Big Point... Things like: interaction, level of need (the patient 'needs' pain relief), belief, expectation, fulfilment (getting the drug!) and hence feeling of reward (because the need for relief is fulfilled), can all be big factors in promoting enhanced anti-nociceptive activity. Note that I could also have said that all those things are big factors in promoting the 'placebo' response rather than promoting 'enhanced anti-nociceptive activity'. What I'm moving towards is the notion, which looks as if it's more or less fact now, that the placebo when considered in relation to pain (and hence nociception) is just the brain's way of switching **ON** the 'pain-off' systems and switching **OFF** the 'pain-on' systems! In other words the biological pathways that can lessen pain are at work when a 'placebo' condition is operating. To me it's the higher brain tapping into the lower brain's networks; it's the bit of the brain that pain researchers find a nuisance and have to go to quite remarkable extremes to get rid of!

Understand and use this stuff and we should be helping some of our pain sufferers to thrive and feel better. Teach them, if at all possible, to learn to 'trick' their 'off' systems to switch 'on' to switch off...? If you see what I mean.

Let's go back to Proglumide, the stuff that's twice as good a painkiller as a placebo when used in the 'open' situation, but when used 'hidden' does nothing at all. The researchers who did the study reasoned that Proglumide wasn't a painkiller at all – it did nothing to the 'bottom-up' nociceptive traffic coming into the brain – but what it did was work on the 'top-down' 'expectation' pathways coming from the higher brain's thinking and assessing of the situation. **Proglumide actually makes the placebo effect work even better!** It'll only work if the subject has some expectation of improvement. Proglumide enhances the biology of expectation! How cool is that, and how cool in the sense that it proves that the placebo can be reduced to a bio-psycho-physical event of some kind.

The statement: 'You responded to a placebo... that means you're a cheating, fabricating, malingering, scheming waste of my time...' is just not true!

You may recall from a little earlier in the chapter that the placebo effect could be stopped by introducing a drug called Naloxone. The example given was for respiratory depression, but it also works for clinical and experimental pain conditions too. In other words, if you give a 'subject' (a normal volunteer) or a 'patient' in pain a placebo drug, its action in relieving the pain can be halted by introducing Naloxone. Naloxone blocks opioid receptors. It therefore prevents our 'endogenous' opioids–our 'endorphins', 'enkephalins,', 'dynorphins' etc. from working. It's hardly surprising that if the 'placebo' mechanism for pain works via the endogenous opioid network that a drug which blocks that network will block the response.

Now, you need to concentrate! Proglumide doesn't influence the opioid receptors at all but it blocks cholecystokinin (CCK) receptors! Proglumide is said to be a CCK 'antagonist' and therefore stops CCK from having its effect. So what's CCK? CCK is a chemical neurotransmitter that has anti-opioid properties, it goes round stopping the opioid and hence 'pain-off' system from working–simply put, it enhances pain-on systems and dampens down or inhibits pain-off systems. So if you **stop** CCK working it **frees** the opioid system to work even more efficiently (less pain). Basically CCK enhances pain, so a drug like Proglumide which **blocks** CCK's actions will reduce pain! Simple.

When a placebo is working, the opioid system is running reasonably freely, busily and happily, dampening down the 'bottom-up' nociceptive traffic and the brain processing of it the best it can... Now, if you block CCK with Proglumide you actually free up the opioid/endorphin system to work even more efficiently. That's why Proglumide enhances the placebo effect.

You could look at this another way, that CCK is actually 'pro-nociceptive', its role is to turn off the opioid system and actually enhance pain, for example, when the individual is worrying about their pain. I hope that you're thinking of how this type of system may be running rather well in our chronic pain patients? Let's hear it for 'Shane' and his family!

Now it's time to take a look at and think about 'nocebo'.

Chapter 8.2
Nocebo

The observation and question is simply this, 'If you can do something to enhance a placebo response surely you can intervene to enhance a nocebo response?'

What's a nocebo response? Basically it can be distilled down to this: give a patient an inactive/innocuous intervention or substance which then makes their pain/problem worse.

To illustrate, this is the sort of thing that researchers do; they tell their subjects that they're going to give them a quite nastily painful stimulus, when in actual fact the stimulus may be some form of touch or perhaps an electrical or thermal stimulus that would normally be mildly unpleasant. The subjects report that these mild stimuli are nasty and far nastier than if they were told they'll be receiving a mild stimulus. Prime the brain and it'll follow like a well-trained pet!

Nitrous oxide, laughing gas, is a powerful anaesthetic and analgesic gas which is well known for improving matters during child birth and dental extraction. Dworkin and colleagues reported, back in 1983, that with verbal suggestion, they could get nitrous oxide to make a subject's pain worse instead of better. The researchers manipulate the subject's expectations – it's likely that a degree of anxiety is involved too and this may be a critical factor!

For a bit of light relief, here are some 'nocebo' type examples from the bigger picture...

1. Grim frowning therapist to patient, Doug,

    'Right Doug, I've had a good look at you now and you know you thought you'd pulled a muscle? Well, it's far worse than that, you've blown your disc, trapped your nerve and it's likely to take ages to get better... It's bad, you've got what we physios call a 'derangement 7 and in my experience all derangement 7's end up having surgery.'

2. Grim frowning clinician to patient Fred, who's in his mid 40's and otherwise fairly fit,

    'Right, I've now had time to review all the x-rays and scans that I ordered and it's hardly surprising you're in a lot of pain. For a start the neck is showing signs of severe degenerative arthritis with spondylosis – that means I'm afraid that you should stop golf right away, because there's a big risk of the spinal cord being damaged and that means paralysis and a wheelchair – if I were in your shoes I would go very carefully from now on...'

3. Patient, with husband coming out of Dr's surgery, she's been given a tube of cream and a prescription for pain-killers and antibiotics... she's chuntering on at her long-suffering husband...

    'How long was I in there for? Barely five minutes? I told him I had pain in my head and it had stiffened my neck. I told him I've not been feeling well and you know, he was looking at the screen the whole time and typing up the prescription... He said hmm twice. He got me to 'open-wide'... looked out the window, when he should have looked down my throat and that was it... said I had a throat infection, he didn't even look at my neck or even feel it. Look if I die of meningitis later, I want you to complain about him...'

4. News headline...
   'CJD risk from red meat... prions to blame...'
   ... Red meat sales take a pounding!

Or...

5. 'Terrorist bomb alerts London...'
   United States diverts its holiday plans to TEXAS...
   ...or a cruise in the Caribbean...

Perhaps we may even be able to relate it to this sort of thing...

This is taken from Paul Martin's book 'The Sickening Mind'. He is discussing the impact of the 1991 Gulf War when Iraq (Saddam Hussein) launched a series of missile attacks on Israel.

'In the early hours of 18 January 1991 Iraq launched the first of several SCUD missile attacks against Israeli cities. Measured in terms of physical destruction, the Iraqi weapons were surprisingly ineffective. There were no deaths through physical injuries in the first attack and only two people were killed by the direct physical effects of SCUD detonations during the subsequent sixteen days on which missiles fell. And yet, on the day of the first attack, the death rate in Israel leapt by 58%. A total of 147 deaths were reported, 54 more than would have been expected on the basis of previous mortality figures for that time of year...

The evidence consistently pointed towards one conclusion: the sharp rise in death rate on the 18th January 1991 was primarily a consequence of severe emotional stress brought on by fear of the Iraqi bombardment...'

Think 'Voodoo magic' and Voodoo death' and you can see that the individual's interpretation of the situation they are in can have dire consequences, not just for pain, but for health too. No wonder the psychosocial yellow flags[1] are good predictors of poor outcome! Stress, as I will discuss, is particularly worth looking at.

Back now to the 'open' and 'hidden' drug administration experiments discussed in the previous chapter. Remember these post-operative patients have a drip tube going into their arm from a hidden pump that is secretly driven by a computer.

When looking at 'nocebo' responses what the researchers do in the 'open' situation is tell the patient that they are going to stop the patient's supply of pain killer via the drip line and pump. In the 'hidden' condition they stop it without telling the patient. The patient therefore has no idea and believes that they're still receiving their morphine therapy.

---

1 - See chapters GE 4.5-4.9.

They then observe the patients and find that those in the 'open' condition, who know their morphine supply has been stopped, quickly report increasing pain and ask for more medication than those who have no idea that it's gone. They conclude that in the 'open' situation the patient's fear and negative expectations of pain increase plays an important role in the outcome.

Back to our friend Proglumide! This time the researchers create a situation that they call 'a post- surgical manipulation that induced expectations of pain worsening'(Beneditti et al 1997). They did the trial on post VAT (video assisted thoracoscopy) patients in a whole variety of conditions – some 'open' and some 'hidden'. In all the 'open' conditions, they told the patients that the injection they were giving them would make their pain worse within half an hour. One group were injected with saline – this being the pure 'nocebo' group. The rest of the six 'open' groups were told exactly the same thing, but were given various strengths and mixes of Proglumide. One of the 'hidden' groups received saline alone and it was to this group that pain intensity was compared.

What they found was that when an 'open' saline injection was given with the message that the pain would be worse within half an hour there was a significant increase in the patient's pain compared to the 'hidden' saline. But fascinatingly, when Proglumide was administered 'open' with same pain increase message – the pain did not increase. In other words, the combination of suggestion of worsening with the administration of Proglumide actually blocked the nocebo response of pain worsening! The Beneditti paper is worth reading for it is a very clever set-up and smart logical conclusions.

The authors again reason that Proglumide works on 'top-down' pathways whose activity is associated with the expectation and the anxiety of pain worsening. It effectively blocks the anxiety generated increase in pain. As discussed Proglumide works by blocking CCK production and it has been demonstrated that CCK is an important neurotransmitter in the production of anxiety. CCK is therefore said to have 'anxio**genic**' properties and effects – take it and it'll make you feel anxious. Synthetically manufactured CCK-like drugs have even been shown to produce panic attacks and CCK antagonists like Proglumide have been shown to have anxiety reducing properties – hence the term 'anxio**lytic**'. 'Genic' means to 'produce or cause' and 'lytic' means to break down or prevent.

A thought just popped into my 'reductionist' head! What if a patient came in to the clinic and we didn't perform very well with them and they were walking out a bit disgruntled and confused, or even a bit more anxious than when they walked in... and you want to have a nice weekend rather than sit worrying yourself sick about their reaction to your rather inept efforts...

'Mr Cardew, oh, by the way don't forget to pick up your Proglumide pill from the receptionist on the way out... it'll stop your anxiety and make your pain-off system work so you won't be worse and want to think about sueing me... ha, ha!

If only! This rather cheeky 'fix-it-quick' teaser is an example of how reducing the complexity of an interaction to just one chemical's effect in one area of the brain is rather naive – to say the least. Unfortunately, there are great many researchers and clinicians who are caught in the spell of such possibilities, they are surely missing the bigger picture.

The message I want to get over is that your interaction with the patient can influence their biological processing system, and if you can influence it, so can they. Interactions change the chemistry far better than the other way round!

The power is within us! (Up to a point!).

I have one more bit to add before this reductionist spin on pain gets too out of hand. It's our friend Fabrizio Beneditti again and it's more about the effect of stress on pain circuits. In the next chapter I go into stress a bit more and I also talk about 'stress-induced-analgesia', that's the common experience of being injured and not feeling very much more than some awareness of an injury, or nothing at all and being able to carry on functioning. Evolution has cleverly endowed us with a very impressive pain-off system, so that even if we're injured we can still function well enough to be able to get to safety and survive. Pain-on only comes later when the panic has settled down. So what about stress-induced-hyperalgesia? The exact opposite! How does that work? It's simple: if the thing that is stressing you is the pain, then the pain is amplified; if the thing that is stressing you requires some vital action to survive, the focus is not on pain – but on the immediate threat and a way out of it and the pain is dulled. It's all to do with what is grabbing your attention at that particular moment. That's why 'Rotwieller therapy' (I still want to tell you about my 'machine-gun therapy' (MGT) but Philippa still says I can't!) is so successful; it quietly takes your mind off things... At a less sick and less brutal level, that's also why reassurance can be a very powerful pain killer and why worry and concern about a pain problem can make it far worse.

Fabrizio's group found that the 'verbal' suggestion of hyperalgesia (that pain was going to get worse) was accompanied by an increased activity of the subject's 'stress' system. More details of this system later, but for now it's enough to know that when an individual is feeling stress it activates two major systems: the adrenaline system, the 'sympathetics' and the 'glucocorticoid' or 'cortisol' system – the HPA axis. HPA stands for hypothalamic-pituitary-adrenal. When a brain is stressed the hypothalamus becomes highly active and in so doing relays impulses to the pituitary gland which in turn releases ACTH. ACTH, you may remember from your school biology is 'adreno-corticotrophic-stimulating-hormone. It gets released from the pituitary into the blood stream and has its effect on ACTH receptors in the cortex of the adrenal gland, which then releases glucocorticoid/cortisol into the blood. It's the other big stress hormone alongside adrenaline and its uses and effects will be discussed later. Importantly, it's easy to measure stress by taking blood or saliva samples and measuring the concentrations of ACTH or cortisol in them.

The researchers found that by administering Diazepam (a powerful anxiolytic/calming drug) they could stop the nocebo suggestion of increase in pain from working – just like Proglumide did. They also noted of course that Diazepam markedly reduces the levels of the HPA axis activity as measured by ACTH and plasma cortisol levels.

Note that Proglumide and Diazepam are not effective pain killers per se. According to Fabrizio, they only work on stress/anxiety networks and so are only of any use in pain states when the patient has high levels of concern about their pain and it getting worse. They reduce the anxiety about the pain and this in turn winds down the 'pain-on' system from above – 'top-down'! This would be an interesting and not too difficult research project. Mick and I are sceptical about this mechanism and believe they may work just as well on low anxiety/stressed individuals with pain. Turn one system down a bit, and it affects another component.

But why worry, far better to examine the patient well, explain things, reassure them, get them to calm down and then use more standard and safe analgesics or other modalities. A human can have their stress system's networks dulled by chemicals, but if they're still not reassured there's hardly going to be any overall advantage, is an important way of thinking here.

I want to finish off this section with a brief overview of the 'pain-on' 'pain-off' circuitry and then mention a little bit about those where these systems may be not working in an any way helpful direction – their systems have become 'dysregulated'.

Chapter 8.3
Pain-on and Pain-off ? ... Respond or not respond?

'One good thing about music, when it hits you, you feel no pain.'

Bob Marley

This is a first foray into the brain...

Control of nociception is achieved via what are often referred to as 'descending control systems.' As we've already seen in the 'Dorsal Horn' chapter there are two systems: 'Shane's family' or 'pain enhancement' and 'Claudia's family' or 'pain inhibition'.

The old pain literature of the 1990's focused on two mid-brain areas which have since become famous – that is the PAG, the 'periaqueductal grey area' and RVM, the 'rostroventral medulla'. The two are strongly connected. The RVM is more caudal than the PAG and is part of the brain stem. Researchers have found that it sends descending nerve fibres to the dorsal horn areas where pain is processed. Figures 8.1 through to 8.4 are simple illustrations of the two areas and how they work. Back in the 1970's, the early researchers found that when they stimulated the RVM or the PAG areas of the mid-brain they could produce relative analgesia. They called this effect 'stimulation-produced analgesia' or SPA for short. Back then, the stimulation they used was electrical and they did their experiments on animals and then on humans. Later experiments showed that they could turn the SPA on with various opioids and turn it off with opioid antagonists (like naloxone). They eventually showed that there were two basic types of descending neuron – there being 'on-cells' whose activity actually enhanced pain (Shane's family) – being 'pro-nociceptive'; and the other being 'off-cells' which dampened the nociceptive activity (Claudia's). You can see this illustrated in figures 8.2 and 8.3.

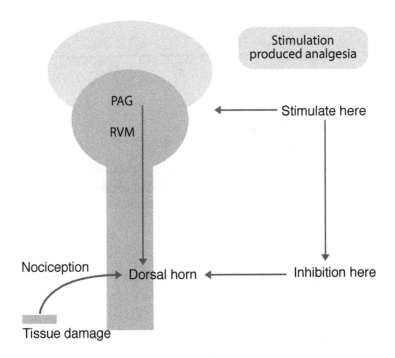

Figure 8.1 Descending inhibition of the dorsal horn.

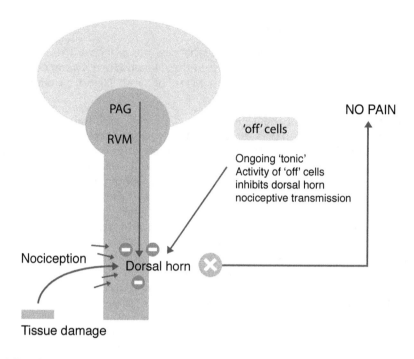

Figure 8.2 Ongoing or 'tonic' inhibition of the dorsal horn

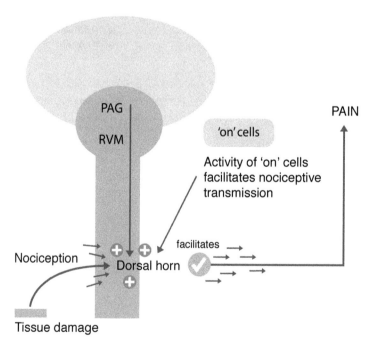

Figure 8.3 Descending facilitation of nociceptive activity at dorsal horn.

Back in the mid 1990's, when I was learning about placebo and endogenous pain controlling systems, I wanted to scream at the researchers for not attaching it all to higher brain centres and the feeling and thinking human being. 'Top-down' was dawning on me, but it hadn't with these researchers.

Here are two situations:

1. You're running for your life and you trip over a tree root and bash your shin... Your attacker is catching up with you fast... pain-off system please!

2. You're sitting quietly minding your own business and you get this shooting pain down your leg for no apparent reason. Your instinctive reaction is to feel rather concerned... 'Pain-on system please – let me listen out for this a while, see if I can make sense of it. I'm sure I read somewhere that shooting pain in your leg for no reason was a common first sign of multiple sclerosis...'

    Oh dear!

Attention and anxiety directed towards an 'important' activity like survival or having sex – drives the pain-off system... Attention and anxiety directed towards a pain or the cause of pain – drives the pain-on system. The person and their 'processing' brain is attached to this lowly and primitive circuit – surely?

Thankfully more recent research has been linking the lowly brain stem 'pain-on/ off' nuclei to processing going on 'above.' For example, the so-called 'limbic' or emotional processing areas, as well as those specialised areas that brain researchers like to label as being concerned with assessing and thinking about a situation and what to do about it. Further, famous areas like the hypothalamus, the thalamus, the amygdyla and the frontal lobes of the brain have all been shown to connect with and influence these pain-on/off areas. Whoops, better be careful, they'll end up finding the whole brain's attached! (Which I reckon it most probably is!)

The next thing that fascinated me and still does is the simple observation that some folk tolerate pain much better than others, some people seem to hurt more easily than others and some people seem to hardly respond to noxious things, that others might find extremely painful. Our individual pain sensitivity varies of course and depends on things like the situation we are in, but it also seems that some people have very poor pain-off systems regardless of the situation. Could it be that many of our patients with on-going chronic pains have a rather weak or ineffective pain-off system?

There are two interlinked sides to this[1] – one is that our genetic variability plays a part – some people are just born with poor 'off' and good 'on' systems while others have the exact opposite.

'I always knew that our Geoffrey was weird; he was born a pain and he never stopped being a pain from that day on...'

---

1 - See Robert Sapolsky's essay 'A gene for nothing' in his book 'Monkey Luv.'

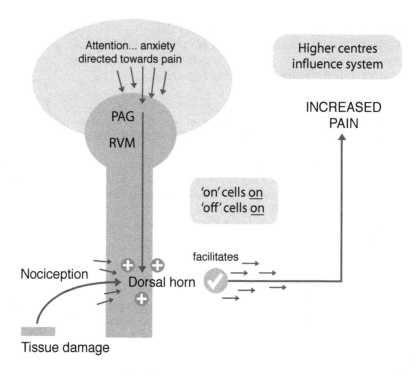

Figure 8.4 Showing the influence of higher brain processing centres or 'Top-down' processing on nociception. The situation illustrated shows facilitation.

The other side follows the thought that maybe the pain processing system is responsive, or sensitive, to training in the developmental stages of the brain. In other words plenty of rough and tumble when we're young, parents who make light of injury and encourage us back into rough and tumble nice and quick – versus very little rough and tumble, a rather physically mollycoddled up-bringing, lots of concern and stress over any injury and a 'big-deal' made over pain. Mix either one of those 'environments' with a gene predisposition (either way) and could you end up with Mr or Mrs 'supersensitive' or Mr and Mrs 'totally insensitive' in later life?

The 'social modeling' literature certainly supports this type of stance (see Klaber-Moffett 1999). The main point is that our processing system characteristics are hugely influenced by learning and past experience when imposed on a given predisposition. The way you and I are wired up relate to the experiences we've had imposed on the genetic programmes that provide the basic instructions and guidelines. As Matt Ridley (2003) tells it, it's 'Nature via Nurture' – never one or the other, always both together.

Let's come back to those placebo 'non-responders' I mentioned back in chapter 8.1. If you ever get into a discussion with another clinician, medic or researcher about the placebo and they roll out something like... 'Of course only 33% of people respond to a placebo,' take it from me, they haven't read and understood the literature properly. They've probably been indoctrinated with the notion that folk who respond to a placebo treatment are: a) not ill or in pain and there's nothing wrong with them; b) neurotic, introvert, suggestible, extrovert etc. c) fabricating their symptoms and therefore not worth bothering with.

This notion of 33% responders (hence 77% non-responders) comes from the work of Henry Knowles Beecher whose famous paper, 'The Powerful Placebo' in 1955, left the medical world with this figure and it stuck. Beecher was an anaesthetist and served in the US army during the Second World War. His situation was one of army doctor having to treat the battlefield wounded many of whom were in great pain. Short supplies of morphine to control pain lead him to treat the patients with 'placebos'. The patients were told that they were receiving morphine, a very strong pain killer, and many of them responded well. After the war Beecher went on to review a series of fifteen trials that involved using placebo medication compared to an active drug and he reported that responsiveness varied in the trials from as low as 26% to as high as 58% – hence the average figure 33% that's so often quoted. Since then Beecher's conclusions have been heavily criticised – mainly due to the fact that he was reporting on trials that had no natural history groups to compare to. Beecher was controversial, and it has been alleged that he was linked to highly unethical human drug experiments, in collaboration with the CIA and interrogation prisons in post-war Germany.

Patrick Wall pointed out that the proportion of placebo responders' shows huge variation and is highly dependent on the way the research study is set up. Responders may be nearly 0% to as high as nearly 100%! Some researchers are obviously better at priming their research subjects and their processing systems in positive directions and others towards the negative!

Another side of this is that you can turn a poor responder or a non-responder into a good responder –all you need is a bit of success to start things off. This is where 'conditioning' can come in.

Researchers have a neat way of creating pain without doing any damage; they tie a tourniquet round the subject's arm at the elbow and thus can temporarily cut-off the blood supply to the forearm. They then get the subjects to clench their fists a few times and the whole thing becomes very unpleasant for as long as the tourniquet is on. Subjects are left to stew with their pain and told to tolerate the pain as long as they comfortably can. Most people manage about 10 -12 minutes. So, you do a base line trial on a naive subject (i.e. never been involved in research trial before) on day one, and say they manage 12 minutes before giving up. The next day you repeat the procedure and give them a drug beforehand along with the notion that it's going to dull the pain – but in actual fact it's a placebo. This time they improve, managing around 14-15 minutes before asking for the tourniquet to be taken off. The placebo works but nothing that fantastic.

The next experiment runs like this: day one get the baseline time for the subject (say, 13 mins); day two give them a good painkiller (e.g. the NSAID Ketorolac) and record again – this time they manage 23 minutes! Day three get them in again and repeat exactly the same with the Ketorolac, result – well over 20 minutes again; day four same again but give them a placebo Ketorolac and they go for 18-19 minutes; day five go back to giving nothing at all to see if the previous experiences have had any effect... they're back to 10-12 minutes.

What's noteworthy from this is that a placebo will always work better if it's used following a session with considerable analgesia.

Patients who have had good previous experience of being 'helped' are very likely to respond to a similar form of help in the future. Placebo research underlines that learning/conditioning isn't just the pill or therapy – it's you the clinician, it's your clinic, it's the whole atmosphere and experience given and the experience that has gone before.

('Make mine a big syringe done by the softly spoken, caring and confident nurse (rather than that Dr with shaky cold hands and bad breath) and I prefer the quiet and warm consulting room out the back please!').

Attempts have been made to see differences between responders and non-responders in their biological reaction to a placebo intervention. For example, low back pain responders showed increased levels of plasma endorphins compared to non-responders. Another group showed that in responders the anterior cingulated cortex of the brain was activated whereas it wasn't in non-responders.

Whether you are a responder or non-responder may simply boil down to your thinking/appraising/expecting/believing/emotional processors - all firing in a unified and biased way - and your brain's ability to make contact and influence your pain-'off' or 'on' activity.

For example, a good placebo response might occur when... you're *thinking* that you need help with the pain you are in; you *appraise* the situation you're in with the Dr as likely to be useful; you feel he knows what he's doing and he's convinced you to *expect* pain relief because you *believe* the drug he's given you is really going to help. You're already feeling *emotionally* relieved.

Or this: you're *thinking* you've come to the wrong therapist, your *appraisal* of the premises is that it's a big grubby and when you see the therapist your feelings are confirmed. You're now *expecting* to be given some kind of examination or treatment that you're not at all keen on and don't really *believe* that it's going to help. *Emotionally* you're feeling a bit wound-up and wishing you weren't there...

Or this: a friend made the appointment for you with the physio even though you weren't that keen. You're thinking it won't be much help but you're appraising the fellow as quite pleasant and he seems to be listening. You're not *expecting* any miracles and you don't *believe* in things like massage and machines to fix the problem you've got. *Emotionally* you're feeling pretty ambivalent about the whole consultation.

In the first two examples the top-down processors are all unified in the direction they're pointing. One is geared for a good result, the other for a no result or even a bad one. The third example is not 'unified' and the patient is being tugged in several directions and therefore not well primed for a good or bad result. Here, the therapist may have to work hard to get him on side.

Good therapists are good at picking up how hard they have to work to get patients 'on-side'.

A great deal of research into chronic pain, in particular on conditions like fibromyalgia, is indicating that an important factor in the problem's manifestation may be that there is a weakened or dysfunctional 'pain-off' system. Using a term from pain-science language – they suffer from pain 'disinhibition' problems! All it means is that the system is very good at allowing pain/nociception up and into consciousness – or as I've been putting it for so long – there's an 'annoying tune' constantly playing in their consciousness. Sadly, the chronic pain is largely meaningless, very common, and a terrible burden. I will argue later that this terribly maladaptive situation may be in some part a consequence of poor early management.

Roger's foot again...

I now come back to Roger's foot (Morton's neuroma). Recall from chapter 8.1 the bloke who was so angry with that acupuncture treatment and the physiotherapist. It was really a wonder that he hadn't already started proceedings against her for malpractice he was so wound-up. Roger's 'top-down' was clearly one-way unified– in a very negative direction ABOUT the foot pain and much else besides. There was no way anything was going to help until I'd done my best to 'set' his brain up to shift to what I call 'treatment acceptance' mode! Behaviour theorists might call it 'readiness to change'. That's a term normally used in relation to 'bad' behaviour – like drug addicts, smokers, drinkers but also applied to some chronic pain behaviours too. Here I want to 'change' Roger's attitude to me, to his foot, to his pain and to whatever form of management I might offer.

So, I listen very thoroughly and I do a very thorough examination. I find the exact pain spot and I can see he's starting to get more enthusiastic...

'How are we getting along with this...?' I quizzically ask.

'I reckon you're the first person who's really listened and got to the bottom of it... I've seen three different Drs now and none of them have been able to find the spot...'

'They've all called this 'metatarsalgia' Roger. It's a funny diagnosis because all it means is that you've got pain (algia) in your metatarsal, metatars-algia... The metatarsal is right here where I'm pressing at the base of your big toe and between it and your next toe's metatarsal. If I was to open this up and we could both wander round inside and have a look we'd see the bones and ligaments, a few tendons from the muscles and little tiny nerves. (I also showed him the bones on a skeleton).

'Some of the old researchers into this condition reckoned that the cause was due to pinching of little nerve branches between the bones and some of the old surgeons reckoned that the nerves there became thick and scarred. These days they still blame the nerve and as a result the pain's often described as 'neurogenic', meaning generated by a nerve and that may well be the case with yours...'

Roger was listening intently and enthusiastically nodding... I now wanted him to see the full extent of the problem... and also understand that I knew what I was talking about... that might sound a bit big-headed but the only way you're going to get someone to listen to you and shift a bit is for them to realise you know what you're talking about... The term 'unconsciously competent' may be better–just quietly get on with doing something really well and it'll all look after itself.

I go on...

'Let's just review what the treatment options are, starting with the most drastic. There are all sorts of operations for this problem, but they're only usually done on quite bad feet – deformed, arthritic and so forth and the operations are usually done as a last resort. So, we've got good news straight away – your feet are good feet, they're not arthritic and you haven't got any odd wonky toes, dropped arches or anything else. If you look at your painful right foot and compare it to your left – they both look the same, you can't see anything bad about them...'

'Now my experience with these sorts of problems is that they usually slowly and gradually get better – the time it takes varies from a few months to a year or more but they still get better...'

Roger interjects... and now looks a bit concerned...

'So that's it then, there's nothing you can do... I've just got to grin and bear it until it goes...?'

I come back...

'There's actually quite a lot we can do – the key thing is we need to create a better environment for recovery and a better environment for the pain to be able to switch-off. Recall just now I said that if we went into your foot where the pain hurts we'd see various bits of your foot... well, we'd also not be able to see anything much going on in the pain spot – perhaps a little inflammation where it's sore or perhaps a slightly enlarged and swollen little nerve, but more than likely nothing much at all... On the other hand, if we could wire up a little device that recorded the electrical activity in all the little nerve fibres where it is sore we could well hear a great deal! OK, Roger, I want you to shift your thinking from something awful going on in there to thinking that what you have is an electrical fault – like an bit of household flex where inside the insulation has been damaged a bit and it's short-circuiting. Looks fine on the outside but it's pretty busy on the inside!'

'An electrical fault'! Roger raises his eyebrows. 'So how could that acupuncture needle have made it so much worse then, do you think she stabbed my nerve?'

'Well, I guess that is a possibility, but we know that you can put small needles into nerves quite safely and it doesn't cause any damage – big needles where you inject something is a different matter. What we do know though is that nerves are normally very robust and can be squashed and moved without much harm – especially those that are in places where they're likely to get squashed and moved – like those under the foot. Nerves in your armpit where they aren't exposed to much physical force are a different matter; they're a lot more sensitive.'

'So I've got a problem that shouldn't be there and can't have been made worse by acupuncture!'

'Whoa! Hang on. Metatarsalgia is well known, it sometimes happens in some people and it's just bad luck. Maybe the nerve can't quite cope with what it's been subjected to and it gets a bit sensitised – we don't know exactly what happens or why, but most people – like you, get it following a bit more activity, or a different activity than they are used to. It only usually occurs in the over 50's and even more in the over 60's and it's very uncommon in youngsters.'

I pause, he nods...

'I'm with you...'

I go on...

'So, the nerve gets physically knocked about a bit more than it's used to and it can't cope. It then starts to become more sensitive – the short-circuit I mentioned. So, every time you squash it, it sends of lots of electrical impulses, they go up your leg into your spinal cord and nervous system and your 'processor' sends it to the part of your brain which says pain in the foot! You then limp to avoid it and get fed up and frustrated. Then you go for therapy and unfortunately you happen to be one of the occasional people who are made worse by a physio with an acupuncture needle...'

I look at him with raised eyebrows and a bit of a grin... he's smiling and rolling his eyes (good I'm getting him onside... he's with me I think...).

'... I'm going to emphasise – that it is highly unlikely that the acupuncture did any bad damage, all it did was cause a local tissue reaction that further sensitised the nerve fibre. I'm now going to be blunt, ready?' I'm smiling...

'Ready, go on...'

'We can't wind the clock back, it was bad luck, that's life, what's happened has happened and we're starting from the situation as it is right now.'

Phew, I've timed it okay... he nods his head...

'You're right I've been getting mad with the bloody foot, the physio, the acupuncture and it's not helping...'

'Good, no it's not. I'm now going to get down to how I'm going to help you get this well on the way and hopefully beat the horribly long times I mentioned earlier. I want to come back to how you're processing this and I want you to try and change your attitude to it. This is why. The brain, our 'processor' – think of it as like a computer for a minute – our brain works a lot of the time by concentrating on things so we can make sense of them; you 'focus' on my conversation, you understand what I say and hopefully it makes sense and it all may help... You focus on the radio or TV in order to hear it and follow what is going on; if you don't focus on it – it doesn't make sense and sometimes you can become quite unaware of the radio or TV even being on... it goes in and bounces right out again...'

'Sounds like when the wife's talking...'

We both nod and laugh... This is good, I've managed to shift him from an angry wound-up sufferer to a relaxed cheerful sufferer...!

'Big point now Roger... when we are wound-up or cross or angry with something – it brings that something into our mind a great deal... it keeps nagging at us and sometimes it really gets us down. The 'processor' gets stuck on it, pre-occupied perhaps and even amplifies the problem. Can you see what I'm getting at?

'I can indeed, if I stay mad with the physio and the pain in my foot, then that keeps my mind on it... that makes me madder and that makes the pain worse and I get madder...'

'Yup – big point is that if you keep giving attention to something it actually makes it more intense... you then notice it all the time... it gets trained into your system like an annoying tune gets into you...'

I pause, he nods, happy...

'Right, so before we 'do' anything therapy-wise – lesson one is that if we can change your attitude and thoughts to the pain, get you less mad with it, get you to even **'make friends with it'** a little bit (I do wincey sort of smile to show him that might be a tad difficult)... we can get your processor to leave-off it a bit... maybe?'

'Seems a bloody hard thing to do when it stabs every time you walk...'

'Right, lesson two is to see if we can make it more comfortable to walk and even get you walking normally again. It's far easier to 'make friends' and tolerate more comfortable pain than it is with 'knife in' pain.'

I then spent ten minutes cutting out bits of sponge and putting it in his socks then putting shoes on... we tried walking in socks, in shoes and even in bare feet with various thicknesses of sponge attached. I put the sponge so it went in the 'traditional' way – across and behind the metatarsal heads... I also tried longitudinal and in a great variety of thicknesses. We soon found that he was most comfortable with about two cms of sponge stuck longitudinally combined with a proprietary soft heel cushion.

I then spent another five minutes or so finding out the best way to walk without tension and limping. Short slow strides were the best to start with but after a while he managed to walk normally – the key was when I commanded him not to tense even when it hurt!

'Relax with the pain Rog... that's better... your frowning and wincing... keep walking and concentrate on your face! Let it go... that's it...'

We stopped and sat down.

'Lesson three is called 'Shut it up!' By this I mean we're going to try doing lots of different things to it until we find what it likes. Shutting a nerve up is all about getting endorphins into the system – the body's natural pain killers and anti-inflammatories and you get them when you do things that shut it up. For example, I can do massage, I can use some of my electrotherapy machines, I can lend you a bit of kit called a 'TENS' machine... we could even do acupuncture!'

We both laugh...

'Oh no, you don't...'

'Right, I'm going to start some of those things in the next treatment but in the meantime I want you to experiment with hot and cold. You can use a washing up bowl if you like – cold water, throw in a few ice cubes and dunk your foot in and out for 10-15 minutes a couple of times a day, or, do the same with warm water... Loads of people say one of these helps but only for a short while... See it like this – if you can shut it up even for a short time, you're doing something that switches it off or turns it down... that means you're shifting it in the right direction. What you need to do is keep doing it and usually it gradually works better and better for longer and longer... you're actually training it or even 'tricking' it to shut up... but, like learning anything new, it needs practice so you have to repeat and repeat and repeat...'

'Will do... no problem.'

'Lesson four, fit people get better faster than unfit people and doing some physical activity helps get the endorphin system going too... I know it's hard to exercise much when you're off your feet but I often find with a bit of shoe fiddling that most 'metatarsalgias' can manage a bike or rower. We need to look at that next time too, but have a little go, don't go mad...!'

So where was the placebo in that? Answer, everywhere! At least the lessons we've learnt from the placebo were everywhere. When a clinician gives a pain killing injection of medication they 'set' the brain to make it work better by simply saying 'This injection will help your pain very quickly...' If the patient is in a great deal of pain the procedure is accompanied by a mass of change – feelings of relief, expectancy, reduced anxiety, hope and so forth. In those situations Drs have it easy.

With the day to day things that I see, those important feelings are far harder to achieve – especially when the starting point (e.g on-going anger) is so far away from where it needs to be. I guess I could have taken him, put him on the couch and said, 'I can feel the imbalance of fluids in your foot, your leg, your sacro-iliac area, and it's even spread up here to the joints in your skull... I'm going to start working by correcting your skull imbalances and then work back to your pelvis... I'm going to use gentle correcting pressures that should be very comfortable... Afterwards you are likely to feel very tired but I expect your pain to melt gradually away in the next few days...'

I can't do that wacky pseudo-scientific stuff, it just doesn't resonate at all well with me. However, I won't deny that people may be helped – because of rapid changes in processing – but the majority of problems, when we really look and listen, have a natural history. So, while blips of improvement can be achieved and seen as miracles by the therapy operators, the overall pattern of recovery rarely deviates and the song remains the same.

What happened to Roger?

Well Roger picked it all up well and got on and it got quickly better in about three weeks but overall it took about three months before going completely. I guided him over three treatment sessions – two in the first week and then followed him up at about six weeks. The biggest thing that helped when I asked him...

'Two things Louis... first, you told me to stop being angry... it took about a week for me to really get my head round it, but that was key. Second, I enjoyed riding the bike and after about three or four days from first seeing you I cycled down to the river to row my punt, but when I got there the tide was nearly out and it was virtually on the mud... I took my socks and shoes off and found that being in the cold mud and in the cold water made my foot feel really good and for quite a while after... You know what, I started going paddling for 10-15 minutes every day and I reckon that really helped.

He changed his top-down processing and he found a great way to get an effective endorphin response going with a bottom-up input on a well prepared and accepting brain!

A last comment, about his diagnosis – metatarsalgia. Note that I went along with it. I gave it a label and attached a very rational and useful story to it in relation to him and what I needed to have him understand and change – with his thinking, his attention, his mood and his thoughts about anything that I could do for him and so forth. Whether this diagnosis was reasonable is one thing, the other is that in reality we haven't a clue what really causes this sort of problem and why it can be so easily exacerbated, but what I said I believe is pretty near the mark!

It's now time to leave the wonders and the very revealing world of the placebo to enter the world of stress and pain in the next few chapters (they're all linked up). I wrote an essay[1] in Topical Issues in Pain 4 called: 'An Introduction to evolutionary reasoning: diets, discs, fevers and the placebo. For those who are interested, I ask why the placebo response might have evolved and I also put therapy and therapeutic interactions in a biological/evolutionary rather than medical context. I also look into this later in the book (chapter GE 3.1 – where we learn from observations of mothers and hurt toddlers and chapter GE 2.2 which looks at evolutionary reasoning).

1 - Download for free here:
   http://giffordsachesandpains.files.wordpress.com/2013/06/06-chapter-ju.pdf

Section 8
Read what I've read

Benedetti F. et al., (1997) Blockade of nocebo hyperalgesia by cholecystokinin antagonist proglumide. Pain: 71:135-140.

Benedetti F. (2009) Placebo Effects: Understanding the mechanisms in health and disease. Oxford University Press, Oxford.

Benedetti F. (2011) The Patient's Brain: The neuroscience behind the doctor-patient relationship. Oxford University Press, Oxford.

Dworkin S.F. et al., (1983) Cognitive reversal of expected nitrous oxide analgesia for acute pain. Anesthesia and Analgesia: 62:1073-1077.

Gifford L.S. (2013) An Introduction to evolutionary reasoning: diets, discs, fevers and the placebo. In Gifford L.S. (Ed) Topical Issues in Pain 4. CNS Press, Falmouth.

Klaber-Moffett J. (2013) Pain: Perception and Attitudes. In: Gifford L.S. (Ed) Topical Issues in Pain 2. CNS Press, Falmouth.

Lawes N. (2013) The reality of the placebo response. In Gifford LS (Ed) Topical Issues in Pain 4. CNS Press, Falmouth.

Levine J.D., Gordon N.C., Fields H.L. (1978) The mechanisms of placebo analgesia. Lancet: 2:654-657.

Martin P. (1997). The Sickening Mind. Brain, behaviour, immunity and disease. Harper Collins. London.

Klaber-Moffett J. (2013) Pain: Perception and Attitudes. In: Gifford LS (Ed) Topical Issues in Pain 2. CNS Press, Falmouth.

Ridley M. (2003) Nature via Nurture. Genes, Experience and What Makes us Human. Fourth Estate. London.

Section 9

STRESS

Chapter 9.1
Acute stress.
Melzack and Selye

Having seen how the mind could influence, not just the processing and appreciation of pain via the placebo and nocebo, but also, actual and quite dramatic physiological effects on the body, my interest was directed towards understanding what I could about the mind-brain-body-brain-mind connections. Back in 1993-4 I had no idea where to start until listening to Ronald Melzack give a talk at a conference in London. The key was stress biology.

Ronald Melzack mentions Hans Selye

Thursday 6th and Friday 7th October 1994, Westminster Central Hall, London, just across from the Houses of Parliament, I attended a two day 'International Conference on Pain' with the subtitle, 'Human mechanisms of cortical and subcortical responses to pain'. The programme looked fascinating and the speakers even more so: Patrick Wall, Ronald Melzack, Jon Levine, Clifford Woolf, Chris Main, Steve McMahon, Bruce Kidd, Tony Dickenson and many others whose work I was to read and re-read for many years afterwards. These were the top stars and brains of the pain world and I was amongst them for the first time. Thrilling!

If I remember rightly, I was also with Dave Fitzgerald a physiotherapy friend and colleague from Ireland.

It was Ronald Melzack who sparked my interest in stress.

Melzack told his own pain story, how one very wet and dark night in the Canadian winter, he was driving home from work and was involved in an accident. He said he had quite badly cut his head and was bleeding profusely – yet he felt nothing, there was no pain at all. He was taken to hospital and still had no pain... the story continued and in amongst it he mentioned 'stress-induced-analgesia', highlighting the importance of understanding the science of stress for those who wanted to really understand the broader impact of pain and its modulation. He didn't say a great deal about stress biology but he did briefly mention Hans Selye, the so called 'father of stress', whose research and publications detailed the state-of-the-art of stress science up until the early 1980's. Melzack, it seemed to me, was also having a bit of a dig at the then sole focus of pain research on nociceptive neurones and 'upward' processing rather than looking at a bigger picture, which included nervous, hormonal and circulatory systems – and systems that were 'downward' or 'outputs' of the brain.

What no one seemed to say, was that pain itself is a 'stressor'. It's not nice and hence makes you stressed!

After the conference I struggled with a bit of a conundrum: if a body is 'threatened' in some way by a 'stressor' it causes the body to mount a stress response, whose sole purpose is to restore normal equilibrium or homeostasis – fine, but part of the stress response may be to actually produce pain... but, pain itself is stressful, it may act as a stressor in its own right... and therefore could cause more of a stress response... and so on in a continuous positive feedback loop! That is just not good biology!

I'll revisit this later, but one ah-ha moment that followed the conference was that while pain may be a stressor in its own right, it is also a unique and very variable part of the stress response that may or may not occur. It clearly depends on the circumstances the individual finds themself in, as well as the nature of the stressor. Environmental threats hardly need pain to occur, but tissue injury may at some point. It became clear that stress responses may be primed to produce pain given a tissue injury and an environment deemed to be safe. On the other hand, as in Melzack's situation where there was a degree of shock and stress, the production of pain was inappropriate. So, a little rule if you like, that pain should always be viewed, observed, studied, discussed and researched in the context of a bigger 'stress-response' perspective. Pain therefore, is a very variable creature; it just doesn't report a consistent level of sensation as medicine, traditional therapy and manual therapy wants it too. It just pops its head in from time to time, as opportunity allows (which is smart evolution)...

Thinking about stress now led me to revisit the International Association for the Study of Pain's (IASP) definition of pain[1] – having never really liked its wordiness. Sounds a bit pig-headed, but the more I read the more I was starting to think that pain researchers rarely thought further out than a purely mechanistic perspective. From a stress and evolutionary biologist's perspective it seemed to me that pain (adaptive pain, see below) can be viewed...

*...as **a variable, conscious product of a stress response whose major purpose is to change the individual's behaviour... when conditions allow... to the advantage and wellbeing of the tissues that are about to be damaged, are damaged, are healing, and/or are diseased or weakened in some way. The advantage of this to the whole organism's survival is self evident.***

Pain, and more importantly, the pain behaviour that derives from it is a tissue requirement, yet it is not always convenient to have it. Pain's presence is dependent on and governed by the circumstances of the individual as judged by its brain! You don't really want a whiny, achy pain coming from a healing twisted ankle when you're being confronted by a gang of thugs who are about to kick your head in... You want to get the hell out of there and fast – hence 'stress-induced-analgesia'. Smart? You bet.

The definition I gave above is my way of understanding 'good' pain, 'helpful' pain or in biological language 'adaptive' pain – pain that has evolved over millions of years to provide a clear advantage for survival. On the tissues behalf it may try to come in when it can, but if you're too busy doing something else that's vitally important, like running away from threatening thugs, or just about to score a winning goal for your local pub footy team, or make out with this new chick you've just hitched-up with... it may not get a look in!

At a rather more mundane level this makes sense of why pain and pain behaviour can easily disappear when we are occupied or preoccupied by something. Think of those things you love doing that require a bit of concentration! Like socialising,

1 - *The IASP definition of pain is "an unpleasant sensory and emotional experience associated with actual or potential tissue damage, or described in terms of such damage."*

watching your favourite footy team, listening to music, making music... writing! Also, think of how the chronic pain sufferer gradually leaves interests, hobbies and socialising behind – and what an opportunity that must leave for pain to manifest.

Unsurprisingly, as we've already seen in the last chapter, evolution has endowed us with an allow-pain-now-it's-OK system and a don't-allow-pain-now-it's-not-OK system. It's Shane (pain-on) and Claudia (pain-off) again!

As I will discuss and suggest later, it is my opinion that a major proportion of pain in the clinical (physiotherapy) setting could arguably be labelled as biologically 'maladaptive' or 'not so good' or 'out of proportion to the damage or degeneration shown'. Whether pain can be labelled adaptive or maladaptive is, I think, a vital clinical question (see NR 1.1)...?

While evolution may have done a very good job for species survival, for some individuals in their day to day lives, it may seem to be nowhere near perfect. Perhaps it's enough to be content with the notion that evolution doesn't give one jot about your quality of life and well-being so long as you've lived long enough, reproduced and made sure your offspring reach maturity! On-going pain is a mere aberration in the bigger survival picture – and if that is the case it is hardly going to suffer many pressures to evolve 'out'. It is only when an issue has significant effects on survival that evolutionary forces have any impact. Luckily for survival the *healthy* sexual, reproductive and nurturing urges come with very powerful inhibitory modules that block out virtually everything but the very worst threats!

Perhaps too, we should make a bit of an allowance for a negative 'cost' that arises from the amazing advantages of brain neuroplasticity when it is combined in parallel with our ability to think, attribute and make sense of what happens to us. Chronic on-going unnecessary pain may be one of the terrible costs of a plastic 'learning' brain.

Let us return...

After the London conference I found and absorbed all I could about Hans Selye and the story, language and science of stress. If I think, David Fitzgerald sent me a copy of Selye's book, 'The Stress of Life'.

The Selye story of how he stumbled into 'stress' is brilliant and of course, is told in quite a variety of ways by different authorities, but here is the main gist of it. (Read some of the books suggested in 'Read what I've read' at the end of the section).

In his early career, probably like all research scientists, Selye wanted to make his mark, come up with some earth shattering findings and get the Nobel prize for them. In the 1930's he was working as a research endocrinologist in McGill University – which was where Ronald Melzack was to start his research career in the 1950's. Selye's focus was on a new as yet unnamed substance that had been isolated from ovarian tissue by lab colleagues. He determined to find out as much as he could about it and started injecting it regularly into laboratory rats. Or, as Robert Sapolsky described it (I think this is the 'folk-myth version' of the events, but it's fun):

'He attempted to inject his rats daily, but apparently with not a great display of dexterity. Selye would try to inject the rats, miss them, drop them, spend half the morning chasing the rats around the room or vice versa, flailing with a broom to get them out from behind the sink, and so on.'

At first there was little response but as time went on the rats he'd injected became sick and some died. He felt that he was on the verge of understanding and describing a new hormone as yet unknown to science.

Being a good scientist he re-ran the injection protocol, but this time included a series of control groups of rats that were injected, not with the new hormone, but with substances extracted from other organs, like the placenta, spleen, kidney and the pituitary gland as well as harmless hypotonic saline preparation. Surprisingly, after some weeks he found that the rats in all the groups became sick and again, some died. What on earth was going on? Selye was at first disappointed with the results as it stymied his hopes of describing this new hormone. However, he reasoned that the only thing common to both experimental groups was the daily handling, chasing and injection-giving and maybe all those injections were toxic in some way too... i.e. all these things were stressors! He went on to run more experiments – placing the rats in adverse conditions for long periods – like extreme heat (in the university boiler rooms); extreme cold, on the lab roof in the winter; in proximity to threatening looking cats; some were exposed to forced exercise and so forth. Here again he noted the same results – the animals suffered and became sick. When he dissected the dead rats he found the following:

- gastric ulcers and bleeding

- enlarged and hyperactive cortex (outer layer) of the adrenal glands

- atrophy of lymph nodes, the thymus gland and spleen (in other words, major tissues and organs of the immune system had taken a hammering).

Selye went on to devote his life to the study of stress and became famous for proposing and presenting what he called the 'General Adaptation Syndrome' or GAS. He also used the term *'the syndrome of just being sick'* which I rather like. I also like his definition of stress: it being *'... the non-specific (that is, common) result of any demand on the body, be the effect mental or somatic'* (see Selye, 1993).

Two important elements arose from Selye's work; one was that whatever the stressor experienced, the body responded in a fairly stereotypical way... hence his term 'General' in the GAS. The other was that stress can make you sick and sometimes may even kill you, and, it doesn't seem to matter whether the stress is physical – as in suffering extreme heat or cold; or psychological, as in being frequently placed near a cat or in a noisy and unpredictable environment.

The GAS that Selye described is characterised by three main stages:

- the stage of ALARM

- the stage of RESISTANCE

- the stage of EXHAUSTION

The rest of this chapter and the following will be devoted to acute stress, Selye's stage of alarm, as well as many aspects of mind-brain-body-brain-mind interaction and connection that fascinated me at that time and since. The stages of Resistance and Exhaustion while pretty self explanatory for anyone who has had to deal with on-going stress of some kind, will be dealt with later (see section 20 and chapter GE 2.3).

Chapter 9.2
Selye's stage of alarm

Take one happy rat and put it next to one hungry cat. What's going to happen to the rat? Yup, it gets very alarmed – scientists crudely measure how alarmed rats are by counting the number of droppings they do. 'Christ, little Roger Rat, what a mess, you must be really wound-up today'... etc. So here's one shit-scared rat. It knows it's in danger and it needs to escape. Thankfully, evolved top-down pathways (psycho-somatic pathways!) turn on all the physiology that is necessary for the rat to make some kind of dash to freedom and survive – it's good old 'flight from 'fight or flight'. Crudely, the rat's brain draws in all the information it can get and assesses the situation, decides it's life threatening and not nice; so, it's brain goes wild in the 'fear/threat' department and very soon afterwards, there's also a whole lot of activity in the 'plan-your-move-to-freedom-and-get-ready-to-do something-fast' departments and off it goes. The emotion – the fear – provides the motivation to produce the best escape option the rat can think of. The result: the brain's all focused up on what's important right now – the cat. So, a quick recce for any hiding place or escape route, and then total focus on the eyes and body movements of the cat – it moves, I move... it stays still, I stay still... it comes forward, I go backwards... cat and mouse (rat)! Meantime the rats' (and the cats' too) heart rate is whisked sky high, adrenaline pumps through the blood stream, blood is diverted from chill places (eating, digesting, thinking about and doing sex type things...) to places that need to function very quickly and help the whole response happen. For example, the musculoskeletal system and the brain and CNS areas that plan and execute it all! Reflex times are enhanced, breathing goes up, pupil's dilate... all good stuff for absorbing as much information as possible and then the quick survival dash.

Expose any organism to a stressor and some form of acute stress response kicks in. To me it's the ultimate example of a mind-body reaction. Everyone's experienced it. It's the middle of the night, you're unusually home alone and thus a little anxious going to bed, dozing but a bit restless through the night, there's an odd and very disturbing 'thud' from downstairs... you're now sat up in bed –completely awake and frozen still, eyes wide open and senses on high alert for the slightest thing... your head is pumping with thoughts... 'What on earth was that?' 'Someone's down there?' 'What the bloody hell could make that weird noise?' 'Shall I turn the light on and go down and look?' 'I need a weapon...' 'I'll use the guitar over there...' 'Maybe I'll just get under the bed with the guitar...'

Your heart is pounding... and if someone really is coming up the stairs with heavy breathing you might even soil yourself... like the excited rat does...

You're now prepared! You're mad, you're totally pumped up with super human strength, you're ready for a fight and if the stink doesn't put them off...

Let's have a bit of a closer look at the acute stress response.

Recall that anything that threatens our lives or our health is eventually a threat to our homeostasis. Homeostasis – maintaining the steady state that allows life to carry on. Threaten homeostasis and you threaten life, little wonder that there are very powerful mechanisms in place that quickly maintain it at just the right level.

A homeostatic mechanism requires several things – **firstly a *monitoring* or sampling system**. For example, when looking at body temperature regulation –

the body has 'thermoreceptors' – which are located in places where 'knowing the temperature' matters. So, they're in the skin, where temperature fluctuations can be massive. Here temperature information is associated with thermoreceptors found embedded in the cell walls of the nerve ends of specialised C and Aδ sensory fibres of the skin (yes, the traditional pain fibre!). I like the term *'peripheral'* monitoring or 'sampling' system here.

Our all important core temperature is famously 37.5°C, but notably fluctuates from here to a low, at around four in the morning, of 36.4°C – is thought to be monitored by thermoreceptors deep in the 'pre-optic' area of the hypothalamus in the brain. They can be described as *'central'* monitors or using my preferred word – 'samplers'. Keeping the body temperature within very tight limits is essential for the adequate functioning of most enzymatic reactions in the body for example. Any major deviation of core temperature quickly causes death. Careful with that cold pack now... you'll get stressed out if you're not careful... and that ice immersion bath, wow, what a stressor that is, right when you're completely knackered after the game too... talk about adding a stressor to a stressor! Talk about a massive extra 'endorphin' release!

Peripheral and central monitoring receptors, with their specific inward (to brain scrutinising areas) bound pathways and relay stations are basically *'Input'* components that serve to inform central 'control' about the current and on-going situation. It's quite neat to see the peripheral thermoreceptors of the skin as an early warning system whose sole purpose in life is not to upset the central monitors deep in the hypothalamus.

'Getting cold hands? – make him go find his gloves – keep the core temperature steady and those central monitors happy...'

Now, **the second requirement is for a *'Control centre'*** – an area that gathers all the information in from the central and peripheral thermoreceptors and then makes a decision about what needs to be done. I like to call this area the *'scrutinising'* centre. For temperature, this area is the pre-optic area of the hypothalamus just mentioned. Any deviation or actual or potential 'threat' to the central requirement needs action and thus **the third requirement of homeostasis – is an *'output'* or *'effector'* system**.

Think about the brilliance of temperature regulation!

It's your gap year. Your crappy old Land-rover, that Gordy's Dad gave you, has broken down in the middle of the Sahara desert. It was quite a cold night but now the sun's coming up. Temperatures quickly whisk up from just above freezing to the high 20's and keep climbing. There are two basic things that happen – you do stuff, and, your body does stuff. The first is behavioural (but is clearly underpinned by physiological activity); you move into shade, you take clothes off, you move into a cooling breeze, you douse yourself in cold water (if you have enough!), you become lethargic and stay still; the second, your body 'doing stuff' is usually classified as 'physiological'; you sweat and your circulation is diverted to the skin's surface so that the cooling effects of sweat evaporation on the skin can be passed to the circulation. If you're hairy, your hair erector pili muscles will relax allowing your hair to lie flatter and therefore not trap as much air – air moving over the sweaty skin facilitates rapid evaporation and hence cooling... If you're a big hairy dog sweating won't work so your tongue lolls out and you start to pant.

The fourth homeostatic requirement that is really inherent in the first three is that of a **feedback system**. So, for temperature, as the temperature goes up as we've just seen, this kicks in a 'positive' control system that engages the physiological and behavioural changes that bring temperature down. If this then leads to a drop in temperature, a 'negative' system then turns these off, but at the same time turns on a 'positive' system for measures to conserve heat – hence move into the sun, put clothes on, jump around a bit, rub your hands together; as well as shiver, hairs stand on end, blood diverted away from the skin and so on. For every reaction or response that occurs in biology, there has to be some kind of mechanism that will control it – hence the prevalence of negative feedback loops and systems. It's hardly surprising that there is a pain-on system and a balancing pain-off system; that there's an inflammation-on system and an inflammation-off system and so forth. (The systems should not be seen as antagonistic but complimentary – always attempting to raise the correct levels of response.) It seems that in most of our patients the pain-off system just hasn't had enough practice! In my lectures I used to wind people up by saying – send the kids outside, let them fall out of trees, get stung by stinging nettles, lots of rough and tumble. Biologically speaking, I'm serious! The point with pain though, is that, unlike temperature, which has to be maintained within a degree or so of 36.8°C, it has evolved to vary its setting. So, we all vary in our 'laboratory tested' basic 'pain' threshold, but we also vary as individuals depending on the situation we're in. Homeostasis therefore is all about keeping the right setting, which can be within tight (e.g. temperature) or loose (e.g. 'pain' threshold) physiological limits, of a given observation for the circumstances the individual finds themselves in.

For me, anything that threatens homeostasis, even in the broadest sense, can be deemed a 'stressor'. By broadest sense I mean anything across a spectrum from minor, but very important, adjustments – as in the temperature changes just discussed, through to injury, disease... to such external 'potential' threats as a threatening gang of thugs. Or what about another extreme, the 35 year old person, who thinks that because their father died of cancer at 70, then every little thing that feels a bit odd in their body means that they've got cancer and are about to die? It seems incredible that the thinking and reasoning compartments of the human brain can do this sort of thing. Yet it does to a great many. And a great many patients, who are in pain, often have a great many (mostly unhelpful) fears that can maintain a simmering pain orientated stress response and with it their pain state. Brains that help us to dream-up unhelpful stuff can be a real nuisance.

Combating the threat from a stressor requires some kind of response. Selye saw it as a generalised response, but when you look at more specific stressors – like physical injury – you realise that the stress response as defined and presented here, also has to have more refined and specific components too.

So, I've always divided the acute stress response into two:

1. ***The general stress response*** that in large part can be considered to be driven by our personal assessment of the situation – that damn brain thing again! How we perceive a certain situation drives a very powerful physiological response – its mind-body – it's top-down! If we perceive a threat, what are the options? Stay and 'fight'? Whack the guy coming up the stairs with your guitar? 'Flight' perhaps? Slam the door closed, lock it, then jump out the window making as much noise as you can to alert the neighbours. 'Freeze'? Remain rooted to the spot and don't make a sound, don't even breathe, try not to even let off a smell and hope the intruder won't see, smell or hear you (you have sneaked the opportunity to get under the bed with the guitar as a weapon). And a piece of advice here, don't have a young baby, child or a pet with you – they just don't get the-don't-move-stay-silent bit... Finally, you could try the 'Give-up' strategy? In he comes and you start pleading; you show him pictures of your kids and your ageing grandma, you offer him money and anything else that might be of use... and he turns out to have a heart after all... he takes your money and family jewels, beats you up, ties you upside down over the balcony... but hey, you're still alive.

To witness human beings pleading with those in a position of power must be one of the most degrading, distressing and awful things... yet sometimes it can work, footballers do it all the time – it's called play-acting, but it won't work if you're confronting a hungry great white shark or polar bear! They just don't seem to understand what you're on about with that grandma, money and kids pleading stuff. I have a cunning plan for soccer refs to be replaced by polar bears with whistles for a season or two!

When dealing with musculoskeletal injury the degree of 'stress-response' can vary massively, as already stated. It's all about how the individual perceives the situation – what meaning they might give to the injury, the pain they have – and the circumstances of it.

'Yeah, I was like snowboarding in this real deep powder man, frigging ripping it... And, then like from nowhere man, the front of the board just dived way out of shape and then I hit this iced up snow, so like, hard man, and my head just whipped like it was on a spring or something'. Neck went off like a frigging ratchet and there I was still alive, yeah, it was cool... neck felt like it couldn't hold my head on... so weird for about 30 minutes.' Next day, this fit and well 25 year old was off snowboarding again and never even thought about it or had any repercussions.

And this...

'So I was at this roundabout looking for traffic coming from the right before I moved off, I was listening to Jimmy Young (old BBC Radio 2 DJ!) and humming along to that 'Spirit in the Sky' song when there was this almighty screeching sound and then this huge bang and jerk. It was a black moment. I knew my life would never be the same again. The car was all dented up, I couldn't even open the boot, and the man who did it started yelling and swearing at me. I was crying, the pain was in my head and neck and I was feeling really sick. That was five years ago, I was 25, fit, well and active, I've not driven or worked since and I hurt constantly...'

2. ***The more specific stress*** response that's mounted to any actual challenges to the body, hence physical injury precipitating physiological reactions, whose aim is to render a first-aid response and then follow-up with as rapid a healing as possible. Such reactions include changes in local circulation, activation and control of clotting and inflammatory responses, changes in blood pressure, in muscle activity, the production of pain and behavioural patterns relevant to the injury (e.g. limping), in immune system activity and in the pain system's shifting responses to suit changing situations for example.

The general stress response in the acute situation powerfully diverts resources towards some kind of 'big' physical action – and away from not-quite-so-essential processes like the healing and recovery processes. This is a sensible tactic that's neatly evolved to prioritise the ushering of resources towards saving the whole organism. The use of resources on less important recovery processes just have to wait until later, when things are safe once more. That stress puts healing and other 'vegetative' functions on-hold, or significantly slows them, needs more research attention. That reducing stress, especially stress that's focused on the musculoskeletal problem and the pain, may increase healing efficiency also needs more clinical and research attention. This fascinating area is discussed at length later in chapter 15.4.

In an acute stress situation the last thing you want is pain slowing you up.

Imagine... So there's this great big buffalo bearing down on you and 'Gordy', on your gap year holiday in the African rift valley (you made it across the desert), unfortunately you've wandered off from the party and got between the buffalo and its calf... you're now making off at sub 10 second 100 metre speed and you twist your ankle... damn... ow... bugger... hop, hop... stop... sit on a log and take off your shoes and socks... ker-thwack! Twit, you're dead and your genes are no longer destined for the next generation. Those ancients who evolved a pain-off system when they were being chased from within an inch of their lives survived to see the new day, even though they may have injured the ankle more than they might of otherwise. It's what Melzack had, 'stress-induced-analgesia' and it's what makes my ~~Machine-gun-therapy~~ Rotweiller therapy so effective too!

Pain, while being a given partner at some point in an injury stress response, can also be a stressor in its own right. If we're greatly troubled by pain and it has a very worrying meaning too, it becomes a source of stress and may by my reckoning, inhibit or dampen the healing response. How we interpret and perceive the pain and the situation we are in as a result, can have a big impact on how we recover and on the potential for maladaptive neuroplasticity. Good therapy surely needs to work hard at reassurance and creating an optimistic perspective on recovery.

So ... REASSURANCE IS A PAIN KILLER.

In summary, note the words in 'bold' – the classic adaptive response to threat includes...

Increased arousal – yes, you wake up very quickly and you don't want to go back to sleep for hours after just in case that threat is still nearby somewhere; you're more alert and super vigilant – all your senses become hyper-responsive and up goes your attention – even if you were never good at concentrating in class, you're now **focused where it matters**; there's **increased 'cognition',** which means that areas of the brain involved in processing the situation and working it out and what to do about it... are on full gas. Hence things like **searching for relevant memories** – 'What do I know that could help me right now? What past experiences have I had that are relevant to this situation? Oh yeah, I remember in that film, Indiana Jones did a good bluff... no, not quite right for now, oh yeah, I remember Crocodile Dundee staring down a buffalo and pointing two fingers at it, it just pulled up and went and laid down... yeah, I'll try that!'

Ker-thwack! 'Dang, can't have done it right!

Sorry! I guess I'm making the point that modern 'Western' man is becoming more and more dependent on film, play station, TV and paper media for potential helpful experiences in the memory banks, rather than the real thing! Sadly, what's spoon fed us via the media, we tend to believe... when often it's a very poor snippet of the fuller picture.

... High threat to life situation – the **pain-off brain areas are up and running** and on full throttle. Later on when you've survived, the lowered threat situation allows the pain-on system to start simmering away.

Physiologically we get... increased blood flow to the relevant areas of the brain and CNS and to the appropriate components of the musculoskeletal system. If they're working overtime they need plenty of oxygen and glucose, hence the amazing diversion of circulation to just those areas that are operating or are about to operate; blood is channelled away from skin where it's not needed, there are increases in cardiovascular tone; in blood pressure and in heart rate. Respiratory rate increases, glucose is mobilised from glycogen stores, pupils dilate, reflexes increase...

Anything else? Yes, something that's usually not mentioned in biology class but which is important here. There's a huge *inhibition* of 'vegetative' functions; feeding, digesting, loss of hunger, loss of interest in sex... in all the processes that 'build' the body, these so-called 'anabolic' processes are all inhibited – growth, repair, healing, immune function... All switched off and dulled down to allow all the body's resources to focus on the one important thing – survival. Thus, because it can drain resources, stress is often said to be 'catabolic' – meaning 'breakdown' metabolically.

Out of this comes a clinically useful statement:

TURNING OFF A STRESS RESPONSE, ALLOWS HEALING TO BE MORE EFFICIENT

The big message here is that if your patient's brain is in a 'high-threat' state – meaning they're stressed up – it's likely to impair the very biology that's needed for healing, recovery and lessening of the pain response.

'Ah, but hang on... I thought you said that stress turns the pain off – stress-induced-analgesia, Rotweiler therapy and all that? Now you're saying get rid of the stress to help the pain away?'

Correct, but think like this – stress, worry, anxiety and anger... all make the ***thing you're concerned, stressed, worried, anxious or angry about*** more intense and more dominating in the mind – sometimes in exclusion to all else. Think of some situations that you've experienced and realise how overwhelming a thing of high concern can be? High concern/stress draws your attention, it's 'me, me, me, me' at all costs. If your concern is for your life, as in an accident or during a session of Rotweiler therapy, your focus is on the threat – the last thing you need is pain – so this situation powerfully inhibits pain. However, think about the patient in pain, where issues like high concern, a bit of anger, wondering what's wrong, how the future might change become the mode of thinking for the individual. The outcome of this situation is that pain itself is the dominant thing of concern and therefore gets highly focused on – amplified, imprinted, remembered.

Here are a few things to mull-over for the clinical situation...

> I can't emphasise enough that it's the patient, and their mind-and-brain's response to the situation they are in, that holds the key to responses like those we have been discussing. Think of the difference between the snowboarder and the car accident victim earlier? No wonder high levels of stress and negativity at pain onset predict a poor outcome! Negative emotions have negative effects at all levels.

> It's worth asking the patient what they understand is wrong with them and ask how concerned they are. A great many who seek help do so because they are concerned and they often have a terribly skewed and grim perspective on their situation. Reassurance can be a very powerful pain killer!

> When it's appropriate, I frequently ask whether the problem they have and the pain they have are constantly nagging on their mind... 'Some people in your situation find that their mind keeps coming back to the accident, to the pain, to that bad consultation they had – is this sort of thing happening to you?' As a clinical aside here – if you know this to be the case then you are also making the patient aware that they may have got into a 'pain thinking habit' and you can start to help them get out of the habit.

> A great many day to day musculoskeletal pains are straight forward and we deal with them without undue concern. How many of us at some time or other twist our ankle and end up in a degree of pain that largely makes sense and we just get on and deal with it? However, I'm sure most alert clinicians regularly hear stories about pain appearing out of the blue, with no obvious or clear incident to account for the degree of pain. It seems quite natural to suspect something more serious and as a result feel anxious! Some sciaticas' for example often come on for no apparent reason. Imagine waking in the middle of the night with marked pins and needles and a slightly dead feeling in your toes, and that by morning a ghastly deep searing toothache pain has developed which no amount of positioning or moving or resting seems to make any difference to?

What about a minor injury that causes a huge amount of pain, as in the early development of some complex regional pain syndromes? Many patients say things like, 'I must be going mad,' or 'No one will believe me...' and the more this sort of thing goes on the more worried/cross/emotional the patient gets.

Think about the context and atmosphere at the time of injury; again think of the car accident and the snowboarding injuries earlier. In this modern age there are huge 'blame' issues, so often with anger and distress directed towards the perpetrators of the situation and there are often financial incentives to muddy the situation still further. All have an impact on how we deal with the situation we are in. I have had many chronic pain patients post-whiplash that have the following issue in common...

'I was waiting to pull out onto the main road and this idiot rammed me from behind, the car lurched forward into the road and a car on the main road then rammed into me. I was OK at the time but completely stunned. Then the idiot who hit me into the main road came over and started ranting and raving at me he didn't even say sorry.'

Saying sorry often diffuses the situation and calms it. It helps those involved to at least communicate and help each other. 'Sorry' though, means admitting you were wrong – something that many find hard to do, just like the words, 'I admit I cheated, adjust the score line...' Also, and thanks here to our perception of the insurance industry, there is the adage that it is always unwise to admit liability in any accident. Certainly a great many patients with accident related chronic pain problems admit to still feeling angry with those that caused the accident (and no apology from them) – and the on-going litigation processes merely add to the stress. I am sure there will one day be a new syndrome called, 'litigation-maintained-pain-anger-stress-and-disability-syndrome'! I'm wondering if there will ever be some guidelines for those involved in an accident that include the request that it's important to calm down and to say sorry if you were in the wrong?

Early stress with injury or onset of pain is often heightened by the words and deeds of those who are supposed to be helping – so called 'iatrogenic' factors. Here I mean the way the patient is dealt with by clinicians – physically and verbally.

This is the car accident whiplash patient telling me what happened several months later...

'I went into A & E the day after the accident, my brand new car was all smashed up, I could hardly move my neck. All they did was ask me where it hurt? Someone then banged on my knees and elbows to see if I had reflexes, they asked me to wiggle my toes and squeeze their hand, they got me to walk up and down. They didn't even x-ray me and some junior Dr, who didn't listen to me, eventually gave me some pain killers and said I'd strained my neck and I'd be fine in about ten days. Oh yeah, that was two months ago. They didn't even get me to take any clothes off – I was mad.'

'POOR REASSURANCE CAN BE A PAIN AMPLIFIER!'

So, if negative emotions have negative effects – so must positive emotions, have positive effects. Yellow flags are the negative and I like to call the positive, Pink flags! (see chapters GE 4.5 to GE 4.8 for the yellow flags and GE 4.9 for the pink flags).

Section 9
Read what I've read

Sapolsky R. (1997) Junk Food Monkeys and Other Essays on the Biology of the Human Predicament. Headline Book Publishing. London.

Selye, H. (1978) The Stress of Life. McGraw Hill. New York.

Selye H. (1993) History of the stress concept. In Goldberger L. and Breznitz S.(Eds.) Handbook of stress: Theoretical and clinical aspects 2nd Ed. The Free Press. New York. (Note that Selye actually died in 1982, which was when the first edition of this book came out. Selye's chapter was clearly added for this 1993 edition and he tells his own story beautifully).

Sternberg E.M. (2001) The Balance Within: The Science Connecting Health and Emotions. Palgrave. New York. (Esther's father worked with Selye in the University of Montreal – in the 1950's and she knew him well as a youngster).

Section 10

THE MATURE ORGANISM MODEL (MOM)

Chapter 10.1
The Mature Organism Model 1: Start with an amoeba

Discovery: 'To see what everyone else has seen but to think what nobody else has thought.'

Biochemist, Albert Szent-Gyorgyi.
In 1937 he was awarded the Nobel Prize for Physiology or Medicine, his achievements included the discovery of Vitamin C.

The mid 1990's saw me reading everything I could on stress, psycho-neuro-immunology, psycho-neuro-endocrinology and anything else that linked a person's thoughts and emotions to changes in body physiology. See the reading at the end of the chapter, especially the 'must-read' material – it is fascinating stuff!

This series of three chapters is going to look at the circuitry and mechanisms of physical threat in the context of a homeostatic or threat response mechanism. I'll also be taking a look at a useful perspective on it all, my Mature Organism Model (MOM).

Physical threat is usually discussed in terms of some kind of injury but I'd like it to also include other potential physical threats, like degenerative joint and muscle changes, spontaneous inflammation in the musculoskeletal tissues such as that associated with rheumatic and arthritic problems, it could even include tissue infection and disease. They are all threats to the adequate functioning of our organism. Some of you may have come across the term 'allostatic load' – it's a term that was coined to explain the way the body constantly adapts to on-going stressors (Selye's stage of 'adaptation') but which can eventually lead to a state of failing health as the 'allostatic load' takes its toll on the system (Selye's stage of 'exhaustion' – remember the rats dying?). The literature tends to focus on on-going 'psychological stress' and the pathophysiological consequences like hypertension and subsequent heart disease. Think of the classic so called 'Type A' personality, the highly stressed company 'executive' who ends up with heart failure. The point for us, working with many 'on-going' conditions like Osteoarthritis, Rheumatoid Arthritis and even on-going chronic pain states – is that they are all allostatic loads that are bound to have long term consequences. My 'Vulnerable Organism Model' (VOM) is of great relevance here (chapter GE 2.3). One key aspect of on-going pain and 'allostatic loading' is that issues like the patient's attitude, reactions to and coping mechanisms will massively increase or decrease the burden on the system. It's one time when we can safely say that the bigger the burden of stress an on-going condition, *and the individual with the condition* brings, the more wear and tear occurs on those systems that are having to continuously deal with and respond to it (see maladaptive stress discussion – in chapter 20).

Central to understanding the MOM is the notion of 'Sample-Scrutinise-Respond.'

Recall from the temperature discussion in the last chapter that the homeostatic mechanism has several components: namely, 'peripheral and central monitoring' systems that sample the state of affairs and which then, 'input' a central 'control or scrutinising' system that, in turn, may 'decide' to mount a response by way of an 'action', 'output', 'motor' or 'effector' system. There seem to be so many terms for the same thing and that is why I have come to favour this: a sensory or 'sampling' system... a scrutinising system... and a response system...?

Let's go back to an amoeba or a similar tiny single celled organism. Oh, and as an aside, it's much better if you're happy with the truth – i.e. the fact of evolution? If you're not sure there are two good books, I would say beautiful books, the first, 'Why evolution is true' by Jerry Coyne and the second is by Richard Dawkins: 'The greatest show on earth – the evidence for evolution'.

Evolutionary reasoning in the clinic will be discussed later, it is incredibly useful.

As an old zoology graduate I find that the issues of evolution and where and how life evolved fascinate me, it's really an on-going hobby of mine and I like to think and talk about it from time to time. I drive my kids up the wall, they say I'm blinkered! Ah, young heads. So if you're now going, 'Well that's biased there is 'The Creation' and all the other thousands of different religions and their 'origin' perspectives to consider and evolution is only a 'theory' anyway.' Well, I'm sorry, the creation myths are many and varied and all societies have one and they can't all be right. If you ask a question someone will come up with an answer, like, does (your) God exist?

Anyway, thank God (ahem...!) I was born into an age when a great deal of good science came along and started to make much better sense of very many things. How life came about and the evolution of life is one of them. Evolution is now a 'fact' and you'll see that the evidence is overwhelming.

Use of the word 'theory' as in, 'The Theory of Evolution' by the way, is in the following sense as defined by the Oxford English Dictionary.

Theory is:

'A scheme or system of ideas or statements held as an explanation or account of a group of facts or phenomena; a hypothesis that has been confirmed or established by observation or experiment, and is propounded or accepted as accounting for the known facts; a statement of what are held to be the general laws, principles, or causes of something known or observed.'

As Dawkins says, this is the definition of 'theory' as used by scientists, the second 'sense' of the word 'theory' from the OED is often that opted for by those who say evolution is 'only' a theory, hence...

Theory can also be defined as:

'A hypothesis proposed as an explanation; hence, a mere hypothesis, speculation, conjecture; an idea or set of ideas about something; an individual view or notion.'

The 'current theory' is that the planets in our solar system revolve around the sun. Not all that long ago though, the theory was that the earth was at the centre of the universe and the sun and everything else revolved around us – the 'geocentric model'. I think anyone who has had a reasonable education will be quite comfortable with the proven nature of this 'current theory' and happily believe it without fear of being severely castigated, charged with heresy, imprisoned and subject to an inquisition by the church, as Galileo was through his support of the 'heliocentric' (sun centred) model proposed by Copernicus.

Please read the evidence for evolution, it is fascinating and beautiful – and please remember that we evolved to have 'moral' as well as 'immoral' characteristics and that no amount of religion over modern human history seems to have successfully made an impact on down-regulating the immoral side of things! The bottom line is that you don't need religion to be good or bad and having religion doesn't make any difference to being good or bad either. If you want a good read, try Robert Wright's book: The Moral Animal: Why we are the way we are.

Now to our single celled animal, the amoeba which we all studied at school[1]. I use a single celled organism as all this is easier to see and appreciate at a less complex level of life. If you can 'get-it' at this level you can then see that all multi-cellular organisms run on the same principles, it's just that it's a little more complicated to achieve the same ends. It also makes me marvel at the incredible capability and complexity of a single celled organism!

An amoeba's life, like anyone else's, is all about staying alive, finding food and sustenance, avoiding injury and dangerous situations and environments, mending itself if it does get injured, and it also has to reproduce. At a nice simple biological level, 'that's life'!

In order to stay alive an amoeba continually samples its environment, scrutinises it and then acts or responds. I like to think of the little fellow going round its watery environment continually sniffing it...

'Hmmm, smells nice over here, I detect some food not very far away... (I can smell its chemicals)... I'll just follow this scent trail a minute'... Sample, scrutinise, respond... starts to move towards the desired food... hold up a minute, there's something a bit odd, I can smell a paramecium (remember them, they look like microscopic chain-saws and they're predators) and they like that watery scum I'm smelling too... better use one of my clever survival dodges a minute. Ok, I'll use the make-myself-big and spherical dodge...' The amoeba responds by inflating a bit like a puffer-fish does when threatened and the paramecium bounces off and runs away... So, there we are an example of the continuous sample-scrutinise-respond process that allows life to go cleverly on.

Let's say though that the paramecium found our little amoeba friend all puffed up and managed to take small chunk out of him (though a bit unlikely as paramecium really feed on smaller things like bacteria). Luckily, the amoeba has an *internal* sampling system that's constantly checking its health status! It basically sniffs itself all the time (sounds like a dog going for its backside smell! Sorry, the image just popped in there!).

Now, biologically 'sniffing' is all about detecting chemicals using chemical receptors that can make contact with their environment, be it external or internal. For checking the external environment receptors are lodged in the amoeba's cell wall – right at the environmental interface. Here chemicals can lock onto specific receptors which in turn may initiate reactions within the cell. These reactions lead to cascades of chemical activity that are often called 'messenger' systems and they ultimately lead to an appropriate physical and/or physiological response. Note that in our lowly amoeba not a lot of scrutinising necessarily goes on – as there may be only one response available! He doesn't have to go, 'Now, I've got ten possible responses here, which one should I choose?'... ponder... hmmm... too late, zap, gulp, gone. But in the more complex higher organisms – from the lowly to the grand, there often are choices, so a bit of quick scrutinising and moderating, if there's time, can give the edge in the staying-alive game.

---

1 - *Type amoeba (and paramecium) into Youtube search for a good look at these lowly organisms.*

It may be worth reviewing the discussion of chemical receptors in section 5 because it is the same here. Note that the principles of communication using chemicals has been beautifully preserved by evolution – hence similar pathways and messenger system 'basics' in the dorsal horn to those in the amoeba!

Sniff a favourable food type chemical and the response is 'follow the chemical gradient until you find the food.' A chemical gradient is rather like when you smell a bonfire or something cooking on a barbeque from a good distance – you get a vague notion that someone's having a bonfire/barbeque somewhere and it's pretty easy to detect where it's coming from – lucky for us we can integrate information not just from smell but we can also see the smoke trail and maybe hear the fire to get a better handle on its direction! Move away, if it's a bad smell, move towards if it might be to one's advantage! It's the same for us as the amoeba.

So some senses are 'is it good' monitors and some are 'is it bad'. Good move towards, bad move away. Most of us like the smell of some flowers and not others? In unadulterated and old-fashioned nature, as it once was, the smell of a flower often leads us to nice sweet fruit... or an edible plant. Or maybe, a bad smell told us to avoid its poisons, or was the plant just trying to trick us into thinking it was poison and hope we'd just go away? If you decide to 'go bush[1]' someday it's best to know your smells, especially if you go collecting and eating mushrooms and fungi. Isn't it true that if we're offered an unusual food or drink to taste – we usually sniff it before putting it to our lips or eating it?

Sensory systems are thus specialised 'sniffing' and 'checking' systems that continuously sample – not only the environment, but also the body itself. The body checking system sniffs in order to ask its ever repeating question... 'Am I ok? Am I ok? Am I ok? ... on and on and on...

Ah, the paramecium's taken a chunk out of the amoeba – smashed up cells walls, tissues mangled, cytoplasm dribbling out of the leak... Chemicals are also released into the cells inner environment that aren't usually there, specific chemical receptors pick up on this and signal the emergency...

All together: 'What's needed? New cell wall. What's cell wall made of? Protein. When do we want it? We want it now!'

Messengers from the damaged area speed off... er, where to? To where proteins are made! Where's that? Well it starts with switching on a gene in the nucleus – remember this being mentioned in section 5? So, chemical messengers switch on relevant genes on the chromosomal DNA in the nucleus of the amoeba that code for the cell wall proteins. This leads to the manufacturing of RNA copies of the gene which take the code out of the nucleus into the cytoplasm to act as a template for the amassing, in the correct order, of the required amino-acids... Enzymes aid the process and once assembled the whole lot gets transported to where it's required and the breach finally gets stemmed (or the amoeba dies). How about that for a stress response? (Greatly simplified)

Key things then: novel chemicals – like smashed up cell wall proteins, receptors that

---

1- *Australian term for surviving in the wild/bush.*

detect them, which then trigger the release of messenger molecules, then a transport system for the message – remember cytoplasmic streaming – a kind of very primitive circulation within the cell? The next requirement is a message receiving receptor, which then triggers an appropriate 'scrutiny' and mounts a response, hence, the gene switching and the subsequent building of an appropriate protein structure. The final 'response' is the transport and instalment at the required site. Appreciate that genes aren't just little codes for programmes that build you and make you from sperm and egg to adult and that's it – they are also busy throughout every second of your life – being turned on and off in order to produce the appropriate proteins for the situation and requirements at that time.

Cytoplasmic streaming in the single celled organism is a quite brilliant circulatory system. As far as I know all cells have it, for example, neurons, which are often incredibly lengthy cells, have an internal bi-directional circulatory system called 'axoplasmic transport'. The axoplasm is gently wafted along clever little highways by minute cillia like processes. Transport in fluid like this is ok, but quite slow and evolution has craftily come up with a much more efficient system. As multi-cellular animals evolved and got bigger, so the requirement for faster communication came about – the result – electricity and nervous systems!

What's fascinating is that all large animals not only have an evolutionary modern electrical communication system, they also have a transport and communication system that uses good old fashioned fluid flow too! Communication using a fluid medium is called 'humoral' communication – think of the way hormones get secreted by the brain into the blood stream and wander around before being picked up by receptors in their target organs and tissues. Or what about the diffusion of neurotransmitters across the synaptic gap in neural communication as we discussed in section 5? Neurotransmitters are also known to wander out of the immediate synaptic environment into the interstitial fluid of the central nervous system – and have quite marked effects at targets surprisingly far away. Old systems that worked well have been well preserved throughout.

Chapter 10.2.
The Mature Organism Model 2: Numskulls and modules

I'm now moving from simple life forms to humans. I hope the reader can appreciate that as organisms become larger and more complex the task of keeping everything that's going on that produces 'life' is rather complicated and needs a great deal of co-ordination. It all needs to happen in the right order at the right time. So it's hardly surprising that as organisms evolved and became more complex the requirement for some kind of 'central' coordinating centre was paramount. At a rather prosaic level nervous systems and the brains of nervous systems do just that – they gather all the information in, scrutinise it and then make an appropriate response.

In this chapter I want to get clinicians to think more about nervous, systems, brains, minds and the individual. An injury is more than just the tissues where it hurts and what is wrong, and so is pain.

Think about tripping over and falling to the ground. Mostly the brain and via consciousness, the individual has all the information to hand about the injury even before it's happened, because, for one thing; via information from the eyes, it sees it coming and for another; via proprioceptive, balance and kinaesthetic inputs that inform about the movements and positioning of the body – it feels it too. The brain anticipates what's going to happen and does its instant best to try and avert the worst. It samples, scrutinises and responds. If you've ever fallen over you'll know that your arms and legs fly out to try and regain balance or prevent too hard a fall and you're more than likely to tense appropriate muscles to try and rebuff the pending impact. Information surges in from sensory systems that monitor what's going on in the environment – hence the term 'exteroceptors' and also what's going on within our body – hence 'interoceptors'.

I've often wondered whether it would be appropriate to think of the brain rather simply as merely a 'stress control centre'? Think of a snail's brain perhaps, rather than your own. As the stress control centre the brain's main purpose would be to constantly take in information related to potential or actual threats and process them all in order to generate appropriate survival responses. That makes the brain's task all about keeping out of trouble and staying alive? Well yes, but life is also all about staying adequately nourished and living in a safe and 'just right' place as well as reproducing.

So, in a rather basic biological sense, in a lowly snail or cockroach sort of sense, a great many of the brain's functions boil down to constantly asking the two survival questions, 'Is it good?' or 'Is it bad?' (Or maybe there are three? – The last being, 'Is there an opportunity to have sex right now?) And then organising what can be done about the situation to the advantage of the brain and the body that tags along with it.

Ah, I suddenly find myself thinking about humans and the many other animals that switch off at night and go to sleep! That stymies the idea that we ask those, 'Is it good or bad,' questions all the time. Our brains just aren't processing 'Is it good' or 'Is it bad' questions when we're asleep? But when we're awake we are – and we're mostly we're processing these questions in response to what's out there in the environment – in preference to any internal issues. However, when we're asleep, the brain can turn its attention away from 'surviving' in the environment to what's going on with its own body. Sleep time is healing and recovery time – so the 'is it good/bad' questions do crop up again, but this time their focus is not environmental (and sex!) but on the body and its well-being.

Good sleep equals good recovery and healing – poor sleep equates to inadequate healing. Sleep time is growing time too for youngsters. Work hard at helping your patients get good sleep is vital.

As you can see, I keep popping into the brain to imagine what it might be asking if it were conscious and I shouldn't really do that because consciousness is a lot more than just a 'brain'. That's why I've mentioned snails and cockroaches and hoped you'd see I was referring to human brains too. Having said that I'm now going to be really naughty and tell you about the Numskulls, which as you'll see, are all about putting a little 'conscious' individual or two or three in different parts of the body to see what might be being 'thought' there. The bottom line is that it can be very useful in explaining things, especially to patients and it's a bit of fun. The top line is that it mocks the notion of consciousness rather. Bear with me and this little bit of stupidity.

Numskulls...

In explaining stuff to patients (and clinicians sometimes) I often get them to see what the Numskulls might have to say! So, who the hell are the Numskulls? They're a comic strip in 'The Beano' comic! When I was a kid in the 60's the Numskulls were in the 'Beezer'. The comic strip is about some tiny human like creatures that live inside the head of Edd Case (a pun on *head case* obviously!) and control his actions.

Here are some of the main characters... **Brainy**, controls Edd's brain; **Blinky**, controls his sight/eyes; **Radar** (originally called **Luggy**), controls his hearing/ears; **Snitch** (originally called **Nosey**), controls his smell/nose; and **Cruncher** (replaced **Alf & Fred**), controls his mouth/taste. Occasionally other Numskulls are seen who control Edd's other body functions including; germ-fighting Numskulls, Numskulls in the stomach, pelvis Numskulls and blood Numskulls.

We can see the typical interaction between the Numskulls in the story "An Alarm clock gives them a shock" which appeared in The Beezer Book 1980. "Our Man" is pictured asleep in the first panel and in the second we see Radar in the Ear Dept. awoken by the sound of the alarm clock next to "our Man's" bed. Using an intercom system Radar sends a message to Brainy that the alarm clock is ringing. Brainy, in turn uses his intercom system to wake up all the other Numskulls and feeds the written message "switch off alarm!" into the suggestion box. We then see "our Man" thinking "Noisy alarm! I'll switch it off. Where is it?" In the following panel we see Radar informing Brainy that the alarm is still ringing whilst Brainy reads a print-out from the computer "Where is it?"

It transpires that Blinky, who is in charge of the man's eyes, has neglected his duty by staying in bed. The other two Numskulls burst into his department and force him out of bed. Grumbling, Blinky opens the man's eyes with a hand-crank whilst Brainy and Radar stow his bedding in cabinets under the eyes. In the last panel we see "our Man" reflecting that he couldn't open his eyes this morning and now he has bags under them, caused by the bedding.

I took that from wikepedia, with thanks...

When appropriate I use the Numskulls to help with appropriate explanations – mostly for patients but sometimes in my lectures too. Here's the sort of thing I do... with a bit of swearing it makes it a bit more adult!

So, imagine we're peering into Edd Case's head as he's falling off to sleep after a hard day surviving. Blinky, Nosey and Radar are tucking into their beds for the night and poor old Brainy is still up scratching his head pondering the day.

'Christ that was some day! That bloody great king sized hamburger caused some problems for the guys down in the guts and all the bloody phone calls of complaint I kept getting from the gall bladder, the liver and even the bloody heart had to ring up to find out what was going on. Bowels weren't best pleased either. Then the lungs phoned in to say they were bored and wanted something to do – bloody cheek! Right after that he went climbing and fell out of a tree into a patch of stinging nettles – stung all over his legs (he had shorts on) plus scratches and bruises everywhere. Bloody phone lines from the legs were on fire... panic out there, there was... tried to get the guys down at the brain stem to tell them all to belt-up for the time being but they hardly shut-up for over an hour. Ah well, it's going to be tough for a little while organising the night shift to sort out the mess down there, at least we can use some of that burger in the gut-store to help the boys keep going. Better just turn on the really deep-sleep button a minute, were going to need a bit of peace and quiet... I'd better just get onto the chief down at the immune system too...'

Off goes the night shift dampening right down all the guys who were busy in the day (guts, lungs, cardio vascular, ears, nose, eyes, legs, arms... Oh and the consciousness bloke who they sometimes have a devil of a job to find...) and shunting resources to the areas where they're needed. Tissue mechanisms quickly get organised to set up the damaged environment so the mending and defending process can begin in earnest (I nearly wrote 'in Ernest'! Reminded me of my Mum's joke: 'Two maggots making love in dead Ernest'...! Sorry).

Night time is when the body can forget about 'wasting' resources on what's going on outside and 'doing' and getting on with repairing and sorting out the body that's basically been trashed during the day. It could be seen as coming down to – day, equals awake, equals stress, equals 'catabolic' (breakdown)... and night, equals sleep, equals no stress, equals 'anabolic'... build back up again (see Esther Sternberg's work).

Clinical/biological thought here. Maybe one possible reason, among a great many others, as to why we might not sleep well is if the night Numskulls have got nothing to do? It's certainly noticeable that most of us tend to sleep better after an active day – there being plenty of work for the 'recovery' Numskull brigade to get stuck into at night. If there's a lot to do requiring a lot of resources, then surely our biology would see to it that none goes to waste on unproductive 'wakeful-state' physiological activity? If there's a lot to do, on goes the 'turn-on-sleep' pathways and circuits and we sleep soundly.

I don't know about you but when I have a bad night I'm for one thing quite restless and for the other, my mind is buzzing. That doesn't sound like it would consume much in the way of energy resources until we consider that the nervous system consumes more glucose than any other organ in the body. Researchers have shown that when the mind is at work doing cognitive stuff like 'reasoning' and working things out – blood glucose levels drop considerably – no wonder it's sometimes such an effort to really think and work something out (e.g. see Kahneman 2011). So logically if you've done nothing physical during the day then there's nothing for 'recovery' physiology to do and in turn no need to switch on the sleep physiology with such enthusiasm.

Good sleep is vital and in order to sleep well the individual must be good at finding a safe and comfortable place. Most of us find it very hard to sleep if we feel even the slightest bit vulnerable, unsafe or uncomfortable. Think of the extremes some prey animals go to so they can sleep well, reproduce and nurture or hibernate; long deep burrows, elaborate nests often in hard to access places... or maybe they just all huddle together! Think of emperor penguins, sheep, gazelles, zebras and us humans even!

Now, in future, if I start giving 'consciousness' status to parts of the body or parts of the brain, or even to the whole brain, perhaps you could think to yourself that Louis is really off on one doing his 'Numskull' thing again.

Right, here's a Numskull conversation going on in the lumbar spine of someone who's got 'wear and tear, triple discs out and spondylosis'...

'You know what Mr C Fibre, it doesn't feel too safe round here at all, I'm really not happy with the situation, I reckon we should turn the sensitivity up big time.'

'Well, Mr Aδ Fibre I was thinking just the same, you know how bad it was when he helped his mate with that slab the other day... cor, bedlam it was. The thing is all the muscles round here are being so pathetic, it's like there's no support, no protection, no backup for the guys doing all the work, everything's just vulnerable... come on, grab that knob over here and we'll turn everyone within hearing distance's sensitivity right up.'

This guy hardly moves and he hurts virtually all the time.

He eventually gets sent to Louis for a graded back exercise programme. Three months later he's worked up his cardio-vascular system (rower, cross-trainer and bike); his walking distance and pace; his 'natural corset' (that's what I like to call the abdominals and the back muscles combined) and his legs and arms. He's also lost half a stone and working towards a goal of losing a stone and a half.

Back to the Numskulls and it's Mr Aδ...

'Mr C... Mr C... Mr CCCCCCCCCCCCCCCCCC...!'

'... Wha, yeah, ah... wow, I was so like deeply away man... what is it? Shit that's so bad manners doing all that yelling down here...'

'You went to sleep again, what's wrong with you?'

'It's me default, mate, it's not my fault it's me default. Hey, when I got this job I was set-up for life.'

'Look what I wanted to say was that you know we had a discussion a couple of weeks ago and we both felt that it was so much more secure here since he'd been getting fitter and we decided to turn the sensitivity knob down, well why don't we turn it down some more?'

'What's the consensus then?'

'Well that's what's pissing me off so much, they're all frigging sleeping all the time, no one's got a bloody opinion anymore.'

'Well, you turn it down if you want, but us lot we're making the best of our default while it lasts…'

What better way of reasoning how getting fitter works so well… ask the Numskulls!

Sample-Scrutinise-Respond Modules… and need states…

This has all led me to thinking about a few survival 'Sample-scrutinise-respond' modules (SSR's) that have evolved and are relevant to how we deal with and respond to injury and pain. SSR 'modules' are ultimately tissue/environment to neural and back out again circuits and can be seen as being heritably 'pre-loaded' for a particular and important purpose.

If you're hungry and I put a Cornish pasty in front of you, among many things that happen, salivation is likely to be one of them. So, sample (sight, smell), scrutinise (it's good), respond (salivate, get ketchup, eat, digest and get a cup of tea)… is an example of a few well entrenched Cornish modules in action.

There's a big problem here though and it's the physical notion of a 'module' in terms of the CNS and brain. The last thing I want you to be thinking is that it is like a printed circuit-board that you can buy off the shelf and slot into the nervous system and later take out and replace if it starts malfunctioning. Having said that, this way of thinking is how a great many of those in brain research seem to wish it would be. It's so seductive to be able to identify the areas and neural pathways of the brain involved in a given condition or presentation. However, immediately you start conceptualising the nervous system as a hard wired series of identifiable isolated and organ like structures problems arise, for example, the reality is that there's massive functional overlap between the various regions of the brain. It's just not like the lungs do this, the heart does that and the liver does this and that… it would be easier if it was for sure, but it's not. Imagine you're abdominal cavity as being one massive organ that can do the functions of all the separate organs we have and that within that one organ there's no clear distinction between which bit does what and you're on the way to grasping the problems of conceptualising the brain as a neat series of anatomically isolated functional units.

That brains do have identifiable anatomic zones is clear, the problem is that teasing out function in one brain will give you a bit of an idea until you come to try and tease out the exact same thing in the next brain you decide to investigate. No one person's brain is functionally connected up the same way as anyone else's. That's after all a major part what makes us individual!

Let's view a SSR module as a unit of 'function' whose precise anatomy is rather variable.

Here are a few...

1. A 'looking after the body' module, it's an, 'Am I ok' (or, 'Is it bad?') module where the tissues and organs of the body are being constantly monitored for any signs of distress. Ultimately if something amiss is detected the module has the capability of not only getting on with an appropriate physiological response, but also producing an aversive sensation, i.e. discomfort or pain which then motivates and becomes part of an appropriate behavioural response.

2. Similar to that we can think of modules concerned with maintaining the classic homeostatic internal steady state, hence attention to issues like body temperature, blood glucose and oxygen levels etc. Modules here are associated with feelings of thirst, hunger, feelings of being hot or cold and feelings associated with lack of oxygen. As you're well aware, those sensations make you do something about the situation. All sensations have an inbuilt variation capability, as they move along an intensity spectrum or continuum, from mild and then moderate to intense. The Numskulls would use a 'dimmer-switch' type device I would imagine, and this is the analogy I often use when discussing pain sensitivity with patients. Full bladders hurt and are good to use as examples (see chapter 18).

'Guys, hey guys, GUYS! GUUUUUYYYYS! I'm desperate for a pee...' The bladder monitoring or Peepot Numskull is getting a bit fractious. Brainy now pips in with harsh whispered tones ... 'Listen Peepot get back in your poxy little room and belt up, he's just about to give a lecture to the biggest audience he's ever stood in front of...' Hey presto, the feeling disappears as Peepot mopes back to his room, re-tightens the flow 'off' taps and takes a bit of an edgy nap. Brainy applies a double precaution not trusting Peepot and turns down the 'need to pee' sensation dimmer-switch.

The lectures now over, the questions have been answered and now... 'HEY Brainy, what about me...!' At last, all the other stuff is done, the pressures off and Brainy starts hearing Peepot yelling away. Brainy softens, lets the 'need to pee' feeling back on again and he makes an excuse to find a urinal.

Pat Wall (1999) argued that pain (like badly wanting a pee!) can be viewed as a 'need' state – it makes you need to do something to get rid of the pain to find relief. Pain drives the relief seeking behaviour. Delve into it a little and there are perhaps two or three basic kinds of behaviour for intense discomfort or pain. Think about twisting an ankle; the first is doing something to try and help the pain yourself i.e. limp, rub, rest, move, stretch, even distract (yell, moan, sing, giggle, twitter on, tense and clench, hold your breath, cross your legs!) – anything – it can be very personal! The second; is to try and get someone else to help you; hence you might look fed up and a pit pathetic and you might cry, limp, moan and groan or simply ask! Lastly, you can in most cultures, actively seek help from a healer of reputation – visit the local witch doctor or healer, your local Dr, physio or chiro-practor... or lastly, simply go and find a safe place and rest up...

3. There must also be strong modules associated with sensing, assessing and dealing with attack and potential attack. There is really no such thing as an organism that has no enemies – even the beautiful and enormous Whale shark that for 60 million years has serenely gone about its mysterious and undisturbed business without any obvious macro-predator. It surely has as fantastic a population of potentially threatening micro-organisms as any other creature. Attackers can therefore be tiny, invisible and microscopic or smaller. Think of bacteria and viruses that want to use you for a feed or as a place of charm to settle down, dwell in, grow a bit and maybe reproduce for a little while. Then there are larger but hidden and not that obvious attackers, like gut parasites, who may also find your insides a somewhat agreeable and safe place to take up residence; and lastly, the bigger and very obvious ones we all have a much better handle on – like Great White sharks, aggressive buffalos and other folks from your own species – thugs, basically. Note that for the little guys, those little attackers we can't see – there isn't so much 'feeling' associated with them as there is for the presence of a Great White shark! Big attackers create fear, – which very much drive our escape behaviour. Fear circuits and pain circuits are closely linked. I hope you're now thinking about feelings associated with the 'little guys' – things like disgust – when you see food that looks or smells off for example. It's all very smartly worked out!

4. There must also be a module that deals with the need for safety and finding safety. For one thing if most prey animals weren't good at hiding up somehow they'd soon end up extinct. Isn't it a good feeling you get when you're safe and tucked up? I've now got this picture of a flock of sheep in my head with thoughts of 'safety in numbers'. It must be such a good feeling to be nicely trotting along right in the middle of the flock, but not quite so good on the outside and really not good at all to be separated, especially with that fox around somewhere...

There are two ways of looking at this nice-nasty feeling stuff and it's a kind of all-round principle of need states that's being illustrated. First, be a sheep in the middle and you feel a nice feeling of relief and pleasure about being pretty safe, but be more on the outside or even separate from the flock and you're desperately wanting to get that feeling of comfort and pleasure that you get when you're in the middle. Second, and a kind of opposite, is to be on the outside and feel super-stressed (anxious and fearful are probably the best descriptors) and want to get rid of these horrid feelings by getting back into the inside of the flock? The principle then is that there are probably always two needs that drive any behaviour – the need to get rid of the noxious one and the need to get a pleasant one back. Do something that's likely to help get homeostasis back on song and you get a pleasurable feeling or, do something that is likely to upset homeostasis and the feeling is noxious or unpleasant. The more effective the stimulus is in restoring homeostasis or reducing threat the stronger the feeling of pleasantness... and the more effective a stimulus is in disrupting homeostasis the more unpleasant the feeling is ... and this is usually pain. Feelings drive or motivate behaviour and pain and comfort are big ones! So into my head pops the common childhood memory of getting chucked into the sea by my mischievous friends, in you go... cold agony... out you come... warmed up and clothes on... ecstasy! And that great feeling of relief you get when you empty a painfully full bladder!

There are a great many other SSR modules that could be considered, for now, I'd like to highlight one more – the important module that's responsible for remembering things and is such an important part of the Mature Organism Model.

Chapter 10.3
The Mature Organism
Model 3: From origins on

It was around 1997 I think. I was on a plane to Denmark from London with Dave Butler to do a five day 'Dynamic Nervous System' course. I can't remember the name of the place we were to be teaching at but it wasn't very far from the famous 'Lego' factory! We landed at Billund airport, that, I can recall. I think Dave was in some big comfy seat down the front of the plane, so I was back on my own in 'steerage'! I've always found that I come up with ideas for teaching and explaining when I'm travelling. I was pondering some new thoughts about getting Danish die-hard manual physiotherapists to understand the bigger pain picture – and I drew a scrappy little diagram. Within ten minutes I had four sketches and I'd called the whole thing the, 'Mature Organism Model' or 'MOM'. I realise that it's a weird name for it but I'll now take you through the diagrams and you'll see why.

The first figure (10.1) is titled 'Staying alive – Homeostasis' as it represents most of what I've been discussing so far – that the human central nervous system (or any other animals' nervous system) is constantly sampling its environment, sampling its tissues and sending the information to the central nervous system and brain. The brain then scrutinises the information coming in and responds as necessary – hence the arrows out of the brain to the word 'output'. Outputs can produce a visible or invisible effect, hence the 'altered behaviour' and 'altered physiology' phrases beneath. The changes brought about are then re-sampled to see if they were any good, and the sampling followed by scrutinising and responding process goes on endlessly. Clearly the environmental sampling is massively curtailed when we are

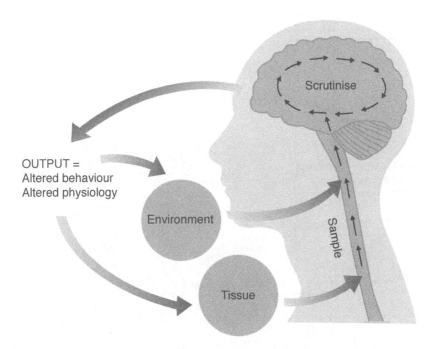

Figure 10.1 'Staying Alive – Homeostasis' Redrawn from: Gifford L S 1998 Pain, the tissues and the nervous system: A conceptual model. Physiotherapy 84(1): 27-36

asleep. The key is the pretty obvious big circle to it all. I think at the time this model was a big reaction to the way pain was being taught – always as a straight line – starting in the periphery and ending in the brain with a bit of deference to 'modulation' and 'pain-gate' on the way. This linear model ends somewhat pathetically, in my opinion, in forebrain cortical sensory processing areas. It's as if we're all waiting for pain researchers to list the structures that do 'pain processing' and make it all conscious and that will be that. Pat Wall had it right when he mooted that it was what the brain might need to do about what it was receiving and what was happening that was important. I agree, but it's also good to know the state of the art regarding where (if there truly is a 'where') the brain processes various sensory modalities that go on to produce sensations – like pain! More later …

The second figure (10.2) shows an injury – hence the 'blast' effect drawn into the 'environment' and 'tissue' areas! Trip over, twist your ankle and fall over; inputs flood into the CNS and brain from the eyes; from the kinaesthetic and proprioceptive sense; from the mechanosensory and damage sensing nociceptive system; from the skin where we contact the ground and the ankle joint as it's twisted and sprained. Stuff coming in from the body is often referred to as of 'somatic' origin. Soma means everything in the 'body' except the reproductive tissues. Another term for the systems involved in this 'soma-sampling' is 'interoception,' which I mentioned earlier and I rather like. 'Interoception' – the body's internal sniffing and sampling system!

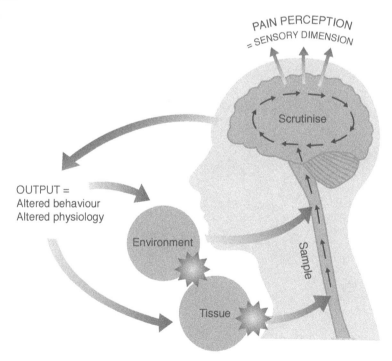

Figure 10.2 'Pain Perception' – The Sensory dimension. Redrawn from: Gifford L S 1998 Pain, the tissues and the nervous system: A conceptual model. Physiotherapy 84(1): 27-36

Figure 10.2 also shows the brain scrutinising the incoming information and producing pain in the 'sensory dimension'. The sensory dimension of pain is the easy one. It gives information firstly about the location of the pain, secondly the type and quality of it, for example it could be very sharp pain or it could be a deep aching quality, thirdly it gives a notion about *intensity,* and finally information about pain's *behaviour over time.* This 'sensory' dimension of pain is where most traditional medics, clinicians and physical and manual therapists feel comfortable and where we'd all like pain to remain and be simple and straight forward and consistent! Just like symptoms for a car mechanic! They have a location to home in on; the worse the symptoms, the worse the problem, the quality of the symptoms convey further information about what's going on and the symptoms are always consistent in quality and over time (yes, unless the car's got a damn electrical fault!). The symptoms pretty exactly reflect what's wrong – the worse the problem, the worse the symptoms in a nice linear-relational way. We could call it 'uni-dimensionalism', or 'mechanical' thinking or how about 'medical' thinking! Sadly for all those who are still locked into mechanical thinking, most manual therapists for example, if you're going to understand pain, you can't cut out the brain and the individual who experiences the pain and what they make of it and, how they respond to it. It's nice and complex! Multi-dimensionalism rules OK! And down with Rene Descartes who separated the material 'machine' of the body from the immaterial 'spirituality' of the mind all those centuries ago. Leaving the medical profession thinking along the lines of 'If we can't find anything to explain your disorder in the body machine... It must be in the mind. Therefore, in our opinion, your symptoms are a confabulation – you're a fraud.' Descartes legacy is often referred to as Dualism i.e. 'If it's not this, it's that. I have always hoped that the MOM would help explain the process and stop this terrible uni-dimensional type of thinking in its tracks!

To Figure 10.3. This figure clarifies why I called it the MOM and it brings in 'the brain' quite seamlessly I think! As you can see this figure shows the brain 'sampling' *itself* for information that may be relevant to organising the output. In order to fully scrutinise the incoming information the 'brain' (well, the human whose brain it is!) sometimes has the opportunity to have a little ponder about it all (psychologists like to call pondering or thinking, cognition). Remember how we said that because the amoeba hasn't got many choices it's unlikely to do any real pondering! To my way of thinking the ability to ponder or deliberate had to have evolved when more and more behavioural options became available to organisms. So maybe the amoeba does have choices and does ponder a little! This way of thinking about thinking could drag the possibility of animal cognition and consciousness back to far more evolutionary 'lowly' animals than we're used to. Just a thought.

If you fall over and hurt yourself, how you respond in terms of behaviour, and how you respond in terms of physiological response, depends very much on what the situation is and the meaning you give to the situation. How you react may be vastly influenced by the brain sampling itself and hence what the brain's got in it! For example: all the responses, all the little quirks of habit that are in your head that you picked up and learnt from your parents, friends and teachers as you grew up and matured, you could call it the influence of your little micro-culture; all the various beliefs and the bits of knowledge you have... it includes all your past experiences,

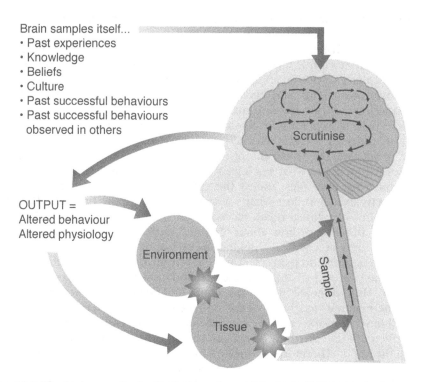

Brain samples itself...
• Past experiences
• Knowledge
• Beliefs
• Culture
• Past successful behaviours
• Past successful behaviours
  observed in others

Scrutinise

OUTPUT =
Altered behaviour
Altered physiology

Environment

Sample

Tissue

Figure 10.3 'The brain samples itself' Redrawn from: Gifford L S 1998 Pain, the tissues and the nervous system: A conceptual model. Physiotherapy 84(1): 27-36

what you did in different situations, your past behaviours if you like; and there's all those things you've witnessed others do, or seen, heard or read about via the media... they can all be sampled before you respond in your own unique little way... Your past experience, wired into your system, predicts how you respond given a new experience...

Here are some different situations... and different responses... that might occur for much the same thing – falling over.

You fall over in the garden... fine, you can take in the situation, take your time, you can feel the pain and when you feel OK'ish, you can you try to get up... no big deal.

Or this... you fall over on the uneven pavement in the street... you feel a real twit and quickly get up and pretend everything is fine... and wander off down the street trying not to limp hoping no one's caught you being so foolish.

Or this... same thing, you fall over on an uneven pavement in the street... you cuss the council and vow to sue them for being so remiss in leaving one of the pavers slightly raised up. Your pain quickly comes on and becomes a major crisis and you make a big scene that goes, 'Christ, oh no, it's broken, I know it is, that's it, I'll never walk properly again, my ankle's going to look all fat and ghastly and I'll always have to wear long trousers, I'll never be able to put on a bathing costume or go on a summer holiday... oh my god, please someone help me, I need an ambulance now... can someone call an ambulance... NOW, GODDAMIT!'

Or this... you trip over and twist an ankle in the middle of a very busy main road, you immediately get up and run to the nearest pavement to avoid being run over... or... you're being chased by a gang of thugs and you fall over – twisted ankle and all, you're up in a flash and running as well as you were before.

Brain sampling adds a bit of colour to the situation! Different brains provide different reactions too.

Our brains are full of information that is just waiting to be sampled given the right circumstances. Life experience, as we saw in the memory chapter is brilliantly welded into the brains' circuitry and somehow from there into our very being, it helps to mould us and make us who we are. It seems that our brains are particularly well programmed to pick up and remember anything that we might find useful for our own survival – for example, our rather macabre interest in other peoples' disasters and misfortunes! It seems smart to learn from others mistakes, to pick up a few tips as to how things should not be done – and so to try and avoid the same trap that they fell into! Don't we just love disasters! Witness the popularity of the ghastly goings on, deeds and deceptions in the 'soaps' on TV, or our penchant for 'disaster' movies. But I like the accident on the motor-way example. You've all done this surely! You're driving along and all the traffic slows down, there's even a bit of a queue forming and you're wondering what's going on ahead. Then you see a police car's flashing light and there's a notice at the side of the road. Accident! You look ahead and it's all on the hard shoulder, all three carriageways are clear and you're thinking, 'Why do people have to slow down and gawp at the accident, they're just rubber-necks and it causes huge tail-backs... I'm going to sail on by and not take a look'. Oh yeah! Five minutes later and you're coming up alongside the crash looking tensely straight ahead... then hey, your rubber-neck swings round to the side of the road and takes it all in... you just couldn't resist it! Don't feel bad, in evolutionary terms, rubber-necking, or 'morbid curiosity' as it's sometimes called, is the right thing to do, it's all part of learning what not to do if at all possible.

I'm not too sure I'd want to go out and witness a hanging or execution mind you, but people did and they probably still do in some places. Witnessing something nasty, rather than being told about it, makes it an even more powerful memory, and even more aversive. Culturally we're not into public viewing of torture or hanging, but I think you'd agree that if the laws of the land said that we had to witness at least one thief execution a year it would be a far more effective deterrent than just hearing that the fellow had been hanged? Don't get me wrong, I'm not a ultra right-wing, totalitarian fascist at all. I'm a very forgiving person[1] and I'm pleased that I haven't been raised in the culture or times when this sort of stuff occurred, but I do see how these things work. Public humiliation, public ridicule... loss of respect... you don't want to go there, you've seen how horrid it is... so behave yourself (up to a point!).

Sampling our own brain to see what it's got in its memory module libraries in respect of getting the best result out of the current situation – for example, our fall and ankle

---

1 - ... and member of the British Humanist Association

injury – has several twists (pun not intended!) that make you realise how adaptable we can be, and, how important memory of our past experiences can be too:

As just discussed, it may be about what we've observed and learnt from others situations and behaviours – the bad and the good. From an injury perspective, in this modern age we observe all sorts of behaviours – that run from the brave (rugby players and boxers), to the melodramatic and the pathetic (like footballers, celebs) and beyond. I'm quite sure that most of us have used just about all of these tactics at one time or another, they all have their uses! It's good self-help-therapy to have a think about where you'd place yourself... and then think why you're like that!

Next, there are our own experiences, and the older we get the more times we are likely to have had quite a few near-misses in life? Here are a few of mine, now sixty years on and done a bit! Aged 17 driving my Triumph Tiger 90 motorcycle (350cc) at about 40mph round a blind bend on a very narrow Cornish country road at night. It's not quite what I was expecting, but the headlights suddenly illuminated a cow full-on right across the road! Holy shit! I jammed on the breaks, the back wheel slid out and I careered towards the back end of the beast sideways and expecting impact. At the very moment I thought I was going to end up smashed into the side of the cow it turned towards me and moved its back end away from the hedge so creating a gap! Through I went and unscathed passed the cow by! My heart is beating quite hard now as I recall it all again.

Motor scooter this time, about a year later, travelling home from college on the main Redruth to Falmouth road here in Cornwall. There's a long blind corner downhill with high hedges and there's a long line of traffic coming up the hill following a very slow tractor. As I start to be able to see further round the bend I see this stupid car completely stopped and some guy's getting out of the car, Holy shit again, just like with the cow there's no escape route – I can't go on the inside of the car as there's a hedge and a door open, I can't go round the outside as there's a bus narrowing the gap to a couple of feet! I'm jamming on the brakes and the little scooter hasn't enough weight to stop it skidding. In amazing slow motion my brain goes... 'Louis, you're going to hit the back of the car, if you try to stay on the bike you'll just smack right into it or go under the bumper... all you can do is jump as you hit and you'll slide along the roof of the car...' I then hit and I jump... up over the car, sailing through the air like Gollum and the Ring disappearing down, slo-mo into the volcanic fires of Mount Doom at the end of Lord of the Rings... but then bang! Right on my head on the cars bonnet and I flip in a forward roll to briefly land on my feet in front of the car... I could have shown off and put my arms up in some splendid conclusion to a fantastic pommel-horse vault and taken the applause from the travellers in the bus, but I fluffed it a bit and stumbled forward onto my knees. As if! I looked at the ground in total disbelief at my good fortune. From a blast of incredible stress (what I imagine bungee-jumpers get?) to the feeling of incredible relief. I stood up feeling almost stoned with elation... 'Yeah, wow, hey, wow... yeah... I'm like still alive, cool...' So why didn't I go smack-splat straight into the back of that car? Simple, my brain has a memory – for everything. That means it has a motor memory, it knows exactly what I'm capable of doing and because I spent a great deal of my younger life playing in the garden, climbing trees and making tree houses and precarious rope walkways between them – I knew I was agile and that was stored in my brain. Later at secondary school I reached quite a high proficiency in gymnastics and I was particularly good at vaulting. So I was agile, I had good timing, I also had driven quite a number of motor-bikes and knew how they handled – so my brain quickly worked out that with the bike I was on and the various other escape routes options available that the hit and jump option was the best bet. So, my brain knew that I was light and agile! Imagine if I was huge, what option then – the jumping for it option might never have even entered the equation!

In reflection, I am very grateful that I had 'real-time' experience here, of motorbikes, of agility, of 'knowing' my own physical capabilities. I fear that the modern 'child' lives, via the dreaded screen, through what amounts to virtual experience. Observed rough and tumble rather than the real thing and I don't think it would have worked very well given that over-the-car-somersault I contrived and survived.

I hope by now the picture is pretty clear – that our brains are sampling the situations we are in all the time and assessing and working out the best strategies to go forward with, given the information that's available. Think now of a baby human – you at four months old say. Your experiences in life are very limited; your developing brain has little knowledge more than of its mother, father and immediate surroundings. A young baby is therefore a **'Naive Organism'**, an organism in the waiting room of learning and knowledge. Before brain development and neuroplasticity was understood many considered the infant brain to be a 'tabula rasa' or 'blank-slate' ready to have its life experience written onto it. It's an easy way to think about it but the reality is that life experience not only gets written onto it, it is also in part responsible for its development too (see Rose 2005).

At this young age the infant is highly dependent on its parents and would soon die without their ability to nourish and protect, but, as time goes on the youngster learns and it is the same for all of us. We slowly imbue our brains with knowledge; about the things and individuals around us, about how they live and behave, what they do, what culture they live in, how they respond to difficulties... and for the most part we take this on and fit in. We know right from wrong in our society, we know what we should and shouldn't do and we begin to know how to look after ourselves without our parents help – we become a **'Mature Organism'**. The Mature Organism is independent and its brain is full of information that can be accessed to help make decisions about any given situation – good, bad or indifferent... 'Is it good? Is it bad?

The very young 'Naive Organism' on the other hand, relies on others to have the knowledge. Left to its own devices the very young naive organism has to rely on primitive reflexes and its very unique and forceful pleading behaviour. Thankfully evolution has endowed us with a 'pleading' related module that makes us respond very powerfully when a baby cries, especially when it is our own.

Before moving on I feel that here is a good place to bring up the issue of what I call the 'raising environment' – by which I mean the environment the child learns from – usually its parents, brothers and sisters, other family and friends and neighbours. I touched on this a little in a previous chapter 8.3. Children learn and mimic adults, as every parent knows when their beautiful little three year old swears in public and says something like, 'Jamie is a tosser Mummy.' Ouch, embarrassing! They also learn and mimic how those around them behave in relation to everyday cuts and bruises, to the experience of aches and pains and mimic the behaviour they see. Have you ever had the guts to ask your patient how their parents responded to pain when they were young? It's not easy but if you turn it round a bit you might ask whether their parents suffered with pain problems and how they responded to their situation. From the perspective of a psychologist we would be delving into 'learnt behaviour' – in part, we learn how to respond to pain, how to behave when we're in pain from others, and in our early years it's primarily from those who bring us up. From a more medical perspective, asking about the family's pain would more likely be enquiring about hereditary! But we also mustn't forget that there's now plenty of evidence for genetic influences on nociception and pain. Nothing is easy!

Well, we're still on figure 10.3! But the whole point of the discussion is to show you how scrutinising, which includes information from the brain's various 'library sections,' adds a bit of colour and context to the situation – a thing that youngsters aren't quite so good at – have you noticed? The colour and context comes from some of the things listed in figure 10.3, most of which I've already discussed – past experiences, knowledge, beliefs, culture, past successful behaviours, past successful behaviours observed in others and so forth. Remember not to just think of memory as just 'facts' there're also beliefs and past experiences and many of these are attached to quite significant emotions.

What this mix of input from the top-down and the bottom-up does in an injury situation is to add the two other 'pain-dimensions' into the mix. The 'cognitive dimension' is basically about what our thinking makes of the pain and injury situation – for example, what we believe to be wrong, how serious we think it is, what our plans are going to be to deal with it, and whether we think it is bad or good and the influence of past experiences. These rather prosaic thoughts hugely influence how we 'feel' about the situation we are in relative to the injury and pain – hence the 'affective dimension' of pain. 'Affect' is about feelings, emotions and our mood state. For example, as a result of pain xyz do we feel fear? Anxiety? Anger even? Stress perhaps? Tension? Low mood? Pleasure! A good general word for most patients is 'Concern.'

In figure 10.4 we can see that the colour and context imbibed and absorbed into the primitive ascending nociceptive alarm signals by the brain and its cognitive and affective dimensions give 'value' to the situation. And that the 'value' given drives the subsequent behaviour. At its simplest this translates to a continuum that runs from one end... 'I know my situation is going to ruin the rest of my life, I feel so angry, so frightened and so anxious that I cannot think... Oh God, I'm going to die...' type thing. To somewhere in the middle... 'I think my situation is bad, I feel anxious about it and I must do something, maybe I should get some help.' Or the other end... 'This situation is not a problem, I feel quite in control, I can deal with it.' Or perhaps... 'Wow, that hurt so bad but I'm feeling totally elated with that experience.'

The 'is it good' to 'is it bad' 'value' continuum is key to turning on and driving the degree of stress response – hence changes in behaviour and changes in physiology that are driven by the relative value attached to the situation. Affect, feelings and emotions drive and motivate our behaviour – hence the affective dimension of pain is sometimes called the **Motivational-Affective dimension** to emphasise this.

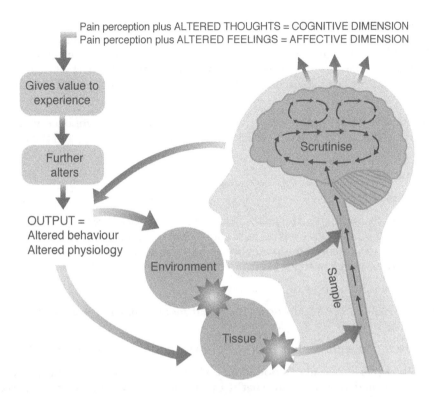

Pain perception plus ALTERED THOUGHTS = COGNITIVE DIMENSION
Pain perception plus ALTERED FEELINGS = AFFECTIVE DIMENSION

Gives value to experience

Further alters

OUTPUT =
Altered behaviour
Altered physiology

Scrutinise

Environment

Sample

Tissue

Figure 10.4 The 'Cognitive' and 'Affective' dimensions of pain and giving 'value' to the pain experience. Redrawn from: Gifford L S 1998 Pain, the tissues and the nervous system: A conceptual model. Physiotherapy 84(1): 27-36

Think about how powerful worrying is in motivating you to sort the thing out that is concerning you.

Clinicians – have you ever done this...?

Patient example – or, an example of the detrimental and powerful effects of worrying!

Friday afternoon, next to last patient at St Stephen's Hospital, London, circa 1982 (I'm barely over a year qualified). This fellow's about 45 years old and has a stubborn on-going sciatica that I've tried everything with, cue, traction! He's prepared to try anything and I'm running a bit late. Quick as a flash he's on his back, harnesses around the pelvis and rib cage and the cranky old machine is winding up to and 25 kg pull, holding for 30 seconds then letting off for 5. After a couple of pulls the pelvic harness has stopped pulling his pants down and he's nicely bound up and feeling the pull. There's no timer on the machine but there's a separate kitchen type timer which I set to 20 minutes. I put the emergency buzzer button in his hand and tell him to press it when the timer goes and I'll come back in and let him off. He nods that he'll be in again on Monday evening. Fine, I finish off with, 'Buzz if you want anything or want it to stop yeah?' He nods and smiles. Great, I whip into the waiting room for my last patient and off I go with her, back on time again, good ploy that...

It's now ten to six Friday night, I'm sitting at home with a Friday night beer watching 'Boys from the Blackstuff' (Alan Bleasdale play on the telly back then) and the phone rings.

'Is that Louis?'

'Yup, who's this?'

'Cleaner love, St Stephen's Hospital. Look there's a bloke here says he's called Barry, we found him asleep on your rack contraption in cubicle 1. My mate Shirley managed to switch it off and undo him but he's struggling to get up. He told us your name so we rang switch and got your number, thought it wise to let you know.'

'Yes, er thanks, is he up now do you know?'

'Hang on... SHIRL'...' she shouts down the department – cubicle 1 is a separate little room used for traction.

'SHIRL', what's happenin' with Barry love?' I can hear her easily through the phone...

There's a long pause. My heart's pounding and I'm feeling shit. My boss Peter Wells is going to be mad with me and what if I've made Barry worse. Christ! Career in manual therapy gone... hauled up for medical misdemeanours... the nightmare module sampling of my own brain... the feeling shit module runs away with itself...

'Louis, you still there love? He's gone, hang on, yeah, Shirl' says he's gone, says he looked crooked and didn't say much. Don't think there's much you can do now really, OK love?'

'Yeah, fine, thanks for phoning, I'll catch you Monday evening if I can...'

What followed that was one of the worst weekends I can ever remember. I was so wound up about Barry – he must have been on the traction for two hours or more. I was used to giving patients a maximum of twenty minutes! I was thinking of all the worst scenarios and wondering what sort of agonies he was going through.

Worry! Un-resolvable worry, the problem took a hold of my brain such that I wasn't able to do anything productive at all. I couldn't even sleep. All I could do was go over and over in my brain what I was going to do. Yep, on Monday morning, get his phone number, and give him a ring and find out... on the other hand that might be asking for trouble, what if he's really angry, what'll I do then? Maybe I'd best wait until he shows up on Monday evening and go through it all with him then? Maybe he won't show up? Maybe he'll start proceedings against me? This isn't looking good for my career either.

Worry and stress like this does your head in until you get it sorted and you're desperate to get it sorted, because the feeling is so awful. I knew I had to get it sorted on Monday. The other option was to run away forever.

Monday came. I could hardly concentrate all day. I was hopeless with the other patients, I smoked about four cigarettes in the toilets, I avoided everyone. I even went to the pub at lunch.

Four o'clock and I'm sighing and holding my breath, out I go into the waiting room, phew, Barry's there, sitting looking out the window, looks quite relaxed.

'Barry, come on through...'

I turn and walk into the traction cubicle and he follows. I turn.

'Hey, sorry about forgetting to take you off the traction on Friday night Barry.'

'Don't worry Louis, it was my fault, I was so comfortable I fell asleep, the most comfortable I've been for weeks in fact. I've been looking forward to coming today for some more!'

He smiled, I was overwhelmed with relief, then I mischievously thought to myself, 'You bugger, you had a weekend actually looking forward to something I thought had made you worse and that you were going to sue me for – and I spent it feeling rubbish.'

The interesting thing about all this was that Barry's pain got a lot better but his basic objective testing signs didn't change one jot. He still had a limited SLR, he couldn't bend past his knee caps without bending his knees and if he bent backwards he got pins and needles in his toes. We carried on with the long sessions of traction... me staying until 6.00pm chatting up the cleaners while he slept for a couple of hours on the traction bed and then struggled to get off it and going out badly shifted... it was the least I could do!

Last bit...

The MOM, in a biological way, is all about bringing the conscious brain firmly and centrally into our understanding of pain. I hope you can see that all the various scenarios outlined are commonplace and I hope you can see why similar physical problems can have such vastly different time-lines and outcomes. In recent years the 'yellow flag' psychosocial factor movement has hugely helped in bringing the importance of the cognitive, affective and behavioural dimensions of pain into the mainstream management of musculoskeletal pain problems.

So, how we think and feel may help or hinder us, how about this... 'Ah, last time I fell and twisted my ankle in the street like this I managed to get three weeks off work and sued the council for £1000... I'll get onto that 'no-win no-fee' company again when I get home.' Help or hinder? This one makes me smile because our instant reaction to this sort of thing is to balk at it and feel a bit peeved, disgusted even – of course it's unhelpful, it's money-grabbing and it is sick! Biologically though it's working on one of the most basic and essential rules of nature, which is, **'Get as much as you can for as little effort as possible'**. I always use the seagull example, which runs –

clever seagull gets up early and makes his way to the area of town whose turn it is for 'bin' day and finds an easy meal from the rubbish bags and bins left out overnight. In fact the gulls round here don't even bother going to bed, they're on permanent night-shift because everyone puts their bins out the night before. So they're at it all night ripping the rubbish bags apart and scattering left-overs and muck all over the street which no-one bothers to clear up or work out how to stop. Talks of seagull culls are commonplace on the waterfront!

Why bother spending hours and hours flying out to sea looking for the odd fish that might crop up. Successful seagull equals the rubbish bag adapted one who expends far less energy getting a gourmet meal than the one who goes to sea. Why are we so surprised by some peoples/seagulls 'grabbing' behaviour? Put it in a biological/ evolutionary context – I might call it the 'Seagull Syndrome' and hey, it's wise action! The 'laziness rule'.

Unfortunately most options in life and biology that proffer some advantage also have some cost attached (see chapter GE 2.2). For example, the 'no-win no-fee' character above may get socially ostracised and criticised for being money-grabbing... hence a social 'cost' – although as this type of behaviour becomes more and more common it seems to be becoming more acceptable. The avoidance behaviour adopted – not going to work, not moving much in order to authenticate the injury and pain – can have longer term costs for tissue health and recovery as well as return to gainful employ and so forth. Costs are almost always there.

Success in life is measured in many different ways, but biologically it's all about staying fit and healthy, making sure you pass your genes on to the next generation and looking after them to make sure they do to! Cruel unfair world! But this is the great legacy we have to come to terms with I feel. If we understand WHY we have the 'uglier' sides of our nature we can work hard to overcome them and live better more humanistic lives[1] (Watson's 1995 book, 'Dark Nature' is of interest).

Here's a couple more 'options' for our twisted ankle that we come across...

'Last time I did this it was sore for a couple of days and within a week or two I was running again, I'll just see how it goes'...

Or, 'Damn, If past experience is anything to go by I better not move this, in fact I better stay put until I get help, I could make it so much worse like I did last time. The surgeon told me I shouldn't have tried to walk on it and that was why it took nearly a year to get better. I think I'll get onto my orthopaedic surgeon and then phone work to say I won't be in for a while...'

What's in our patients' brains and the strategies they adopt can drive a sane physiotherapist nuts! Unfortunately in this modern age we live in there is so much information; so many different opinions, so many different therapy models and strategies for pain, and dare I say it – so much bullshit – so much so that it is getting very hard to peddle good, rational, evidence-based recovery strategies. Yes, human brains nowadays are on information overload, and mostly they're all full of pseudo-scientific

1 - **humanistic** - *of or pertaining to a philosophy asserting human dignity and man's capacity for fulfillment through reason and scientific method and often rejecting religion.*

garbage when it comes to health. Amazingly, we still all muddle along well enough to perform our biological obligations. Maybe I should calm down...

A couple of clinical messages from all this...

As discussed in the placebo chapters earlier, the nervous system has to be shifted into a good 'preparatory' or 'acceptance' state before any therapy or rehabilitation begins. It's 'top-down' before 'bottom-up'! Examples of how I 'prepare' the patient in front of me's brain for recovery are scattered throughout this book.

Don't be seduced by the notion that acute onset pain is a wholly tissue based phenomenon – manual therapists in particular seem to love to make things 'just tissue' or 'mechanical' in nature. Biology doesn't however – for every pain we have there's a 'sample-scrutinise-response' reaction at all biological levels – this means that there are instantly central mechanisms, emotional and cognitive reactions, trawls through memory banks, and a plethora of output responses too. What I am saying again is that for every patient who comes in, including all acute pains – don't just consider the problem from a one dimensional tissue based perspective! For every pain you assess don't forget, there's a brain attached to it and you can talk to it via its owner!

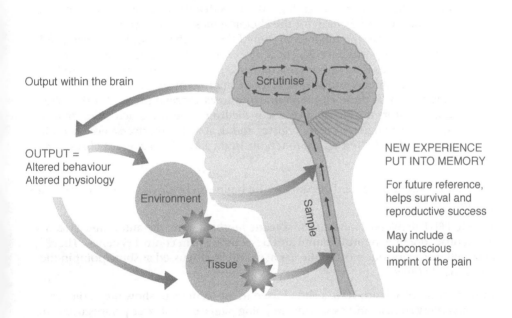

Figure 10.5 The new experience put into memory – the possibility of a 'pain memory' Redrawn from: Gifford L S 1998 Pain, the tissues and the nervous system: A conceptual model. Physiotherapy 84(1): 27-36

The next figure (10.5) is all about putting the new experience into memory. I've already discussed this at length in the memory chapter and given plenty of examples. One thought here is to note that all our most vivid memories are accompanied by strong emotions. So, if you want to remember a pain it's best if it's accompanied by high levels of worry, concern, anger or any other form of 'distress.' Your thinking and reasoning can be one of the causes of these high levels of distress but you may also find that clinicians, practitioners, lawyers/solicitors and your friends and family add a good deal to the mix too!

I want to finish this 'circuits' chapter with some of the components that figure in these INPUT – SCRUTINISE – OUTPUT or SAMPLE – SCRUTINISE – RESPOND processes.

'Interoceptive' input/Sampling mechanisms are all about telling the brain what is going on in the body:

> Using fast 'electrical' pathways, in other words via the sensory nervous system – classically it's 'nociception' but there's more to it than that as I'll discuss in the chapters that follow.

> Using slower circulatory systems, sometimes termed 'humoral' communication, which simply means via 'fluid'. Damaged or diseased tissues and immune cells in these tissues release chemical messengers into the blood stream whose distant targets are further 'blood-sampling' sites in the brain! Examples of chemical messengers that do this are the cytokines/interleukins and prostaglandins. It seems that the brain has blood 'sniffing' sites that constantly monitor the chemical messengers it contains. Where? Known sites are the tuber cinereum of the hypothalamus, the pineal gland and the area postrema adjacent to the caudal 4th Ventricle. Note that the hypothalamus is an important brain area involved with scrutinising and reacting to threats and stressors, as are brain stem areas. So, it's hardly surprising that these blood monitoring areas are right there! Another site that monitors the blood of course is the liver – the great 'detoxifier' that is so well groomed to screen, register and deal with any adverse goings-on in the blood and, then squeal to tell the brain about it via afferent fibres in the vagus nerve.

The SCRUTINISE centres and circuitry in the brain will be discussed in later sections (16-18).

The OUTPUT networks embrace the somatic motor system; the autonomic systems; the neuroendocrine, neuroimmune and descending pain control systems. There may well be others, but most of the list here will be discussed at some point in the following chapters.

Lastly here there's figure 10.6, a slide I used in my lectures to show the audience how complicated pain and especially on-going pain can be if your perspective is to remain wedded to a 'find-what's-wrong-and-where-it's-wrong and then treat it type of approach. The (S?) circles on the figure represent where you might start looking with pain – yes, the tissues, the sensory fibres, the CNS, the processing—brain modules, memory mechanisms, output systems and mechanisms—and so forth. In frustration, like a few patients would like to have done, you might cut the limb off where the pain is located. Unfortunately the chances of phantom limb pain are very high. Ah, cut the head off then? Exactly, you're starting to now see that the brain has to be included.

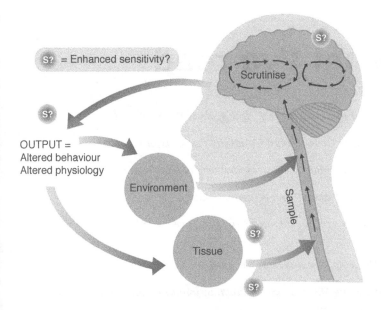

Figure 10.6 Over time, the 'source' of pain and sensitivity becomes widespread and therefore virtually impossible to apply biomedical reasoning to or a biomedical 'targeted' approach to.

Finally here...

'To me the idea of a continuous sensory, input, scrutinise, output, sense again, input again, scrutinise again, output again and so forth type system in some way defines a stress or threat related system. It's an on-going loop of information that is more or less constantly checking what's happening. I think that if you really look you see that these on-going information loops are the very essence of life and staying alive. Sex circuits are 'the other' story, and that's all about keeping your own genes going down the generations – or drifting along on 'The River out of Eden' as Dawkins so superbly puts it.'

Section 10
Read what I've read

Coyne J.A. (2010) Why Evolution is True. Oxford University Press. Oxford.

Dawkins R. (1976) The Selfish Gene. Oxford University Press. Oxford.

Dawkins R. (2001) River Out Of Eden: A Darwinian View of Life. Phoenix. London.

Dawkins R. (2006) The Blind Watchmaker. Penguin. London.

Dawkins R. (2009) The Greatest Show on Earth: The Evidence for Evolution. Black Swan. London.

Kahneman D. (2011) Thinking, fast and slow. Penguin Books. London.

Martin P. (1997) The Sickening Mind. Brain, behaviour, immunity and disease. Harper Collins. London.

Mithen S. (1996) The Prehistory Of The Mind. A search for the origins of art, religion and science. Thames and Hudson. London.

Rose S. (2005) Lifelines: Life beyond the gene. Vintage. London.

Sobel D. (2010) Galileo's Daughter: A Drama of Science, Faith and Love. Fourth Estate. London.

Sapolsky R. (1997) Junk Food Monkeys and Other Essays on the Biology of the Human Predicament. Headline Book Publishing. London.

Selye, H. (1978) The Stress of Life. McGraw Hill. New York.

Selye H. (1993) History of the stress concept. In Goldberger L. and Breznitz S.(Eds.) Handbook of stress: Theoretical and clinical aspects 2nd Ed. The Free Press. New York.

Sternberg E.M. (2001) The Balance Within: The Science Connecting Health and Emotions. Palgrave. New York.

Sternberg E.M. (2009) Healing Spaces: The Science of Place and Well-Being. Harvard University Press. Cambridge.

Wall P.D. (1999) Introduction to the fourth Edition. In: Wall P.D., Melzack R. (Eds) Textbook of Pain 4th Ed. Churchill Livingstone. London. (This chapter was also reproduced in Topical Issues in Pain 4).

Watson, L. (1995). Dark Nature. A Natural History of Evil. Hodder and Stoughton. London.

Wright R. (1996) The Moral Animal, Why We Are the Way We Are. Abacus. London.

Section 11

NOCICEPTIVE MECHANISMS

Chapter 11.1
Nociceptive mechanisms 1: Fibres and impulses....

I'm going to go into a few aspects of mechanisms associated with physical injury and I want to try and keep the bigger MOM picture in mind. I also want to try and keep it easy. Remember the mantra here is, 'sample-scrutinise-respond' or sample/input – scrutinise – respond/output.

If you have a tissue injury, say you cut yourself, quite a lot happens. The nervous system, samples- scrutinises and responds. The immune system may be involved, sampling-scrutinising and responding... and local mechanisms in the tissues, that again involves sampling-scrutinising and responding, will kick into action too.

Think about it and this 'sample-scrutinise-respond' phenomenon happens everywhere – right down to the level of the individual cell that, after all, has to look after itself just as much as an organ or a whole organism does.

Figure 11.1 overviews some input mechanisms whose ultimate targets are what I like to call the 'stress control centres' of the brain. (Yes, criticise me, the diagram is linear... but it's in the context of the MOM...). The stress control centres are where all the 'threat' information travels to and gets scrutinised before deciding on an appropriate response. Note that the immune system not only deals with its 'immune-related' issues in its own rather profound and intelligent way, but also likes to keep the brain informed too. Immune messengers which, classically consist of a wide variety of cytokines are able to reach and inform the brain about tissue damage, infection, immune activity and immune stress.

Numskulls again, 'Oy, Brainy, we've got a serious bacterial infection down here, can you organise a temperature rise for us a minute. Oh, and we'll let you know when things are looking better... and... could you let us know anything that might be helpful from your side of things if you get a minute...'

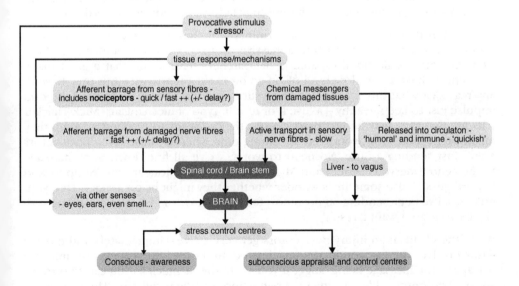

Figure 11.1 Some of the 'Input mechanisms' to the Brain (or rather the 'Stress Control Centre')

Note the two way traffic, immune-brain and brain-immune, and note that bacteria don't like high temperatures – so raising the heat is actually an offensive response – more later, in the evolution chapter!

In the figure, the provocative stimulus – which could be a cut if we're thinking skin, or could be any physical force sufficient to cause damage if we're thinking muscles, ligaments and tendons, or inflammation relating to degenerative change if we're thinking 'wear and tear' – leads to some kind of response in the tissues – 'tissue mechanisms'! If there's an injury – its mayhem, there are smashed up cells, torn blood vessels and blood's everywhere. Some authorities have described it as an 'inflammatory soup' which I rather like. It's more minestrone than cream of mushroom though. Whatever it is, there's a new chemical environment for our sampling system – the massively branching and far reaching terminals of the nociceptive system. A system, which in this particular injury area, has probably not been doing that much in terms of 'injury response' for a great many years! You may be 50 and this could be the first time you've cut yourself or injured this particular spot! Now it's got a large dose of novelty!

The normal life of a nociceptor appears to be... well, just doing nothing – at least in terms of any major electrical activity. But we now know that nociceptors are important 'trophically', I don't want to get too down on them! It seems that without the slightest bit of electrical activity these remarkable little fibres continuously sniff and sample the tissues their terminals embrace and if there's a need for anything the nociceptors help in providing it or if need be, help in activating others to provide it. The humble day to day and electrically lazy nociceptor thus has a rather nice philanthropic 'secretory' or endocrine side to it. It's a carer!

It's well known that nerve injury leads to poor health in the denervated tissues – a fact that's usually put down to lack of normal use, but may also be due to loss of our caring nociceptors and the nourishment they help to provide and co-ordinate.

So, an individual nociceptor, whose terminal branches average a spread of about 1cm in diameter, but may reach to a massive width of 4.5cms in human skin, have Sample-Scrutinise-Respond capability. Researchers have found that a great many nociceptors have a very low level of on-going electrical activity – but they haven't any real idea what this is for. One suggestion was that they need to send the odd impulse just to keep healthy – a 'use it or lose it' type of mechanism? Mick Thacker tells me that they may be just practicing so they're ready to respond anytime they might be needed. I've wondered for a long time whether these firing nociceptors aren't just sending a little 'No need to worry, we're all fine down here' message to the central nervous system and Mick agrees. Nociceptors are the 'Support and Report' guys! I also sometimes wonder whether they might be on a rota – 'Hey, you, wake-up, I've been sending off my report for weeks now and you've been doing sod-all, it's your go, I want a rest...'

When there's been an injury nociceptors get very active – immediately and quickly – this involves the fast conducting myelinated Aδ fibres firing off massive impulse barrages – the message being 'suggest you avoid this as much as you can to prevent any further injury'... like picking up a pan whose handle is red-hot. The message is clear and very precise 'Stop! Avoid you prat!' It's very 'sensory-dimensional' – there's intensity, location and quality that produces a reflex avoidance – 'Drop the friggin' pan...!' I like the example Ronald Melzack used once: if the very hot handle you pick up belongs to a very precious bone-china tea-cup, you do your level best to jostle and fumble it to safety as quickly as possible, rather than drop it straight away. It's amazing how quickly the brain can administer a hierarchical rule that chooses value over injury! Anyway, Aδ fibres are key components of the body's very quick tissue/injury saving/try not to make it worse than it need be type device.

The most populous nociceptor however is the C fibre (in some nerves that supply the skin, over 90% of the neurons are C fibres!). It's maybe worth noting that they seem to wisely congregate in areas where tissue damage is more likely.

A 'C' fibre is very thin—one thousandth of a millimeter—and hasn't any myelin (but does have a coating of Schwann cells, but one that doesn't produce myelin). As a result it is a very slow conductor of electricity. Impulses average about 1 metre per second, in contrast to the big Aβ myelinated sensory neurones which can fire at up to 100 metres per second! Remember from sections 4 and 5 – these big fast fellows can become involved in producing pain given some dorsal horn changes.

C fibres are slow trudgers and are traditionally linked to the post injury 'second-pain' that comes a little while after a knock or an injury. To me, their very positive role at the tissue level is in supporting the healing. They not only sort out appropriate pain to produce the best pain-behaviour for healing (via informing higher centres), but also provide a variety of chemicals that help the recovery process. C fibres are the samplers and brain/CNS informers of the damaged tissue situation as it slowly moves from damaged and weak through frail and modestly functional to strong and fully functional again[1].

If you are interested in tissue focused pain you may find C fibres fascinating – tons of research has been done on them and there's plenty to read. I'm going to cover a little about what fascinates me about them and some of it is from the work of two big nociceptor fibre researchers called Robert Schmidt and Hans-Georg Schaible. They did lots of interesting but fundamentally nasty experiments on cat knee joints and published it in the 1990's. They looked at the impulse activity of cats' joints in four different conditions. The first two conditions were of normal knee joints – one at rest and the second while moving. The second two conditions were the same except that before recording they artificially induced an arthritic-like inflammatory response in the knee joint by injecting a substance called carageenan. It's an extract of seaweed better known for its uses as a 'personal lubricant'! Anyway, they called these now hugely inflamed knees 'arthritic' because they mimicked an inflamed joint flare up. In all the four conditions they recorded impulse activity at rest and when the joints were moved. Further, when they moved the joints they did it in two ways – nicely and nastily!

If you're really upset right now by the seeming cruelty let me tell you that they anaesthetise the cat while all this is going on. It's important to realise that your nociceptors and tissue mechanisms (and the cats) keep going even when bombed out under anaesthetic.

As we've already said, some C fibres (also called type IV articular afferent fibres)

---

1 - Mick Thacker tells me that as a point of interest there are now increasing examples of C fibres generating the fast burst response and Aδ doing the tonic or 'on-going' stuff! Interesting!

have resting activity regardless. In these experiments it was found that in the **healthy resting knee joint** 36% of the C fibres were popping impulses away all the time! The Aδ fibres (also called Type III articular afferent fibres) had about the same proportion. Aβ fibres, not surprisingly, also had on-going activity – presumably relaying information about the position of the joint, but that was only 10% of them. The rest, the great majority were electrically silent.

Now, when they **moved the normal joint in a nice gentle** way – around 90% of the Aβ fibres fire, the 'hey brain we're moving like this' message. Surprisingly, around 45% of Aδ fibres and 30% of C fibres were firing too! Pain fibres aren't supposed to fire with nice innocuous movements, or at rest...? What's this all about? As yet, I don't know of anyone who has tried to address this or even proffer an explanation. I wonder if one of the problems is that researchers into pain only look at these fibres in terms of 'abnormal', or 'damage' or 'pathology'.

Clearly the fibres that fire at comfy rest and with comfy movement are not what can be called 'high-threshold' nociceptive fibres. High-threshold means that it takes a lot to make the nerve fibre fire. Grab a fold of skin from the back of your hand and start pinching – you feel it OK, but at a certain very firm pinching point it comes on all nasty. That's when high-threshold nociceptors fire and in so doing inform the brain to stop you doing it. Clearly not all the traditional Aδ and C fibres are high threshold: there's a spectrum that runs from those that don't fire; to those that like to keep a bit of firing going on just for the hell of it; to those that fire with nice movement; right out to the ones that fire when things get nasty. There's a 'wide dynamic range!' Remember that? Thinking biologically rather than medically should make us come to expect these things I think. What we need to know is where these 'low threshold' Aδ and C fibres relay into in the cord and CNS – which might give more of a clue as to their function. Or would it?

Could they be relaying 'potential-threat' messages perhaps? After all, any movement could be leading to a damage situation so best be ready just in case eh? Sadly, tissue paranoia maybe a near default requirement for survival! That most of my movements are thoughtless and totally pleasant doesn't help the argument at all here.

If the normal cat joint is now moved in a nasty way – all the Aβ fibres fire! It seems that there is a special 10% population of these fibres that only respond to noxious movement! Another about 30% of the Aδ and 30% C fibres also fire. The end result is that the nastier it gets the more fibres join in and it doesn't seem to matter what type of fibre! Forget everything you've been told about pain fibres and start again! Well, sort of...

In the carageenan inflamed joint – things change dramatically and again, in all types of fibre. When the inflamed joint is at rest the number of Aβ fibres firing doubles – eh? They're not nociceptors. They're not supposed to detect inflammation? Well, they did in Robert and Hans-Georg's cats. And Aδ fibres, traditionally associated with the very sudden pain at the time of injury, here, 75% of their population are firing – that's double the number firing in the normal joint! A massive 83% of the C fibre population are firing – which is what we'd expect, but hang on, what about the remaining 17% of them, why aren't they firing too? Maybe they haven't been doing their daily exercises? You know there's laziness everywhere you look in biology!

Now moving the inflamed joint – in both an innocuous and noxious way – brings virtually all the population recorded by the researchers into the picture. However, there are still a small number of fibres in this inflamed state that don't respond whatever is done – 3% of the Aβ and Aδ and 7% of the C fibres!

Maybe the researchers just didn't wait long enough?

Let's sidle a little sideways now...

C fibres that remain electrically inactive in *non injured, non inflamed* or *non pathological* tissues have been called 'sleeping nociceptors' and are generally assigned a pure trophic function as discussed earlier. If you missed it, that means they're sampling, scrutinising and responding without sending impulses. It is also likely that they are maintaining a rather slow and delayed conversation with the CNS – via chemical communication which I'll return to later.

Sleeping nociceptors have been studied in some detail and it seems that they are very common – up to 50% of cat knee joint C fibres are said to be of this variety. The number is far higher in visceral tissues – here the bladder has been well studied. Sleeping C fibres can however 'wake-up' and fire and the key to this is inflammation. Researchers observe that in the presence of inflammation sleeping nociceptors take about 2-3 hours to come out of hibernation. The speed that inflammation develops in a specific tissue is likely to be a factor in this timing.

Speed of inflammation development interests me clinically. Have you ever noticed that after the initial nastiness of an injury it's sometimes not too bad pain wise – you know you've injured it and it hurts a bit to move, but gradually the pain builds and builds over the next few hours until you get the constant aching pain? Sometimes it throbs a bit too and if its muscle or joint related, can stiffen. Clinically this type of pain is deemed inflammatory in nature and is often associated with noticeable swelling and an increase in temperature that's detectable if the injury is not too deep in the body. This delay in onset and slow build-up of discomfort nicely fits with the observed 'waking-time' of C fibres in parallel with the slow build up of inflammation. It's really a reflection of an increasing afferent barrage from the tissues – a massive increase in the impulse activity coursing out of the tissues and into the CNS.

The clinician may also have observed that the delay in pain and stiffness can be quite lengthy – a typical back injury sufferer might report a bit of awareness after a straining activity and later on feel a little stiff perhaps – eased a bit by a hot bath – but the next morning they just can't get out of bed? To my way of thinking this slow build up is a reflection of two things: first, the type of tissue, for example, collagenous tissues like ligament, tendon and disc material (tissues that have a very poor blood supply and a sparse immune and cellular support network) and are therefore very 'slow' metabolically, giving rise to a feeble and slowly developing inflammatory and healing response. Secondly, deep tissues like those in the spine and viscera – are likely to have mostly non-responsive sleeping fibres and hence be relatively 'insensitive' in the normal state. This is a 'tissue' level mechanism that may explain the little or no awareness of injury/pain at the outset in many back pain situations! (Don't forget central 'modulation' of course and poor central representation of deep structures too).

Also in collagenous tissue like tendon, ligament and disc, compared to say skin, there's a far lower density of sensory fibres anyway. The slow post-injury build up of inflammation causes the slow waking of these sparsely populated sleeping fibres and hence the long delay in letting 'you' know what's happened! Normal discs, for example, are virtually devoid of any innervation except in their very outermost annular layer and even that is very sparse.

Another issue to consider is that once a tissue has 'recovered' from an injury this delayed response and slow-build-up phase of symptom development seems to be skipped in subsequent injury events of the same tissue. This time when a re-strain occurs the pain often develops far more quickly, missing out the slow-build-up-symptom response. Could it be that the nervous system retains a memory or sensitivity from the previous injury? I think it's bound to at all levels. Those fibres responsible for the injured tissue (and the 'pain' representational CNS 'circuit') never fully drift back to their original sensitivity state and this includes the sleeping fibres that are unlikely to ever fully go back to sleep. They simply don't forget. This may be wise action: because yet another consideration is that healing of collagenous tissue is for one thing very, very, slow; and for another, is by scar formation and therefore never gets back to its original state. It is therefore less substantial than it once was; the supporting nervous system knows this and wisely maintains a degree of alertness. Drifting fully back to sleep is not allowed and a modest 'ready-for-action' 'pain memory' is neatly filed away for on-going and future protection!

Maybe it doesn't, but I'll bet it does and I think that's smart biology. The problems arise when the sensitivity and the circuit remain active or remain too sensitive for the strength and state of the tissue. Let's just say for some, that the nervous system can sometimes be a little bit too wet and wussy... if it's given the opportunity??

Numskulls again... It's 'C fibre' prattling on after a disc injury...

'Oh my God, should I go back to sleep or not, what should I do, he's so damn nervy my guy, I'm getting mixed messages, one minute he's ignoring it the next he's being super cautious... I don't know whether I'm coming or going... best err on the cautious side and stay sensitive until he makes his mind up...'

There's another thing that I think makes sense, and that's that as tissues slowly age and degenerate their sleeping sensory neural populations become slowly sensitised – it stands to reason that as tissues gradually lose their youthful vitality their sensory carers rouse themselves a bit and pay a bit more attention. No wonder we all become a bit more 'aware' of our joints, muscles and bits and pieces as time goes by.

A nerdy part of me always wondered if anyone knew how many impulses were being generated when we're injured, and thanks to our two nociceptor researchers, Robert and Hans-Georg, I found out.

What we can infer from what they tell us is that once a tissue is inflamed ordinary C fibres start firing more. The sleeping C fibres wake up and they all become continuously active – it's a message that is demanding attention and hence assistance from above! Numskull again... 'I don't care what you're doing up there it's bad down here and we'd really appreciate it if you'd get him to stop pratting about and look after us! ... Heeeeelp!' There's nothing worse than a pleading little C fibre.

I'm left wondering if the 7% of C fibres and the 3% of Aβ and Aδ that aren't even firing when the cat's joint is inflamed and moved in a noxious way may have eventually woken up given enough time? Researchers typically don't hang around too long doing their recordings – and the length of recording time is rarely given – as is the case here. The bottom line is that it's no big deal, what's important is that lots of different fibres fire and when there's inflammation and noxious movement it gets a whole lot worse – not only in terms of an increasingly active population of fibres but also in terms of the numbers of impulses that are being generated.

Robert and Hans-Georg found that in the normal cat knee joint at rest approximately 2,300 impulses every 30 seconds are generated by the various fibres noted. Move the normal joint to and fro and the impulses roughly double to around 4,400 per 30 seconds. Inflame the joint by injecting our sexy lubricant carageenan into it and the impulses jump to 11,100 when at rest! That's approximately a 5 fold increase – an impressive barrage! No wonder there's a constant aching going on. Move the inflamed joint and there's a massive 30,900 impulses being generated – that's roughly a 7 fold increase. Apparently recordings from some individual fibres show an impressive 100 fold increase in their firing rate! Wow! I think we can safely conclude that the 'Numskull' messages from the tissues are something like... 'THIS IS URGENT!' 'WE NEED HELP!' 'DON'T MOVE ME!' and even 'DON'T TOUCH ME!'

Or are they? I flip to what I observe in the clinic and assumptions like this don't always quite hold. Sure, in inflamed tissue – especially in skin that's been cut – the nasty ache and the nasty sharp pains that accompany any movement or touch in the area, make you hold it all still and be very careful when moving it. But some acute 'strain' and 'sprain' type injuries, given a day or two, with obvious swelling and inflammation – aren't always that achy and the patient can move the injured area reasonably well. Sometimes the patient even *wants* to move it. More on this later in the 'Pain' chapter (GE 3.1) The key is that it's what the central nervous system does with the barrage of impulses that is so important, and, we may be wrong to assume that all 30,900 of the impulses are relaying a 'make it bloody hurt' message. There may be a population of optimists in there saying, 'Look, I think that lot of you are over-reacting a bit, let's just calm down, stiff upper lip, what-ho and take stock of the situation.' The optimist message is inhibitory of course! For every biological reaction in one direction there's an opposite controlling one, but the slippery nature of the beast is that there's usually some kind of uneasy battle going on between the facilitators (his family!) and the inhibitors (her family!) and it's this that's likely to be a big factor in explaining why some folk hurt far more than others with similar injuries.

I've got a funny feeling that it wouldn't be surprising to find that some C and Aδ fibres are actually inhibitory... a role traditionally reserved for Aβ fibres.

Sorry, deviation... Oh, here's another... what's to say that one persons ache at rest is X amount as a result of 11,100 impulses and another persons ache at rest is rated the same but a result of only 2,300 impulses! So for all of those who want to say 'All pain's in the brain', me and Mick Thacker understand what you're saying, but we think you're wrong; this impulse barrage is just as much a part of conscious pain as the processing of it by the spinal cord and all levels into and back out of the brain.

Time for a change... because we're shifting now, from fibres and impulses to chemicals.

Chapter 11.2
Nociceptive mechanisms 2: Chemicals and inflammation

Let's get back on track... There's been an injury and we're in the tissues seeing what's going on...

Some nerve fibres may be getting worked up, not thinking they need to demand pain, but rather thinking they need their cell bodies to quickly start making some useful chemicals to help improve the dangerous damage situation. If you injure your ankle – the terminals of sensory nerve fibres in that tissue are about half your body length away from their cell bodies up in the nerve root of the lower spine – that could be around a metre. That's one hell of a long cell, check-out figure 11.2!

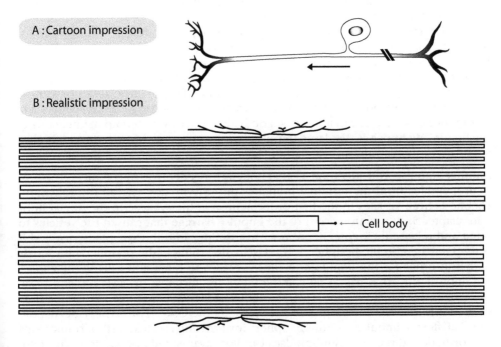

Figure 11.2 The length of a sensory nerve fibre. Adapted from Fig 11.2 - Devor M (1999) Unexplained peculiarities of the dorsal root ganglion. Pain. Supplement 6:S27-35.

In order to stay healthy down at the terminal end (the fibre terminals are highly likely to have suffered some damage in the injury) and to keep its target tissues healthy, the fibre has to manufacture and transport the chemicals and structural products that are required. In order to do this there must be a good communication and switching system between the far ends of the nerve fibre and its very distant cell body. Remember that the nerve fibre cell body up in the spine is where the nucleus is, and the nucleus is where the DNA is, and the DNA is where the genes are... that need to be switched on to make the proteins that mend the cell that feed the tissues that dah de dah de dah de dah....that lay in the house that Jack built! (Sorry, the lilt of that bit made the old nursery rhyme pop into my head!)

So could it be that some of the fibres sending impulses from the tissues are merely alerting their cell bodies that they'd better turn on some genes and get manufacturing quickly? The last thing the situation in the injured tissues needs is for the stock of chemical products already stored in the C fibre terminals to run out. These 'essential products' include structural proteins and specific receptors and ion channels that are important in the mending and sensitising process in the terminals. There are also secretory chemicals needed for 'neurogenic' inflammation which aid the recovery and healing process. These include various neuropeptides, the most famous being substance P – I believe 'P' stands for 'Pig' where it was first discovered! There are others, also with weird names relating to their early elucidation or their structure, these include calcitonin-gene- related peptide – CGRP for short, vaso-active intestinal peptide (VIP!), galanin, somatostatin (SOM), neurokinin A (NKA). The only way these products can get from the cell body, where they're produced, to the terminals, where they are needed, is via the special cytoplasmic streaming that nerve fibres have. It's called axoplasmic transport (remember this in the amoeba?). Axoplasmic transport can be very slow, being measured at rates of only a few millimetres per day, to surprisingly fast, being up to 40cms per day! That's maybe about two and a half days from my foot to the cell body in the dorsal root ganglion! It's a bit slow, so the sooner someone can tell the cell body that it needs to step up manufacturing the better. My hunch is that large impulse barrages passing through the cell bodies stimulate protein synthesis (see p20 of Meyer et al 2006).

Another impulse consideration is that they are needed to trigger the release of neuropeptides from the terminal branches into the tissues. Recall the release of chemicals from vesicles in the first order neuron at the synapse in the dorsal horn – in chapter 5. It was the arrival of the impulse barrage that caused the vesicles to burst and release their contents of neurotransmitter into the synaptic space and it is the same here in the periphery. The fascinating thing in the peripheral terminals is that in order for the impulses to cause vesicles to burst and release their load, the impulse direction has to be coming down the terminal towards the end – see the arrows in figures 11.3 and 11.4. In other words they have to go against the flow of impulses that are coursing their way towards the CNS! For sensory nerves the 'normal' flow of impulses is from periphery inwards and is called 'orthodromic' – it's the 'orthodox' direction! But impulses can flow against the normal flow and these are termed 'antidromic'. How does that work? The exact mechanism isn't known as far as I'm aware, but it does occur and can be produced artificially by stimulating the 'wrong' end of the neuron! Researchers do this and it helps them identify both ends of the neuron they want to study and the target of the neuron they are interested in. There are two origins of antidromic impulses discussed in the literature: first, those whose origins are in the central nervous system, the so-called 'dorsal root reflex'; and second, those whose origins are in the periphery.

The term 'axon-reflex' may be familiar. This is the better known peripheral mechanism of neuropeptide release that is often discussed in relation to 'Hunter's response' and the 'Triple response'.

If you expose your hands to freezing temperatures the reflex physiological response is to constrict all the blood vessels to your hand, sending blood coursing away from your skin and deeper into your torso. Your body is allowing your fingers to chill in

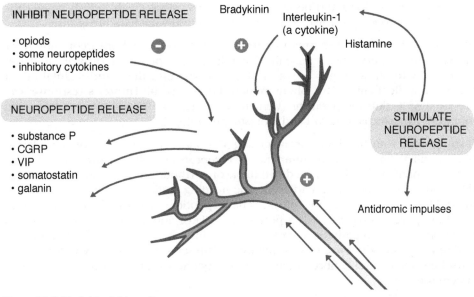

Figure 11.3 'Antidromic' impulses.

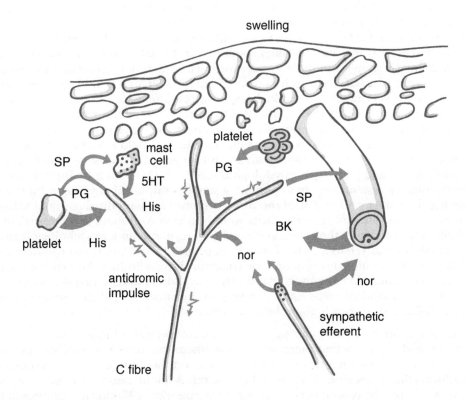

Figure 11.4 'Antidromic impulses' Adapted from Fields H. (1989) Pain. McGraw-Hill. New York.

order to keep its blood and hence its vital organs warm. (Yeah, selfish bugger the fingers, I want to keep warm). This is a sympathetically mediated response.

Were you a Norwegian fisherman or Inuit hunter, both of whom frequently work gloveless in the very cold, your chilled hands would open their surface capillaries periodically to allow surges of warm blood to pass into them and maintain their viability and flexibility. This phenomenon, known as the Hunter's response, can elevate a 35^{0}F skin temperature (virtually freezing) to 50^{0}F within seven or eight minutes! Fantastic adaptation and fantastic physiology!

If you plunge your hand into near-freezing 35^{0}F water it's ghastly – you stimulate C fibre terminals in the skin via temperature receptors and off they fire. Impulses go down the branches and then on down the axon 'orthodromically', but some may go down one branch and up an adjacent one heading 'antidromically' to its end (see figure 11.4), hence, causing the release of neuropeptides, in particular here substance P (SP in figure). Substance P is a potent vasodilator and as such is antagonistic to the efforts of the sympathetic nervous system. This substance P release is thought to underlie the periodic wave of vasodilation in Hunter's response. I wonder if there must be some central C fibre initiated inhibitory effect on the sympathetic nervous system too.

The triple-response is characterised by a three phase reaction to a skin scratch – first and within a minute or two, a reddening, then slowly the red line spreads out into a flare and finally a localised swelling – called the 'wheal'. You can do it to yourself – use a sharp point like the point of a compass or the tip of a sharp knife. I've just scratched my forearm and it's taken about two and a half to three minutes to start to redden. By ten minutes there's a very slight flare and by fourteen minutes a slight wheal. Time yourself and see how you compare? Everyone is different here and some have a very rapid and marked response resulting in a quite massive wheal. What fascinates me are the individual differences – especially with my on-going inquisitiveness about why some people react more or suffer more in response to injury and indeed, why some go on to suffer long term. Could it be that in those who inflame more or who suffer more pain and for longer, in response to injury, have a more marked and prolonged physiological reaction? Or could it be their 'control' or dampening systems are not as potent? A simple study observing, quantifying and timing the nature and extent of the triple response across individuals, and within individuals in different circumstances would be easy to do and quite revealing I think. You could note the extent and rapidity of response under psychological and/ or physical stress versus a state of relaxation or meditation. You could compare the reactions of chronic pain sufferers, or compare those who have known 'immune' related conditions like rheumatoid arthritis. I wouldn't mind betting that most will show quite a marked variation depending on the situation and that some will be more influenced by psychological stressors than physical and vice versa.

If there is a difference it would suggest some kind of central influences on peripheral events, and we know that there are. This is where the 'dorsal root reflex' may be a factor, or at least offer a hint that there may well be more central-to-peripheral pathways than we realise. Take note, because this is our first excursion into 'output' pathways from the central nervous system to the periphery. Making just one possible link between the central nervous system – the scrutinising system; the brain itself, the higher centres that make us who we are and what we think and feel, our psychology – and what is going on out there in the lowly tissues!

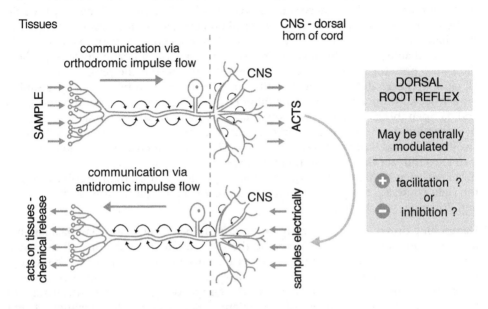

Figure 11.5 The dorsal root reflex.

The dorsal root reflex is illustrated in figure 11.5. The important factor here is significant activity in the dorsal horn of the spinal cord – and we know from section 5 that this can be massive. It seems that antidromic impulses can be generated in the dorsal horn terminals of C fibres and then dodge off down them to their peripheral terminals when there's a lull of incoming orthodromic impulses! (For dorsal root reflex references see: Cervo and Laird 1996; Sluka and Westlund 1993; Sluka et al 1995; Lin et al 2000; Meyer et al 2006 p26-7). Some of this research has shown that if you dampen down central activity in the dorsal horn following an experimental 'knee arthritis' like that described with carageenan in chapter 11.1 – there is a significant decrease in peripheral inflammation – reducing swelling by half and further, the joint doesn't become so hot and the level of sensitivity is significantly reduced too. *This emphasises the importance of an efficient central inhibitory/excitatory control system* – not just in getting the peripheral balance just right for best recovery but also in suppressing an activity when other matters may be of a greater priority. 'Look mate, you're going to have to run like you've never run before... the last thing we need is a swollen and stiff knee right now... you better get going and we'll deal with it later, promise... (If you survive!)...'

Dampening the dorsal root reflex looks like a vitally quick tissue inflammation/ swelling dampening route that's put to use when the environment is getting threatening and physical action may be required.

You may be surprised to know that in animal experiments where experimental arthritis is produced in one knee joint, there will also be some mild inflammation in the unmolested opposite joint! Further, if the nerves of the normal joint or the inflamed joint are blocked from working – this doesn't occur. I will return to some more central to peripheral nerve mediated effects like these when discussing the role of the sympathetic nervous system on peripheral events, but for a moment consider that thanks to this nice little 'control' connection, the central nervous system is able to go 'no thanks, not right now, can't waste time starting a healing process, others things too pressing...' OR … 'OK no problems you can start the process now, we're all clear up here, all threats dealt with and gone, it's safe to become a bit disabled for a while... swell away... but if anything crops up I might have to intervene again and dampen things down...' As always, there may also be the potential for under or over-reaction too... So, bear this in mind when confronted with a patient who has a swollen joint and is being really inactive... perhaps they need a bit of excitement and a run around, set the dogs on them perhaps! I know, that's a bit over the top, but my experience is that when I urge patients to get going more than they have and in the right context... the swollen joint does improve after a bit of 'Tobleroning'... (Up and downing, see chapter 13.1).

Dampening down is all to do with strong dorsal horn inhibition (Claudia's family). So, doing anything that helps decrease the excitement (for example, all the usual 'bottom-up' tissue based techniques you can think of), but also increases the top-down inhibition and decreases the top-down excitation – like reassurance and less concern/attention – can only be helpful. The far end of this top-down spectrum is to frighten the living daylights out of the patient... then re-check the swelling!   Don't forget to think of top-down as an important aspect of changing tissue physiology. That's the big message here!

Remember the poor old dorsal horn processing is up against that seven fold increase in afferent barrage produced by the moving inflamed joint!

What we are actually looking at is a system that doesn't just come on and run its course until healing is done – the whole process is bound to be a stop-start one. Clinically it would be good to know what the 'best conditions for most efficient healing' are and be able to facilitate them. While this area is surprisingly poorly addressed by research, it is well worth speculating on I think. For those of us who latch on to an evolutionary way of reasoning, we could get carried away and go, it's bleedin' obvious! I'll address this more rationally when reviewing the effect of stress on healing later on (e.g. chapter 15.4). It's fascinating.

Chapter 11.3
Nociceptive mechanisms 3: A few questions discussed...

What's physiological and pathological pain?

Unsurprisingly, what is known about what goes on in the tissues after injury is confined to the very early stages, and most research, again unsurprisingly, has been done on skin wounds – because they're easy to make accurately , easy to access and easy to observe. Although this may be said, it is perhaps rather different from the public's perception of what medicine really knows. Little do the public know how complicated things like healing really are and little do they know the rather modest amount medicine actually understands about it all. We are all guilty – and a big fault is with our basic clinical education curriculum for focusing on pathology over and above 'normal' recovery mechanisms.

From the nervous system's perspective, as we've seen, injury causes its peripheral sensory fibre terminals to start firing rapid impulse volleys from more and more fibres, but a second thing occurs and that is sensitisation. Sensitisation means that the fibres, when stimulated, now fire a lot more easily. They don't require as much of the stimulus to make them fire.

This is easy to demonstrate! First of all lightly touch the top of your head – you feel an innocuous touch sensation nicely and precisely where you're touching yourself. Now, whack the top of your head a few times as hard as you can bring yourself to and then wait a couple of hours. I suggest you go off and do something else for a bit. Now touch the top of your head again in the same light way as you did before. If you're normal what should happen is that the same stimulus now produces a feeling of unpleasant soreness – simple allodynia as we discussed in chapter 4. If you've got the courage, try belting your head again with the same force that you used before! Idiot! What you should now find if you're awake and not being distracted by someone with a Rottweiler is that this now hurts one hell of a lot more than it did originally – hyperalgesia (but see chapter 4)… and that the pain carries on for a good while after you hit yourself. In other words, the pain isn't straight-forward on-off, it's on… slowly off. There's a degree of stimulus-response relationship… but it's not wholly mechanically patterned.

The old pain literature, and I'm talking when I was first reading it back in the early 1990's, often described two types of pain – 'Physiological pain' and 'Pathological pain'. It usually caused me to make my usual, 'These guys have never listened to patients or even thought about their own pain experiences' type statement, but, having said that, it isn't such a bad place to begin.

'Physiological pain' is really 'laboratory pain' – by this I mean, that if you take a human and put them in a laboratory with nothing much going on, you find that with mild stimulation they report mild sensation; with moderate stimulation there's moderate discomfort and with extreme there's extreme; it all fits nicely and it's just as we'd all love pain to be as clinicians. Manual therapists love it when the pain is on and off in proportion to the stimulus given. It might be called bend-your-finger-back-hard pain. The findings also fit beautifully with the intensity of the impulse barrage.

Now 'Pathological pain' is injured or pathological tissue pain – where small stimuli hurt, moderate stimuli hurt a lot and intense stimuli hurt like hell and the hurt carries on after. Clinically this is sharp pain associated with some kind of mechanical force. What's often forgotten is the on-going background achiness which is usually present if you really ask. So, injury related pain can have a mechanical pattern when you consider the sharper pain, but also has a background discomfort to it too – that more than likely relates to inflammatory and healing goings on in the tissues and hence the mighty 'afferent barrage', plus maybe a bit of spontaneous nerve activity too.

Take an individual out of the laboratory and into real life and so called 'physiological' or 'laboratory' pain can show many colours and the simple relationships described above start to break down. Someone steps on your toe while pushing past you in a queue...

'OW, you idiot, look where you're going... '

Your new girlfriend/boyfriend is going with you to dance class and steps on your toe... 'Oh, sorry Louis....' 'Hey didn't feel a thing, don't worry, keep going....'

You're in the last minutes of a rugby match, you're winning and you're at the bottom of the ruck, 'Biffo' steps on your foot to put you off... you didn't feel a thing.

You're a soccer centre forward, you're in the opposition's penalty area with the ball and the last defender is buzzing all round you, he lightly steps on your toe... There's a big 'agony' scene, a quadruple roll on the floor and hey, you've been awarded the penalty... Well I never, that's cheating isn't it? No, it really hurt.

When's someone going to make a film about pain behaviour? I might write to David Attenborough and get Derren Brown along too... I would love to be the film's consultant please?

(An aside – what about a pain questionnaire where the last question is: 'When you're in pain do you respond more like a rugby player or a football player?').

Laboratory pain requires a 'neutral' environment... real day to day pain gets hugely modulated by the central nervous system – by what you and your brain and body are up to at the time and by what they've done in the past too.

To explain modulation to patients you can use the 'light stroking' example! Basically you can ask the patient to note the different feeling and sensation they might get when lightly stroked on the front of their thigh by: a) a complete stranger, b) someone they're very fond of and in the mood for and c) when it's totally unexpected. Then you can note how the circumstances, the context, the meaning, the mood that they're in all have an influence on what the nervous system does with the touch sensation... and you've also got to be aware that sometimes some people find that a lot of pain is very stimulating and very nice!

For the remainder of this chapter and the next I'd like to discuss these questions:

1. What causes the nerve fibre terminals to become more sensitive?

2. What causes aching pain?

3. What about postural pain?

4. Is there anything that controls all this in the tissues?

5. Does fluid movement in the tissues affect pain and stiffness?

What causes nerve fibre terminals to become more sensitive?

It's all very similar to the Shane and Claudia tale, except this time it's all about the far end of Shane! Recall from section 5 that impulses are due to ions flowing through ion channels and the resulting changes in electrical potential of the axon membranes of nerve fibres. Impulses are electrical, or 'ion-flow' in nature but the stimulus that causes them is not. So, at the sensory nerve fibre terminals (or perhaps more correctly nerve fibre 'beginnings') in the tissues we can think of the transformation or 'transduction' of one form of stimuli into an electrical one. Thus, mechanical forces, various chemicals and changes in temperature are the three main stimuli that need to be 'transduced' to produce an electrical impulse. Hopefully from chapter 5 it is obvious that what is needed to produce this transformation are a variety of appropriate receptors associated with ion channels. No receptor-ion channels present equals, no action!

There's a neat figure of the various types of receptor in chapter 5.3 earlier (it's fig 5.10). The temperature receptor is not illustrated but in principle it has the same basic components as the others – it's a protein complex in a cell wall that changes it's configuration (opens its little 'gate') when warming or cooling are applied to it – which then allows a flow of ions through the cell membrane. Here, the key for opening is a temperature stimulus. In the old pain literature temperature receptors were called 'vanilloid' receptors or 'VR1' but they're now referred to as 'transient receptor potential' ion channels, hence TRP (often followed by the letter V and a number 1,2,3 etc to indicate subgroups).

The terminals of sensory fibres in the tissues are thus 'detection' agents by dint of their particular receptor population. A list of the various known receptors is getting longer and longer as research progresses (for starters, see Meyer et al 2006; Julius and McCleskey 2006 and McMahon et al 2006). For the clinician it is enough to know that there are receptors for all the various inflammatory chemicals, for example, those for: serotonin (5HT receptor), various prostaglandins (e.g. PGE_2 receptor), histamine (H_1 receptor), bradykinin (B_2 receptor), all the various cytokines (IL- receptors, TNF receptors, LIF receptors etc), inflammatory 'acidic' conditions (ASIC receptors), adenosine and its derivatives like adenosine triphosphate (ATP) (P2X receptors) and so forth and there are many more. There are also receptors for neuropeptides, mechanical stimuli and temperature (various TRP receptors) as mentioned. As research continues it is found that individual receptors can be influenced by a variety of different 'agonists'. Agonists are chemicals that activate or produce an effect whereas 'antagonists' block or prevent an effect. The TRP group of receptors that are associated with temperature detection will also respond to the presence of capsacin – the chemical in chilli peppers that causes the 'heat' sensation of a hot curry! The capsacin binds onto the TRP receptor and it opens. Little wonder that if capsacin is a temperature receptor agonist the sensation we get from it is processed as 'hot'. This is a good example of how precise the nervous system can sometimes be in giving us information... but also how it can be fooled too!

Other agonists of the TRP receptors include acidity (the presence of protons), and some research is starting to propose that they may even be involved in mechanoreception. Surprisingly, little is known about mechanoreceptors! Or if you're a bit cynical – unsurprisingly – because it's of little interest to a drug company who's sponsoring the research... unless of course they can find some drug that blocks mechanical receptors! Now that would be interesting! Can you imagine taking a drug that stopped all physical sensations: can't feel your clothes, can't feel the pressure on your bum when you're sitting, can't feel any movements, can't feel the ground when you walk, can't feel stretching... weird thought, weird drug – but logically it's perfectly feasible and there's bound to be some scientist out there who wants to find it, describe it and patent it to make millions. Misguided reductionism, but there you go. I bet the side effects are amazing?

To drag this into the clinic for a moment, thinking mechanoreceptors in relation to pain means tenderness, pain on palpation, and pain on active and passive movement and pain on any type of physical test performed. For example, static rotator cuff muscle testing for pain response, neural tension testing and so on. You simply can't have those sensations without mechanoreceptors that provide the transducing capability for converting mechanical pressures into electrical nerve impulses. I'll discuss this further in the nerve root section in relation to mechanosensitivity, as in a positive straight leg raise, a positive upper limb tension test or a positive 'nerve-compression' test. These tests are often used to 'prove' nerve involvement – but my clinical experience tells me that there are a great many 'neurogenic' type pain problems where these tests are quite unrevealing and often normal. If you appreciate that there could be very few mechanoreceptors in a sensitised nerve this makes perfect sense. To have pain doesn't mean that there has to be mechanosensitivity.

Just as we discussed in the dorsal horn chapter, receptors may be in three states: 'closed', 'open and active' or 'refractory'. If receptors are refractory they are in an unresponsive state and need to be activated or 'woken' up before they will respond. One of the keys to bringing about changes in peripheral sensitivity relates to the activation of refractory receptors as well as to changes in the properties of receptors and ion channels that are already functional. The overall effect is just like in the CNS – ion channels and receptors effectively increase in numbers, by coming out of a refractory state and becoming functional; and, those that are functional subtly change their physical make up to become more easily triggered. In a longer time frame of days or even weeks, the synthesis of more receptors and ion channels way up in the cell body and the subsequent transport and installation down to the nerve terminals can further the sensitisation process.

How does it all work?

Well, a major line of research headed by the likes of Steve McMahon and David Bennett has focused on the role of 'Nerve Growth Factor' or NGF (McMahon and Bennett 2006; Donnerer et al 1992; Reichling and Gold 1996). NGF is so called due to its importance in the preservation and health of nociceptors during development. It's a relatively simple protein released by target tissues that help growing and undifferentiated small diameter nerve fibres find their way to their target tissue, help to specify what type of fibre they become and also provide a vital nutrient for their very survival. NGF is the 'John Innes' compost of the nerve world!

However, in the world of the adult and the world of pain and injury NGF is viewed as a regulating chemical as well as one that causes pain and one that can directly sensitise nociceptor terminals. It does this by changing the conformity of the resident receptor and ion channel populations as well as by egging on other chemical reactions and nearby immune cells (e.g. mast cells) to produce more 'algogens'. 'Algogen' is a posh word for chemicals that are involved in pain and 'changing the conformity of' means that NGF triggers changes to the receptor or ion channel proteins so that they work more easily! You may remember the term 'phosphorylation' from chapter 5 – it simply means the adding of a phosphate group to the receptor or ion channel protein – and in so doing makes the receptor or ion channel more sensitive and more efficient. This is probably how a refractory receptor is primed in order to make it functional. 'Egging-on' is a simple way of saying that NGF can influence anything that has NGF receptors (trkA) – and mast cells, among others, are riddled with them. NGF is a real 'fat-controller' (you'd know what I mean if you've read the Thomas the Tank Engine books when you were a kid!),having the ability to make:

- ... the genes of mast cells switch on to produce their specific products, or in posh, 'induce the expression of'... for example... a whole bunch of cytokines, or interleukins, which are mostly pro-inflammatory

- ... mast cells start dividing and proliferating...

- ... mast cells spew out packages of chemicals, or 'degranulate' and hence release their contents – which includes pro-inflammatory histamine and serotonin

- ... the inflammatory precursor chemical arachidonic acid to convert, via a complex cascade of intermediary stages, into various leukotrienes (they're inflammatory chemicals related to prostaglandins). Leukotrienes in turn then attract neutrophils to the area... and so it goes on!

The bit I like about NGF is that it acts as a messenger from the tissues to the DNA in the cell body of the nerve fibre. Once there it induces genes to 'express' and thereby up-regulate the production of various neuropeptides and receptor and ion channel proteins.

When there's been an injury a whole mass of chemicals are released from the smashed up tissues which then go on to stimulate and arouse immune cells that are resident there (immune cells hang around in just about all tissues of the body, in particular the skin). The injury chemicals also attract more immune cells from the blood stream.

Mast cells and macrophages in the injury and inflammatory environment release NGF which then gets absorbed into the nociceptor fibre terminals by way of a receptor called TrkA (Tyro kinase A receptor). This receptor actually grabs NGF, sucks it across the cell membrane and spits it out inside – a process called 'internalisation'! NGF then gets wafted away and sometime later, via 'retrograde' axoplasmic transport, ends up at the neurones cell body in the dorsal root ganglion of the sensory nerve root. Once in the cell body NGF initiates a cascade of chemical messenger systems that ultimately leads to the 'translation' or 'up-regulation' or 'expression' of various genes for various neuropeptides and receptor or ion channel proteins. The list produced includes substance P, CGRP, BDNF ('brain derived neurotrophic factor!'), the temperature receptor (TRPV1), sodium ion channels and bradykinin receptors. All these then get transported back to the neurones terminals by 'anterograde' axoplasmic transport. The neuropeptides eventually get spewed out of the nerve terminals and play their role in inflammation and healing. Once installed in the membrane, the ion channels and receptors influence the sensitivity state. Quite a journey!

Now, the clinically interesting bit: in experimental work on rats it has been shown that in the cell body there is an increase in neuropeptide content within 12-48 hours after the induction of inflammation in its paw[1]. By 5 days a 'dramatic' increase in neuropeptides has been noted in the peripheral nerve axons supplying the paw. Sodium ion channel increases in the cell body take 4 days. So, we're talking around 4- 5 days post injury for increases in the cell body related to an injury of a rats paw to be detected. Considering the slow rate of axoplasmic transport – it could be several more days after that before these products reach the peripheral terminals – in other words there's quite a time delay involved here. In the clinic we often hear histories whereby the patient tells us that they remember overdoing something, or straining in some way but that the pain only got really nasty many days later. In others, there is often no recollection of an injuring incident until the patient is asked to go back a week or more prior to the onset of symptoms. Delay in pain onset and delays in increases in sensitivity may in part be explained by this slow mechanism. Nerve pain, in particular which I deal with in the 'Nerve root' section of the book, often shows delays in onset of symptoms following injury.

I have now discussed two mechanisms to explain delays in pain and sensitivity onset and increase; as here, relating to the slow transport of neuropeptides and ion channels from the cell body to the peripheral tissues; and earlier, relating to the tediously slow reactivity of deep collagenous tissues and the gradual waking of sparse populations of sleeping nociceptors.

In summary: in order to understand what makes a sensory nerve fibre like a nociceptor, more sensitive than normal, it's important to understand what makes it sensitive in the first place! Hopefully, it is now easy to see that sensitivity is all about receptors and ion channels, and that it is via these specialised cellular components that a chemical, a mechanical force or a variety of temperatures can bring about an electrical impulse. Normal sensitivity, in any given sensory fibre, is solely down to its resident receptor and ion channel population and whether or not the receptors that

---

1 - *The researchers inject a chemical that stimulates inflammation – remember carageenan? Another one that's particularly good at stimulating NGF production is called 'Freunds Complete Adjuvant' or FCA.*

---

are there are functional or refractory. Sensitisation which occurs following injury is the result of a very complex biology, but ultimately the process is down to the following four things:

- refractory receptors and ion channels becoming responsive – in effect, this makes more of them available

- already active receptors and ion channels becoming more reactive and more easily triggered – they're phosphorylated and have conformational changes!

- new receptors and ion channels being made in the nerve fibre cell nucleus and then transported to and installed in the terminal branches

- the complex and every changing chemical environment in the damaged, inflamed or healing area.

Sensitisation means to fire more easily and to fire more to a stimulus. From a mechanosensitivity perspective this means that a normal light touching force or a normal gentle movement force produces a massive increase in firing over the normal reaction. Clinically this translates into tenderness to palpation, to painful reactions to stretch, movement and pressures that are produced by various 'physical' tests that we do when we examine and treat. This type of pain is often given the label 'mechanical pain' by physiotherapy and manual therapy. I would rather it was called mechanosensitivity because this term gives the nod to the fact that it is the result of very complex chemical and neuro-chemical reactions. The term mechanical pain unfortunately carries the baggage of a mechanical problem with it. For example, something 'out', or 'not moving correctly' and often side steps the likelihood of underlying 'chemistry' or inflammation that gave rise to it in the first place. It's a terrible term in my opinion.

In the good old days, in the 1980's and early 1990's, a great many sciaticas were deemed to be 'stuck nerves' and have 'AMT' or 'Adverse Mechanical Tension' of the nerve and as a result many patients were subjected to huge stretching forces by therapists. Review 'Trevor's slump' in section 2! While stretching repeatedly over time, to try and achieve some increased flexibility is not a problem with me. But trying to do it in one treatment session is a problem. Because collagenous tissues just do not suddenly stretch and maintain the increase in range, unless of course they are torn by the force applied, which I'm sure they are occasionally! Also, clinical reasoning that deems a problem to be 'mechanical', suggests that the use of force is necessary to somehow 'fix' it.

One last thing while we're here... you may recall the discussion of receptive fields in the central mechanisms chapters? And, that changes in receptive fields of dorsal horn neurons was a variable beast, capable of waxing and waning in response to inhibitory and excitatory controls. Changes in receptive field size also occur in the periphery. As discussed, a single human C fibre has been shown to have the potential to have a receptive field of as much as 4.5 cms. It appears that terminal branches can be sleeping or active and thus have the potential to vary their receptive field size – presumably by the mechanisms discussed. Terminal branches are like the branches or roots of trees, if the trees are near each other their branches/roots overlap – so too the branches of nerve fibres. This means that if a focused stimulus to one small spot is applied, then more than just one fibre can be stimulated and of course, the larger the 'active' area of each individual fibres receptive field becomes, the more overlapping that will occur. So, in the non sensitised state a strong pressure with a small pin-prick may, say, stimulate three fibres even though there may be branches in that area from a further ten nearby fibres whose branches are in a refractory state. But, once inflamed and the branches sensitised – the potential for the full complement of ten firing becomes possible.

Is that it then? Well no, in 1997 Coppes and colleagues published their research into the innervation of damaged discs and provided evidence that there's an increase and in-growth of nerve fibres into the damaged areas! So dumb tissues that normally have very poor, or like discs, virtually non-existent nerve supplies become 'connected' and maybe the brain now finds a little space for them in its sensory mapping areas and maybe that's how and why a disc can cause so much grief...? Many years ago I wrote a chapter on Evolutionary Reasoning in Topical Issues in Pain 4 book and in it asked the question 'Why should the disc bother to hurt?' I'll mention this again in the Evolution chapter but for now it's good to contemplate why on earth a tissue like a disc – which has a virtually non-existent biological turn-over and hence an appallingly slow healing response and recovery potential – should want a better nerve supply? Why make a tissue have a greater potential for pain generation when protecting it is hardly going to help? What might be better, rather than think that nerves and innervation are all about sensory information and pain, is to think support for healing. This fits, because in parallel with the re-innervation, damaged parts of discs may also demonstrate increased vascularity. New blood vessels grow in. It can be seen as an attempt by the body to at least try and 'bodge' something and attempt to do it at a faster rate than it otherwise would! The pain is just an unfortunate cost of the tissue being innervated! I'll discuss another aspect of this in the Evolution chapter.

Increasing damaged tissue innervation density is hardly likely to be confined to discs and one is suspicious that it happens in all tissues. I have a reference to muscle injury in rats showing a doubling of density of C fibres within twelve days of the injury. If we think trophic support and protection in parallel it all makes a bit of sense. But it also shows us how things can go awry and be far more sensitised than need be.

Chapter 11.4
Nociceptive mechanisms 4: More questions: Aching pain and Postural pain

What causes aching pain?

For years this was one of my favourite topics, especially when I was on a bit of a high horse about manual therapy's obsession with mechanics and mechanical pain. My gripe was this – yes, patients do come in with 'sharp' on-off pain. On, when you move to a certain position, and off, when you move away from it. Often it's quite repeatable and not infrequently the sharp pain gets less and movement range improves. It's just like a fresh cut on the back of your knuckle, fine when the finger is straight, but very sharp when you move it, but keep doing it and it soon feels freer and less painful, even though it may be bleeding again!

Now, with these on-off type pains, if you really listen and ask, there is nearly always a background discomfort going on and it's usually a low-grade aching pain. In some patients this is so low they discount it, in others it's very obvious and the patient comes forward with it straight away.

Joe has come in with nasty right sided mid cervical pain of three days duration. He can hardly move his neck more than 10 degrees to the right without a nasty sharp pain, but other movements are free, and he's comfortable when in neutral.

(A classic case of manual therapy 'mechanical pain' – and often deemed to be a 'blocked closing of a facet joint' that requires some kind of thrust/unlock manipulation?).

'Standing here now without moving, what do you feel?'

'Nothing.'

'Nothing at all?'

'Yeah, nothing!'

'OK, I want you to think about what you feel on the left side of your neck and then compare it to what you feel on the right.'

'Well, yeah, it's different...'

'Yes?'

'Well there's a little niggly awareness if I really think about it?

You get my drift?! Hopefully some of you will be thinking – ah, but Louis' being a nerdy pedantic pain himself and what he's doing is opening the 'pain gate' to consciousness of this guys neck – if he did that to me I'd probably feel a bit of an ache when there isn't any. I agree, but you need to try it on yourself and see whether you can manufacture a niggly background ache in your neck when you're standing still. I can't but maybe you can, and that's OK, but I believe that a great number of acute 'sharp' 'on-off' pain presentations do have an ache component – and that this ache component is a reflection of a 'chemical' process going on. The thought of doing a forceful thrust manipulation on an inflamed tissue doesn't fill me with much joy I'm afraid. My view is that this sort of treatment is nothing short of primitive and totally un-biological. Better see it like this – that the pain has a mechanically patterned element to it caused by a chemical sensitisation processes. If you wouldn't 'thrust' an acute and inflamed twisted ankle then you shouldn't do it to the acute and inflamed neck or spine pain problem either. (If you would 'thrust' an acute ankle I'm amazed you've got this far into the book!).

From a peripheral mechanism perspective an on-going acute problem 'ache' is likely to relate to on-going 'spontaneous' activity in sensory/pain fibres sub-serving the area. On-going ache here is likely to be caused by inflammatory algogens whose on-going presence makes the nerve fibres continuously fire. These algogens are 'excitatory' agents and if any one of them is dripped onto the end of a pain fibre it will fire a volley of impulses. The list of such chemicals grows and grows but here are a few: interlukin-1, hydrogen and potassium ions, histamine, bradykinin, serotonin, ATP and noradrenaline. Some of these chemicals have a dual role in that they can also cause the fibre to become 'sensitised' as described in the last section.

Explanations of on-going aching also needs to take into account ectopic impulse generating mechanisms in damaged peripheral nerve (see Nerve root sections); spontaneous central activity/central circuits – as in central mechanisms (sections 4, 5 and 6) as well as any issues that may facilitate the activity impacting consciousness – think things like attention, worry and fear about pain, annoyance with pain and so forth... Things that 'conscious-ify' symptoms! And one last one, the crafting of quite normal on-going tissue impulse barrages into pain by central mechanisms. Here, it's as if the processing and interpretation of normal processing has for some reason been shunted away from 'normal' sensory processing to being processed as 'pain.' Think of any hypersensitivity syndrome and you'll get what I mean. It's normal input being processed as 'threat,' something which is common to the Vulnerable Organism (chapter GE 2.3). I have in mind a patient, with no history of any physical trauma, who found light touch anywhere on her body – distressingly painful.

What about postural pain?

I love this because I thought about postural pain a great deal back in the 1980's working in Australia at Geoff Maitland's practice. Many of the chronic pain patients we saw had the diagnosis of 'RSI' – Repetitive Strain Injury, or 'Kangaroo Paw', because it seemed that Australians had it so bad. Even to the extent that when back in the UK, when we were first assessing a patient who had RSI-like symptoms we would politely ask them if they had any Australian blood or even whether they might have been to Australia recently and caught it? Sorry, only kidding, but it is good to rib those guys a bit for not even being able to get it together in an office let alone a cricket pitch!

OK, here's the easy experiment to try. See how long you can sit or stand perfectly still for. Simple, most people are quite happy to sit around all day long, eat, drink, watch TV, chill do nothing achieve nothing, just age a bit and let the clouds go by. But you've got to stay totally still for thirty minutes.

Not so simple I reckon. Take a time lapse film of folks just sitting around doing nothing and there isn't such a thing as being still – everyone's more or less constantly shifting and moving. If you can remain motionless for say fifteen minutes that's some achievement. Folk who learn meditation can sit very, very, still and those that practice for a life time may learn to be able to hardly move for many hours. It requires a great deal of practice. The other folk who are good at this are the 'stay-still' artists as I call them. You may have seen them in the street – usually dressed a bit weird, jokerish, faces and hands painted silver or white... just standing there not moving, frozen solid. They're actually referred to as 'Living Statues', do a search for them on the internet if you don't know what I'm on about! But here's a picture of one (figure 11.6) I find it so fascinating and can't help just gawping at them trying to see if they're going to move, but they don't, they barely seem to breathe. My point is that being completely still is something amazing. It's hard to really imagine doing it.

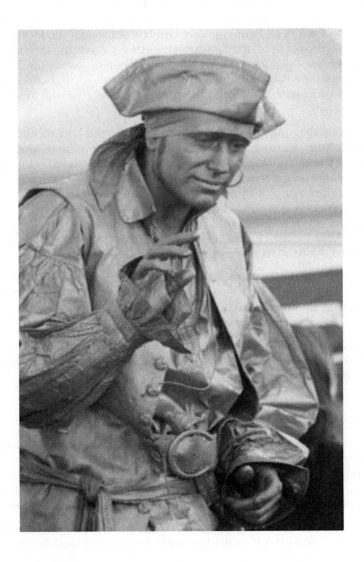

Figure 11.6 A 'Living Statue'.

Being completely still is a form of torture as far as I can see. Even sitting about or staying in bed day in day out becomes a source of distress as anyone who's been a bit poorly will know. So, stick humans in offices with fluorescent lighting and no windows, give them a keyboard and a screen and tell them to type the stock-market share values into some ghastly spreadsheet day in day out for a month or two. Not only is the task meaningless and mind-numbing but the being still and constantly concentrating is too. Even sleeping, though it is amazingly still, is plagued by some degree of movement for most of us. Getting comfy can be quite an art!

What's it all about? For me, and I emphasise, from a *tissue* perspective, one of the biggest deals is linked to ischaemia, lack of blood, a little discussed tissue-issue! Life is blood, life is oxygen, it is nutrients and it's clearance of toxic waste products too. Tissues need to flush in and out regularly. Death is ischaemia – no blood, no oxygen, no nutrients and no removal of toxic waste products. Witness the disastrous effects of circulatory diseases – that is ultimately gangrene, death of tissues and loss limbs and loss of life. Evolution therefore must have endowed us with an ischaemia reporting system that is processed in order to produce ischaemia relieving mechanisms and behaviours.

Sitting for a long time puts pressure on the tissues of your bottom and being in any position for a long time is going to be either squashing or stretching every single tissue that isn't moving. Pressure, stretch, compress, whatever – they all make it hard for circulation to get to the tissues and eventually they're going to want to have a flush-in and flush-out... If they don't get what they need and want, it seems wise that they're somehow going to send a message to the CNS that'll make you improve their situation. So, you clench and rub, you shift and move you stop what you're not doing and you get active. The feeling's pleasurable, the discomfort goes and the tissues are happy again... Hey, new rule: PAIN MAKES YOU MOVE!

Sub-conscious brain body monitoring Numskulls reporting to brainy.... 'Brainy, Brainy, come in Brainy... We're getting big inputs from butt, knees, back, base of neck and across shoulders – they're all getting really short of good quality blood down there... request a quick lift-off... Over ...'

'Brainy here, listen whingers, those guys can survive for days without a good blood supply, tell them to stuff it and wait 'til later, I'm like busy big-time on this GTA game with my mate Leonard...'

'Doh! ...'

(GTA stands for Grand Theft Auto for all you non computer gamers).

It does appear that tissues can survive well on a less than ideal blood supply – hence the relatively tolerable level of their pleas when they're becoming ischaemic. Think about it and you realise that for our hunter-gatherer forbearers to hunt and stalk effectively, or hide effectively – they will have needed to stay very, very, still, sometimes for long periods. Little wonder that we have evolved 'ischaemic tolerance' then!

What little research there is tells us that ischaemic tissues release a great many of the algogens we discussed in inflammation earlier e.g. prostaglandins, bradykinin and serotonin.

A major clinical thing is that if we believe that good posture is sitting with a good lordosis, with the computer all set up so the eye level is at xyz cms above below and around the screen or whatever and your head has to be just like this and your TMJ just like that and your feet all angled at three fifths of four fifths of frig-all – then we're inadvertently giving ischaemia a big leg-up. The best sitting posture is what we all do without thinking about it – we wriggle and MOVE, we slump and lean forward, we lean back and we put our feet up, we sit upright and we twist, we cross our legs and we sit on our feet and don't ever tell me that this is WRONG. I despair at those treating acute back pain that insist their patient maintains lordosis (go to www.giffordsachesandpains.com for the McKenzie debate, it's old, but little has changed in the underlying philosophy as far as I can see). To me the McKenzie postural advice is the equivalent of splinting/increased tension/fear of movement.

Being comfortable in a chair is of course very nice but there should be a big warning label on it that reads 'SITTING DISEASE IS A MAJOR CAUSE OF ILL HEALTH – YOU MUST REGULARLY GET OUT OF THE CHAIR AND MOVE – PREFERRABLY GETTING OUT OF BREATH.'

I think it's amusingly ironic that pew seating in churches is probably the most uncomfortable ever invented...

'Well, I gave going to Church a try, but no soon as I sat down in the pew my body told me that it would be far better if I walked right back out...!' Think about Muslim worship as having something to offer the lazy westerner? It gets you out of your chair onto the floor, it gets full knee, back and hip flexion and feet extension, you move a fair bit and you get to do it four times a day... I'd recommend a bit more... Plus sell the settee...

So in with church pews and Muslim prayer exercise rituals and out with crazy ergonomic and mechano-anatomical postural rigidity fascists. But if you do have to sit for long periods find the most comfortable way of doing that for you... but get out of the chair regularly. Movement is life... ischaemia is degeneration and death. I sit for long periods writing this and my method is two pillows under my little bottom and one more behind my back. That is all free advice, and it's taken six million years of evolution to sort.

If you've ever fallen asleep with your hands above your head and woken up wondering what happened to your arms you've experienced acute nerve ischaemia. It doesn't actually hurt; you just lose the part of your body that's supplied by the nerve that's stopped functioning. The perfect virtual amputation!

In human pain studies ischaemic pain is used as a pretty easily standardised and non-damaging way of creating pain in volunteers. Most people have had their blood pressure taken at some point in their lives – the cuff pressure basically stops the circulation in your arm and then the pressure is gradually released – it's not particularly nice but it's a tolerable and OK sensation for most people. You wouldn't call it 'acute' pain by any stretch of the imagination.

What pain researchers do is put a cuff around your arm holding the pressure at a level that stops the forearm circulation and then get you to work the muscles of the forearm by repeatedly gripping your fist. Now this soon becomes painful and nasty whereupon the researchers start pratting about with their 'variables' – like 'I want you to start counting backwards in threes from 1,999 as fast as you can until I say stop. If you get it wrong I want you to go back and start again...' Most folk find this stressful and the researchers now find out about your reported level of pain when you're under cognitive stress and you're attention is elsewhere... It's really a 'weirdo' way of finding out what GTA players already know... that when you're mind's focused on something powerful, bodily pain issues get side-lined for a bit – and in the old days this was all of great value to hunter-gatherers who's lives depended on their ability to put up with a bit of pain in order to make a bit of a gain!

Ah, but it doesn't always work like that, pain distracts and your cognitive efficiency takes a massive slide, you fumble the numbers... and the pain can be worse than it otherwise would be. It may all depend on the deemed importance of the stressor... GTA is far more highly rated than counting awkward numbers backwards. On the other hand a bit of pain endured while frozen still for the kill might change matters somewhat.

Now, if you do the same thing every day – say plucking chickens, or shearing sheep, or sitting at a computer, or hitting thousands of golf balls (Rory Mcilroy) or tennis balls (Andy Murray), or driving a taxi or a truck... you get my drift?... You can either get used to it and adapt, or, start finding it more and more uncomfortable and in the background it starts to establish those consciousness accessing circuits... maybe to the point that even thinking about it starts the pain... Small repeated little beginnings lead to ghastly chronic established pathways and misery... it's called RSI/overuse syndrome just like 'postural syndrome' is sitting too long... or something similar.

But, surely if you do something over and over it harms? Too little is just as bad as too much? Obsessional athletes who can't stop training end up injured and burnt out? Yes, correct, it's the 'Goldilocks' syndrome – not too much, not too little but just about right... for you. And everyone seems to be different in what is just right for them. The trouble is most peoples 'just right' is way off what it should be or what it could be. We live in an age of medical information being terribly biased to the caution and seek advice side of things.

Chapter 11.5
Nociceptive mechanisms 5: Tissue explanations for pain behaviour...

Is there anything else that controls all this in the tissues?

As is typical of the medical approach to research all eyes and resources have been focused on what makes pain worse, not what naturally makes pain better or controls it. Read any article or treatise on pain and tissue mechanisms and it'll be 99% 'pain-on' or 'inflammation-on' stuff, like it was super pathological rather than a 'normal' process... Luckily for pain science, Christopher Stein and colleagues (Stein et al 1997) forged the way and found that opioids were present in peripheral tissues and that there were opioid receptors all over the place... on sensory fibres, sympathetic post ganglionic fibre terminals and immune cells, especially in damaged and inflamed tissues. It seems that when there's some kind of wound or inflammation present refractory opioid receptors that are already present are activated... and, their production in the sensory cell-body is 'up-regulated' (that's up in the dorsal root ganglion) and they are transported down to the fibre terminals via axoplasmic transport... just as the pro-inflammatory and pro-sensitivity products are.

It's all good biology providing a balance between 'on' and 'off' chemicals in the periphery. You have to come to expect these things. The trouble is researchers are focused on the 'knowing what goes wrong means we can intervene to put it right' paradigm... rather than also going for... 'if we know how the body puts it right, maybe we can intervene and give it a leg-up' paradigm. Hey, ho.

The basic findings are that opioids do everything (having lived through the hippy period of the late 60's and early 70's I always knew that... nobody listened to us...):

- they reduce the excitability and sensitivity of nociceptive fibres

- they dampen the propagation of impulses

- they inhibit the release of pro-inflammatory peptides like substance P from C fibres and noradrenaline and neuropeptide Y from sympathetic terminals

- they thus reduce and control inflammation as well as plasma extravasation and vasodilation – hence they are anti-inflammatory and anti-oedema/swelling

- they elicit local analgesia and dampen the local immune response

- they inhibit bradykinin and hence prostaglandin production

They spoil the party...! Now that's not what happened when I was a hippy...!

It looks as if a major source of tissue opioids is via activated immune cells that are already present or from those that arrive via the circulation soon after the injury has happened. Examples of your local immune cell opioid 'suppliers' are the 'T' and 'B' lymphocytes, mast cells, monocytes and macrophages.

Opioids, and we mustn't forget the powerful anti-inflammatory/healing suppressing stress hormone, cortisol, can of course arrive from the circulation, although Stein and colleagues doubt this. Cortisol is released into the circulation via the 'HPA' axis from the adrenal cortex, and some opioids, (e.g. β endorphin) are released into the circulation from the pituitary as well as the adrenal gland (e.g. enkephalins). Both can be seen as playing a direct part in 'gate control' of pain in the tissues as well as stalling the healing response in stressful situations where resources are better put to use elsewhere.

It seems that 'stress' and the subsequent release into the circulation of corticotrophin releasing factor and cytokines may be factors in causing the release of opioids from immune cells in the tissues. Certainly stress has an impressive effect on healing, see chapter 15.4 later.

Stein's group were interested in the use of synthetic opioid drugs like morphine for the control of peripheral inflammation, for example in inflammatory arthropathies or following knee surgery and found that to be most effective the drug had to be introduced directly into the joint.

It seems that 'local' stress, i.e. injury, is key to the release of local opioids and hence local control of inflammation and nociceptor activity... hence, indirectly, the control of pain via its influence on nociceptor activity.

One thing is fairly clear, a healthy immune system looks vital!

Can fluid movement explain changes in pain behaviour?

All refs below found here:

Gifford, L S (1995). 'Fluid movement may partially account for the behaviour of symptoms associated with nociception in disc injury and disease.' In: Shacklock, M O (ed) Moving in on Pain. Butterworth-Heinemann, Australia.

Gifford, L S (1995). 'The influence of circadian variation on spinal examination.' In: Boyling, J and Palastanga, N (eds) Grieve's Modern Manual Therapy, Churchill Livingstone, Edinburgh.

These articles can be downloaded for free from: *www.giffordsachesandpains.com*

Way back in 1995, some consistent clinical observations of pain behaviour stimulated my interest. And a very common one, with acute low back pain, pain flare-ups related to 'degenerative' joint disease and some muscle and joint strains, was stiffness and pain on first moving after rest; followed by a rapid improvement. The 'back' patients often found it very difficult to get out of bed or a chair and that the longer they had been idle, the stiffer and more painful they became.

One key finding that interested me was the significance of morning stiffness in the diagnostic criteria for inflammatory arthropathies like Rheumatoid Arthritis, Ankylosing Spondylitis and Polymyalgia Rheumatica. It seemed that the severity of joint inflammation was strongly linked to the duration of morning stiffness. My observations were that it was common for the patient to report stiffness when moving after rest, and, just like the inflammatory arthropathies, anti-inflammatory medication often helped quite dramatically. The difference between the two groups was merely the length of time of the period of painful stiffness, my patients being usually only a few minutes or, in the case of severe low back pain, a maximum or around half an hour. Any longer than this and my suspicions were raised as to more serious joint pathology.

My own earlier research into circadian (24 hour) variations in movement range, which I'd done for the Adelaide course in 1985, had shown clear morning stiffness in flexibility of quite a few of the movements I measured. Classic forward flexion to touch toes showed the boldest pattern but with great variability between the few subjects I did. The whole thing was really stimulated by my own forward bending variability – hardly reaching past my knees on rising in the morning but within about thirty to sixty minutes I could easily reach to my ankles. A hot bath instantly freed me up which then made me think that such a quick result had to be due to changes in muscle tone and/or a decrease in sensitivity of the back of the legs where I felt the restriction. The restriction feeling had a very nasty 'go no further' tight feeling about it for quite some time.

Further, I measured my subjects through the night; I woke them up, got them out of bed, did the measurements and they then went back to bed. The 'stiffest' time for finger tip to floor flexion was around 6am and quite a few of them started to free up before they got up 'properly'.

I also measured lumbar flexion using goniometry and later compared my results to those of Adams et al 1990 who 'creep-loaded' individual lumbar 'motion segments. Creep loading goes like this: if you take a ligament and attach one end to a clamp so that it's dangling vertically, and then attach the dangly end to a weight, you will find that over time the ligament gets gradually longer. It 'creeps' and over time fluid is expelled. Adams et al took fresh cadaver lumbar spines, sawed out a lumbar motion segment, i.e. a vertebrae-disc-vertebrae devoid of all muscles but keeping the ligaments and discs intact and clamped the lower vertebra in a vice. The top vertebra was loaded to simulate the amount of force that would occur with sustained bending and then it was left to see what would happen. They found that an individual lumbar segment would increase in range by about 2-3 degrees. Extrapolating this to all the lumbar motion segments gives between 10 and 15 degrees of movement, which surprisingly actually agreed with my rather tin-pot goniometer measurements. I found a mean variation of lumbar flexion to be around 13 degrees; and that all were stiffer first thing in the morning on rising. Fluid expression from the discs due to loading on rising looks to be a key factor although changes in tone/and or length of the back muscles can't be discounted as a parallel factor and one that's likely to show quite marked inter-individual variability I would think. You may be interested to know that muscles very quickly shorten if immobilised in a shortened position. Gossman et al (1982) showed that within a few hours of immobilisation the number of sarcomeres in a muscle starts to decrease (see chapter 13.3).

In my study I asked the subjects about feelings of stiffness and found that 76% of them (they were all in their 20's) recorded feelings of stiffness that coincided with the times of least range of movement. Morning stiffness is almost a normal experience for most of us! Bradley and Tennant (1992) noted that 65% of over 50 year olds reported feelings of morning stiffness. As Bywaters (1982) neatly said, *'Man starts as a jelly and ends as a stiff!'* It could well be that in the presence of tissue abnormality, like degenerative changes, or internal disc disruption, muscle injury etc. that the normal feeling of stiffness becomes amplified.

Let's return to fluid movement and in particular the disc, the so called 'largest avascular structure in the body' that relies on fluid movement in and out, and hence on our physical movement, for nutritional supplies and sewerage activation. Discs are known to imbibe fluid over night and we grow in stature. The youngest amongst us may grow as much as much as 2% of our body height, the oldest only 0.5% and the average for us middle aged folk is 1%. If you decide to go into outer-space you can even reach 3%. You're now turgid!

Due to osmotic gradients vying with physical pressures there is a constant flow of fluid. Take pressure off the spine and the osmotic pressure wins out, the disc fills, becomes turgid and the spine stiffens up – ask your kids? Ah, they don't report struggling to get their pants and shoes on in the morning do they...? Good point.

This happens not only for disc but for all musculoskeletal tissues too. Think collagen, poor circulation and osmosis versus pressure (that's squashing, as in the back of your bent knee when you're praying to Mecca... and stretching, as in the front of your knee when praying...). If you're like me (60 now), and squat for any length of time, you'll 'Ooo' and 'Ah' a bit when you get back up. Fluid movement may be a component of the stiffening.

So, as we age or with injury, physical stress, ageing, dare I say 'wear and tear'... the collagenous tissues change – they become more 'osmotic', because of all those inflammatory/healing/degeneration related chemicals. For those who did a bit of biochemistry, osmotic pressure directly relates to the concentration of molecules, the higher the concentration – the higher the osmotic suction force produced. That's why we're taller in the morning and that's a major mechanism causing swelling following injury/inflammation.

Think about the injured disc: poor nerve supply, poor circulation, incredibly sluggish response to it all, slow gradual increase in a few inflammatory/healing related chemicals, slow activation of its sensory fibre population; sleeping nociceptors wake up... and hey, its morning already and he's got to get out of bed... 'Arghhh... can't move...' Last night he was a little aware he might have strained his back, but now it's completely seized! That is a very common experience for humans. Do you think it happens to the cat or dog too?

So: slow activation of the pain system, plus build up of chemicals means a more turgid than normal disc, if the annulus is still intact, which equates to pain and painful stiffness... but hey, you're a mm or so taller! If you do manage to get up and move, the disc gets compressed and turgidity lessens... the annular fibres are less stretched and there's maybe a little less nociceptor activation when you move... It can take a few minutes or maybe if really fired up as long as half an hour. In Ankylosing Spondylitis when in an inflammatory phase the 'in disc or in spinal segment' inflammatory activity is likely more widespread and more intense, hence longer to free in the morning.

Now, it's not just inflammatory chemicals that attract fluid into the tissues via osmosis. There's a chemical called hyaluronic acid (HA), a member of the glycosaminoglycan family, that has hydrophilic, or water loving properties. Not only does it attract water, it appears to grab it and actually slows and resists its flow, it thus makes fluid more viscous. HA 'lubricates' and is in all collagenous tissues and there's more of it in damaged and healing tissues because it's manufactured during inflammation. The more there is the more fluid it grabs and the more it resists its flow. Back in the mid to late 1980's Engstrom-Laurent and Hallgren (1987) and Lindqvist et al (1988), showed that HA actually passed out of the tissue into the circulation (via the lymph system) when we got moving in the morning. Measures of blood plasma show low levels before rising and a doubling once the subject measured gets up and becomes active. Lindqvist et al also looked at RA sufferers and showed that they had 8 fold higher levels of HA, which rise even further on rising!

So, early morning getting going movement... HA out of the tissues, along with fluid... along with other algogens (inflammatory chemicals that produce pain), along with many other by-products of metabolism (thinking 'sewerage' helps), the sensory sampling fibres go 'ahhh' thank goodness for that...' and although a bit nasty to start with, we feel a whole lot better.

Movement – the great 'flusher', don't just do ten little reps three times a day... get out of breath and do for your body what it's designed to do... get the heart and cardiovascular system going... get out of breath, feel all those endorphins come and all the adrenaline go... and keep that HA on its toes too.

Earlier in this chapter I wrote up my traction treatment disaster... As well as forgetting about this patient I maybe should have listened to his symptom pattern? And expected a struggle off the couch post-treatment?

Thinking disc it may be important to see that for this stiff-move-freer-rest-stiffen pattern it's likely that the normal 'young' hydrostatic mechanism should be fit and well. Thus, any breach of the outer annulus, via fissures to the interior, is likely to spoil things. Many ageing discs have plenty of fissures, the annulus is disrupted and the nucleus becomes annular like. It is well known that the ageing disc becomes less hydrated. Sudden breaching of the annulus, as in 'classic' disc herniation, is likely to upset the hydrostatic mechanism. It is not uncommon for patients back pain and stiffness patterns to change when they develop sciatica. For example, they often report that their ghastly difficulty getting moving in the mornings and after rest... is the one thing that has improved!

I've suspect I've 'blown' a few patients' discs in my time... and caused sciatica... anyone else want to come to the confessional with me? What's the culprit? Ah, forceful manipulation... the yearn for the click... and repeated extension movements after centralisation (as per Mckenzie doctrine)... wait a day or two or five and it can turn into full blown sciatica. That's a story for the nerve root section of the book.

Lastly I cannot leave this section guilt-free without including a mention of central processing and individual reactions to pain. As I've described here, this 'stiffness' pattern can be given a reasonable tissue explanation, but surely there must be central factors aiding and abetting too? While rapid changes in symptoms using simple movement and simple home exercises can be reasoned via changes in fluid volume and the washing out of inflammatory algogens from the area the sustained improvements and quick 'resolution' often gained cannot. This so called 'discogenic' pain thus improves and disappears far faster than any tissue biological changes could ever account for. It's a safe bet to take that the anatomical state of the disc when painful as compared to two weeks later when the pain has resolved, will be exactly the same... and the same or worse, but definitely not better, months or years later.

Nothing's been anatomically fixed – perhaps a bit of a scar bodge job, but probably we can assume that:

a) The physiological environment around the sensory fibres could have changed? Fewer, or no algogens of significance, for example and maybe far more endorphins were secreted because the immune system got in there and did it's thing; thanks in part to a healthy reduction in problem related stress caused by the therapist-patient interaction and a subsequent increase in well-being and sense of control?

b) The sensitivity of the 'sampling' fibres (C, Aδ etc) returned to normal, i.e. their firing threshold increased.

c) Spontaneous impulse activity decreased – due to less algogens being in the vicinity and more endorphins ('gate control' in the tissues). Altered population of ion channels and receptors in the terminals – via down-regulation of genes responsible for channel and receptor proteins in the dorsal root ganglion – hence less efficient transduction and therefore less nociceptive traffic.

d) Central inhibitory effects, some of which will reflect 'chemically' down to the sensory/sampling nerve fibre terminals. For example, by quelling the dorsal root reflex and antidromic impulse activity.

e) A great deal of this could come from changes in the way the individual with the problem deals with the situation. Lowered concern, feeling more in control, getting going again, functionally and work wise. Pain less of a problem... not thinking about it... they're starting to get more confident with the back... etc. Think about it and you see the brain changing sensitivity and firing via... endocrine, neuro-endocrine, psycho-neuro-immune... as well as via impulse directed influences... sympathetic post ganglionic... dorsal root reflex... central inhibition etc.

f) It's clever stuff. Fascinating...!

Sympathetic nervous symptom thoughts next!

Section 11
Read what I've read

Adams M.A. et al., (1990) Diurnal changes in spinal mechanics and their clinical significance. Journal of Bone and Joint Surgery: 72B:266-270.

Cervero F., Laird J. M. A. (1996) Mechanisms of touch-evoked pain (allodynia): a new model. Pain 68: 13-23.

Coppes M. H., Marani E., et al., (1997) Innervation of painful lumbar discs. Spine 22(20): 2342-2349.

Donnerer, J., Schuligoi R. et al., (1992) Increased content and transport of substance P and calcitonin gene-related peptide in sensory nerves innervating inflamed tissue: evidence for a regulatory function of nerve growth factor in vivo. Neuroscience 49(3): 693-698.

Gifford L.S. (1995) The influence of circadian variation on spinal examination In: Boyling, J and Palastanga, N (eds) Grieve's Modern Manual Therapy, Churchill Livingstone. Edinburgh.

Gifford L.S. (1995) Fluid movement may partially account for the behaviour of symptoms associated with nociception in disc injury and disease. In: Shacklock M.O. (Ed) Moving in on Pain. Butterworth-Heinemann. Australia.

Julius D., McCleskey E. (2006) Cellular and molecular properties of primary afferent neurons. In S. McMahon and M. Koltzenberg (Eds) Wall and Melzack's Textbook of Pain (6th Ed). Churchill Livingstone. Edinburgh.

Lin Q., Wu j. et al., (2000) Neurogenic inflammation following intradermal injection of capsaicin is partially mediated by dorsal root reflexes. In M. Devor, M. C. Rowbotham and Z. Wiesenfeld-Hallin (Eds) Progress in Pain Research and Management, Vol 16. IASP Press. Seattle.

McMahon S.B., Bennett D. L. H., et al., (2006) Inflammatory mediators and modulators of pain. In S. McMahon and M. Koltzenberg (Eds) Wall and Melzack's Textbook of Pain (6th Ed). Churchill Livingstone. Edinburgh.

Meyer, R., Ringkamp M, et al., (2006) Peripheral mechanisms of cutaneous nociception. In S. McMahon and M. Koltzenberg (Eds) Wall and Melzack's Textbook of Pain (6th Ed). Churchill Livingstone. Edinburgh.

Reichling, D. B., Gold M. (1996) Gate control begins in the primary afferent. The inflammatory perspective. Pain Forum 5(1): 45-50.

Schaible H-G., Schmidt R.F. (1988) Time course of mechanosensitivity changes in articular afferents during a developing experimental arthritis." J. Neurophysiol 60: 2180-2195.

Schmeiz M., Schmidt R., et al., (1994). Sensitisation of insensitive branches of C nociceptors in human skin. Journal of Physiology.

Schmidt R. F., Schaible K. M., et al., (1994). Silent and active nociceptors: structure, functions and clinical implications. In Gebhart G. F., Hammond D. L. and Jensen T. S. (Eds). Proceedings of the 7th World Congress on Pain, Progress in Pain Research and Management. IASP press. Seattle.

Schmidt R. F. (1992). Nociceptors and their sensitization: Discussion. In Willis W. D. (Jr). Hyperalgesia and Allodynia. Raven Press. New York.

Sluka K. A., Westlund K. N. (1993) Centrally administered non-NMDA but not NMDA receptor antagonists block peripheral knee joint inflammation. Pain 55: 217-225.

Sluka K. A., Willis W. D., et al., (1995) The role of dorsal root reflexes in neurogenic inflammation. Pain Forum 4(3): 141-149.

Section 12

THE SYMPATHETIC NERVOUS SYSTEM

Chapter 12.1
The sympathetic system: Nociception and oedema

Where does the sympathetic nervous system fit in?

I will review the sympathetic nervous system further when discussing the brain and output systems. For now I want to address some 'peripheral' aspects of this system. This is because research into the tissue mechanisms of pain always includes some 'sympathetic' system components. It's a bit of a historic thing, in that there's always been a fascination with the so called 'sympathetically maintained pain' states and with medicine attempting to reduce very complex pain presentations to mere sympathetic 'dysfunction'. The result, frequently and quite sadly, has been the adoption of an approach that seeks to destroy a system that is really rather badly studied and understood. You may have come across patients who have had a 'sympathetic block', a 'stellate ganglion block' or even more radically a 'sympathectomy' – ultimately it's butchery of one of biology's most profound and evolutionary long-serving homeostatic control systems. From more refined research in the last fifteen to twenty years it looks as if this much maligned system, that has taken the brunt of the blame in complex and difficult pain states with labels like 'causalgia', 'reflex sympathetic dystrophy' and 'sympathetically maintained pain' – actually isn't as guilty as was once thought.

For starters, the key to understanding the sympathetic system's role in pain is to appreciate that the sensory system – and C fibres in particular – can become highly sensitised to the sympathetically generated and secreted peptide 'noradrenaline' – which is also called 'norepinephrine' if you're using American terminology. Noradrenaline reaches the tissues in two ways: firstly, it is secreted directly from sympathetic fibre terminals in the tissues and secondly, from the adrenal medulla via the circulation. So, if the nociceptive/afferent peripheral fibres contain active adreno-receptors then adrenaline and noradrenaline become capable of causing nociceptor activity and hence pain and that's the long and short of what can sometimes be a very complex biology.

I'll come back to pain issues, but what I'd really like to promote is the role of the sympathetic nervous system in a positive rather than a pathological way. Why don't researchers start off looking into a system's normal and positive role? It baffles me. Well it does and it doesn't – all you have to do is realise that every research project is tailed by a drug company, looking for the next best intervention to patent for whatever is under study.

Just about every tissue in the body has a sympathetic supply – take skin, joint tissue, gut, blood vessel, muscle, you name it – and put it under an electron microscope with appropriate staining, you'll find masses of sympathetic nerve fibre networks and terminals. Remember Robert Schmidt and Hans-Georg Schaible from section 11 and that they'd counted the number of nerve fibres in the cat's knee joint? They included the sympathetic fibres in their counting and found 500 in the medial articular nerve and 515 in the posterior articular nerve – that's respectively about 60 and 100 more than the number of C fibres they found in each nerve.

Sympathetic fibres and terminals receive impulses from the central nervous system.

Remember, when an electrical impulse gets to the end of a nerve fibre it will cause it to spew into the tissues, whatever chemicals are in vesicles that may reside there. The sympathetic system is therefore an 'output, efferent or 'effector' system of the brain and CNS. SNS fibre terminals in the tissues act as micro-endocrine like organs whose main purpose is to secrete appropriate chemicals for day to day healthy function as well as to provide tissue healing support when damaged, diseased or injured. They're very like C fibres in this respect except unlike them they don't send impulses from the tissues to the CNS, as far as we know! Mick Thacker told me that the sympathetic fibres in the tissues – the unmyelinated 'post-ganglionic' sympathetic fibres, are in fact, virtually identical to C fibres!

I rather like the statement by Kasandra Hanna and Adam Katz in their 'Update on wound healing and the nervous system' article (2011).

'Innervation to the skin is predominantly sympathetic, and continually releases neurotransmitters and neuropeptides to maintain homeostasis in terms of sudomotor, pilomotor and vasomotor function. These functions are mediated by acetylcholine, norepinephrine, calcitonin gene-related peptide (CGRP), neuropeptide Y (NPY) and vasoactive intestinal polypeptide (VIP) among others.'

They then go onto discuss the critical role these neuropeptides have alongside those secreted from C fibres (e.g. substance P and CGRP) in wound healing and inflammation.

For example:

- they attract leukocytes (white blood cells) and lymphocytes to the wound site

- they make neutrophils 'degranulate' (explode their contents out)

- they provoke resident (i.e. things that are already there in the tissues) and normally dormant macrophages into action

- they promote the production of nerve growth factor (NGF) in mast cells, fibroblasts and keritanocytes (the NGF is yet another attractant for leukocytes and as we've already seen, it promotes the regeneration of nerves in the wound area – which in turn release more neuropeptides which may then promote further wound healing).

It seems that a sympathetic and C fibre presence is essential to tissue health and adequate healing.

These authors then review the 'animal model' research into the role of neuropeptides and healing. 'Animal model' means that researchers produce a disease in a rat or mouse similar to one that is found in humans. Diabetes is one such disease that can successfully be reproduced and studied in the humble mouse. It's well known that diabetics suffer poor peripheral circulation. Wounds in their distal extremities take a long time to heal and frequently ulcerate. In diabetic mice inspection of ulcers, that follow wounding of the distal hind legs, reveals no nerve fibres at all in the epidermis and dermis within 1 cm of the ulcer edge – that's quite a large distance for a mouse's leg! This is similar to that observed in ulcers of humans with diabetes.

Comparing the healing time of the diabetic versus normal mouse they found that it took 51.7 days for the diabetic and only 19.8 for the normal. **It seems that lack of a nervous system has a profound effect on healing.** To support this it was found that treatment of the wound with neuropeptides (in this case substance P) dramatically accelerated the healing. This fascinates me because it is very rare that you find research that actually finds that healing can be speeded up.

Researchers have also found that by a bit of clever genetic engineering they can 'knock-out' mice genes in order to stop them functioning and producing their protein product. The 'neuropeptide Y receptor knock-out mouse' (wow!) – is unable to produce receptors for NPY and therefore can't respond to NPY, even though it may be present. In these mice there is significantly delayed healing time. It was also found that adding NPY to a wound in a normal mouse helped speed up healing. NPY, as noted above is a neuropeptide produced by the SNS. It looks as if one of its roles is in promoting angiogenesis i.e. the growth and regeneration of blood vessels into the damaged area.

Calcitonin gene related peptide (CGRP) knockout mice also show a delayed healing. CGRP is an important pro-inflammatory and pro-angiogenic (promotes new blood vessels to grow) neuropeptide as well as having vasodilatory properties – hence its importance in reducing ischaemia.

If we look at the literature in the right places it is possible to find plenty of material that supports the positive effects of, rather than blames the role of the poor old sympathetic system, at the level of the tissue. For physiotherapy this is important because we're dealing with tissue healing, tissue recovery and tissue health in our day to day work – without some kind of 'medical' intervention.

It's important though, that we follow the sympathetic fibre tracts back into the spinal cord and up into the brain – where we find that they come to 'rest' in our stress control centres – the threat monitoring processors! Here, again, is yet another connection between what's going on in the mind, brain and the body that good therapists may have huge positive influences on and hence on the very wellbeing of any vulnerable tissues under our care.

Peripheral circulation control and oedema

Before getting back to pain and inflammation, let's not forget that one of the main roles of the sympathetic system is to control the peripheral circulation. A great many sympathetic fibres actually hitch a ride and course along with blood vessels to reach their destinations. They also innervate them too. Noradrenaline release causes the smooth muscles in the blood vessel walls to contract, hence narrowing the diameter of the blood vessel and slowing or even stopping the blood flow. If you get really scared you go very pale – the sympathetic nervous system has shut down the circulation to the skin and diverted it to where it's most needed – the musculoskeletal system for some physical action!

Nearly twenty years ago now, Helmut Blumberg and colleagues described, pondered and intervened in four rather interesting cases of acute RSD (i.e. reflex sympathetic dystrophy, what would now be called 'complex regional pain syndrome'). The fascinating thing about the cases was the dramatic onset of marked peripheral oedema, and that by using sympathetic blocking they were able to quickly resolve it. One blocking agent they used was guanethidine which you may be familiar with. Guanethidine is taken up into sympathetic nerve terminals and forces the noradrenaline out of its transmitter vesicles there. Guandethidine therefore deprives the fibres of their noradrenaline stores and in so doing blocks their action – it makes them impotent! Guanethidine is administered via injection into the venous system of a limb while a tight tourniquet is applied to it.

Case histories

I'll describe two of the cases and part of the third. The first is quite straightforward. A 37 year old normally healthy male bangs his elbow doing some housework. Not noticing any injury in particular he blithely carries on for an hour, then has a nap for a couple of hours, wakes up and finds to his horror that his hand is massively swollen and he's lost sensation in it. Lucky for him three days later he ends up in Helmut's special lab and they put his arm in elevation and observe it for a couple of days noting no change. They then did the 'block' and there was an immediate decrease in swelling! They did two more blocks at four day intervals and by the eigth day his swelling was gone and all function was back to normal.

The next case relates to a healthy 15 year old school girl who banged the top of her right foot. There was no skin lesion but during the night she developed diffuse pain, warmth and swelling in the foot that increased over the next twenty-four hours. The foot became paralysed. X-rays showed no bony lesion and all 'lab' findings were normal. Phlebography/venography (dye injected into the veins and an x-ray taken to see if all veins are patent) proved normal. Over the following two months various medications were tried and she was eventually found to have severe diffuse osteoporosis in the right foot. She was now diagnosed as having RSD and eventually ended up with Helmut and his team. They decided she needed continuous 'sympatholysis' via spinal anaesthesia. In other words they wanted to completely block her sympathetic system for a couple of days, and the only way to do this without destroying it was to neurosurgically implant a spinal catheter. They placed the catheter at the tenth thoracic vertebrae and regularly introduced the spinal anaesthetic bupivacaine to maintain a situation of complete paraplegia, complete loss of sensation and complete loss of any sympathetic activity! That 'sympatholysis' was occurring was indicated by an increase in temperature of the skin on the tip of her big toes, from 26 to 36 degrees on the affected foot and from 23 to 36 degrees on the normal foot. 'Paralysing' the sympathetic system, stops it's outflow, it's 'efferent' activity; and completely relaxes all the smooth muscles in the blood vessels of the lower abdomen and lower limbs affected by the anaesthesia – hence an increased blood flow and warming of the foot/toes.

Fifteen minutes after the start of sympatholysis the swelling started to diminish and this continued over the forty three hours of the procedure. One day after the treatment some swelling returned but after a further day or two this spontaneously went. After eight months there was no return of swelling and her motor and pain problems when standing gradually resolved.

Interesting! It seems to show quite powerfully that the sympathetic system is responsible for controlling circulation and mucking it up occasionally. I'm pretty convinced that we physios see 'sniffs' of this type of stuff in our day to day work with quite a few patients. I've a patient who's on treatment now for a recovering peripheral nerve problem and his left ankle has quite marked oedema for example.

A few comments for the sceptics though. In the first example, the elbow guy, they could have been lucky in that there was spontaneous remission – just when they intervened. Also, even though the guanethidine block is not very pleasant , having something done to help – an impressive procedure/intervention in this case , may lead to the feeling of relief – hence reduced sympathetic tone and hence the positive result (via a 'top-down' mechanism). Wouldn't it have been interesting to have tried hypnosis, deep relaxation or even anxiolytic drugs in the two day observation period? Anxiolytic drugs reduce anxiety, you may have heard of beta-blockers for example. These act by blocking 'adrenoreceoptors' – those receptors that adrenaline and noradrenaline act on.

In the second case there was clear evidence of loss of sympathetic tone, as evidenced by the marked increase in temperature of the big toe skin surface, but the intervention bupivacaine – produces total paralysis, hence all afferent and motor systems too – so it's hardly a system 'specific' intervention. Another consideration whenever impressive case histories are presented like this – is that there is never ever any coverage given to other similar cases who failed in the approach being publicised! These folks never like to spoil their sensational successes by going, 'Well actually we saw thirty-five patients and only these four responded well...' It's like those TV reality programmes that take unwilling, unhealthy people and make them fit and happy using a 'celebrity hypnotist' or celebrity 'life-coach-dietician-etc.' What they never reveal are the numbers of folks who failed to live up to the goals set or never responded and were rejected by the programmers. But, don't get me wrong – if I had the problems these cases had I'd be quite willing to have the intervention offered.

I'd just like to mention one of the other two cases – it's similarly spectacular to the two discussed but this one developed skin blisters within days of the onset of his leg oedema following an operation for a retroperitoneal haematoma (a big clot in the abdominal cavity). My point is that if something upsets the circulation to a tissue, then that tissue can very quickly become unhealthy. Clearly, an upset nervous system can upset the circulatory system – but so can prolonged postures, lack of movement and lack of cardiovascular fitness.

Swelling and oedema – dissected...

Let's now look at the swelling mechanism in relation to these cases. It looks like an incredibly maladaptive circulatory reaction.

A spinal reflex is usually understood as some kind of sudden or unusual input from the tissues creating a very quick local response. Step on a drawing pin and your foot pulls away, tap a patella tendon with a reflex hammer and your quads contract to jerk the knee forwards. It's all to do with peripheral-spinal-peripheral circuits that 'think' for themselves, they don't require other parts of the nervous system to tell them it's OK to go right ahead or no, not right now. They are 'sample-scrutinise-respond' loops that can't be stopped; although you may have read the claims of yogis who can deeply meditate, have someone let off a loud gun next to their ear and have no reaction, for example, no blink reflex, no increase in heart rate or change in blood pressure.

Right, so if you cut yourself this is a local medical emergency – our 'interoceptors' (nociceptors and all the other fibre that sample the tissues!) fire off their messages into the CNS and out pops a very quick sympathetic reflex message... 'Stop the bleeding, clamp off the blood vessels to the area NOW...!' In the healing literature this first phase emergency process is called 'haemostasis'. The impulses reach the smooth muscles of the blood vessels in the locality and they contract, thus squeezing the lumen of the vessel closed and slowing or even stopping the circulation. While the meditating yogi is bleeding to death, us normals are happy to have our reflexes stop the flow and lend a hand to the sucking and licking we're also doing to ease the situation (saliva has very useful antibacterial and anti viral enzymes and immune components). Once the coagulating process has done its job – (remember platelet plugs and fibrin clots?)... the next requirement is to get the inflammatory process underway. Ironically this requires quite a marked change in the local and immediately surrounding area – 'vasodilation'. Think of an almost completely deflated balloon as the normal state of the local capillary network and vasodilation as when it is blown up a bit... The effect of this increased pressure is the physical stretching of the capillary endothelial cell network so that gaps appear between the cells. These cells are also stimulated by inflammatory chemicals to contract in size, further widening the intracellular gaps. The result: a local outflow or leaking of fluid plasma into the damaged tissue area, along with a variety of blood borne chemicals and cells whose presence is vital to the efficient working of the early recovery process. This is a 'swelling' component of inflammation and, let it be emphasised, is a very positive biological process. The vasodilation and increase in vascular permeability is further aided and abetted by chemicals released from the damaged tissues and local sensory (e.g. C fibres) and sympathetic nerve fibre terminals too. For example, platelets release histamine and serotonin, and C fibres and postganglionic sympathetic fibre terminals release neuropeptides, many of which are vasodilators and promoters of vascular permeability and hence – of plasma 'extravasation.'

For vasodilation to occur there has to be a subtle pressure differential between the pre-capillary (arteriole) and post-capillary (venule) ends of the capillary network i.e. relative vasoconstriction at the 'post' end and relative vasodilation at the 'pre'

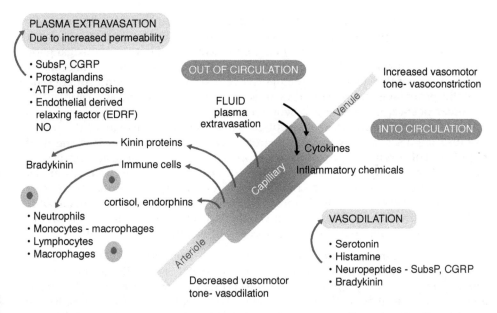

Figure 12.1 Some of the activities that go on in and around the capillary when the tissues have been injured.

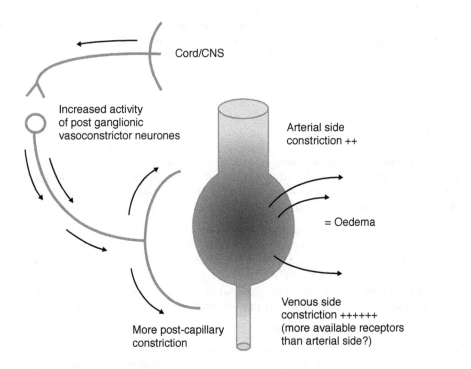

Figure 12.2 Illustration of how pressure is controlled in the capillaries when an injury has occurred.

end. (See figures 12.1 and 12.2 for summaries of this and capillary interactions.). How does that happen? We come back to Helmut and friends. Apparently, pre and post-capillary zones of the vascular bed are innervated separately by postganglionic sympathetic neurons and therefore provides the potential for independent regulation of the calibre of the vessels. In the figure I've re-drawn from Helmut's paper, note that the postganglionic fibre is drawn as branched, one to the pre-capillary side the other post-capillary. One may wonder how this could work but remember that it's not so much the number of impulses arriving but the reactivity of the muscles to those impulses that creates the degree of contraction. They key is simply the population of adrenoreceptors that are expressed there. The more adrenoreceptors that are there, the greater the contraction is likely to be. Since the post-capillary/ venous end contracts far more than at the pre-capillary end it stands to reason that there is a far greater population of adrenoreceptors there[1]. The result of this differential between the arteriole and venule end is that the capillary bed pressure increases and it 'balloons' out, fluid is forced out and hence – oedema!

When you were a student you probably learnt that oedema is not good – hence 'RICE' for the treatment of acute wounds – Rest, Ice, COMPRESSION, Elevation... and take those anti-inflammatory pills too... The idea is that you try to resist the inflammation and resist the swelling as if it's a bad thing. Well, evolution's been doing its thing for millions of years and it's worked out a good way to deal with wounding – it's called healing! With 'RICE' the goal appears to be to try and knobble its 'set-up' phase! Evolutionary reasoning (more later) requires us to always ask what's helpful or good about any observation before condemning it! Inflammation clearly sets the scene for tissue recovery – providing the best environment for new tissue growth; for preventing entry and multiplication of threatening micro-organisms; for the re-growth of damaged blood vessels and nerve fibres (let me underline here – even in a simple skin cut – some nerve fibres and terminal branches are bound to have been cut through – so that there is no getting away from nerve injury); for creating just the right amount of pain or discomfort in order to get the best pain behaviour requirements when chance arises... and so on. But it's all a fine balance and sometimes a component of it can get out of hand, or, maybe fail to work properly. The key clinical judgement should always ask the question – is the response I'm observing adequate, inadequate or over-the-top? Just as we can have maladaptive pain, so we can have maladaptive swelling and maladaptive inflammation too. Also, and vitally, it's important to reason that on the one hand there may be too much pain/swelling/inflammation/healing physiology... and on the other, too little.

So what's good about oedema? One proposal is that it helps to dilute the concentration of inflammatory chemicals and other breakdown products from the clearing up process going on. Oedema dilutes and therefore reduces their toxic effects. Clever! I'd also add that anything that is swollen feels pressured and becomes uncomfortable which in turn makes you do something about it! A swollen twisted ankle – it goes all stiff and uncomfortable, so you self massage it and move

---

1 - Mick Thacker tells me that there's emerging evidence that this expression may be reversed in CRPS – creating a bigger contraction at the arteriole end and thus inhibiting flow to the tissues!

---

it, you squeeze it and put on a 'compression' stocking and it feels a lot better as the oedema reduces. Clever!

So, swelling reduces the concentration of inflammatory chemicals – and at some point it gets to the stage where it needs to be moved on or washed out. The discomfort cleverly makes you do just that and it's all neatly shifted into the lymphatics and eventually back to the venous system. The process repeats itself of course and patients need to understand this as a positive and smart process – not a worrying one!

'Louis, is that you?'... 'Er, yes, it's half past midnight... ' 'Louis, well, Oh my God, the swelling's all come right back again... what'll I do... Dr ... Ambulance...?'

No wonder wearing compression bandaging feels good for a while but later starts to become annoying. Think carefully before telling patients that they **must** keep the compression going constantly, evolution dictates that lack of oedema for too long is not good – get the bloody thing off, let it swell, tell your patients a bit of up and down swelling is good, 'normalise it' rather than make it an issue to worry about. A bit of massage and moving is good and a bit of compression bandaging is good too – but take it off when it doesn't feel good and let it swell and dilute!

Any volunteers for a three month plaster immobilisation?

Now, back to Helmut and colleagues theories for their patients' massive and inappropriate oedema...

- a local lesion generates a nociceptive barrage into the CNS that sensitises the appropriate segmental 'spinal circuits' (see section 5). The subject gets some pain...

- the result of this spinal circuit excitation is an abnormal discharge pattern of sympathetic vasoconstrictor fibres, especially those to the venous side of the capillary bed. (Don't forget the lateral horn of the spinal cord is bang next door to the dorsal horn and that connectivity between the two is massive!)

- the oedema is generated because of the biased effect of the vasoconstrictor activity to the venous/post capillary side rather than the arterial pre capillary side. Blood can flow in but cannot get out, the balloon goes up, the fluid is forced out and the tissues swell...

- increased pressure within the oedematous tissues then excites and activates further the local nociceptive population producing more afferent barrage that further maintains the sympathetic vasoconstrictor tone...

Normally swelling is pretty much contained to the rough vicinity of the lesion – but in Helmut's patients the swelling was massive, a whole forearm and a whole leg – way out of proportion to any pathology or injury. My question is: could the observed 'over-reaction' be a function of their central sensitivity state? A massive Shane and Claudia and beyond type 'scenario'?

Let's think a bit more about this...

First, could the nervous system be pre-sensitised somehow – vulnerable to over-reaction? Later I'm going to discuss the 'Vulnerable Organism' model (see Graded exposure section) in some detail, but it's relevant to mention it here. My observation is that when an organism is 'low' – meaning, out of sorts, ill, diseased, stressed, running on low batteries, struggling to cope, starving, or generally weak for some reason – it hurts more easily. As I've already discussed, our sensitivity can vary, depending on the situation we are in, but also may relate to our general sense of well-being. It's certainly clear that we have a centrally placed sensitivity adjusting module somewhere in the hypothalamus (more later). You've all been there – you're poorly with flu, you've got a temperature and you stumble out of bed and knock into a chair, you're already aching all over and now this hurts intensely and far more than it would when you're normal and feeling well.

In the typically 'medical' way of presenting things, we don't know too much about any previous history, or the life and circumstances of Helmut's first example, the bloke who just banged his elbow, or the 15 year old who 'just' banged her foot, but the third example, the fellow who'd had an operation for an abdominal cavity haematoma was actually pretty poorly with renal failure and had been on dialysis for some time. He was certainly in a 'vulnerability' state.

Now, here's me with my clinical hat on again – I don't know whether all you experienced therapists have noted that there is no such thing as a complex patient presentation that hasn't some kind of a complex past? Their history is frequently laced with disasters, traumas and difficulties of both the physical and social/psychological kind and there's plenty of stress and plenty of stressors. To distil a complex past, into a bite-worthy nugget, is to simply state that vulnerability arising from past physical/ and or psychological trauma may well predispose the nervous system to entering a more sensitised state, or, that a state of maladaptive sensitivity is more likely or more easily achieved. I'll discuss the opposite, i.e. 'hardening' or desensitising, in the vulnerable organism chapter later (chapter GE 2.3). The important other side of this is that a great many humans go through traumatic situations and cope really well, some may even get hardened to them and report how their hard times helped them become a better person. How different individuals respond to different stressors is quite remarkable.

So, what I'm saying here is that in considering the reason for an over-the-top swelling reaction it is important to consider a maladaptive central sensitivity state, or predisposition to it, and then consider the reasons why it might be there. Here, I'm underlining listening to the individual's history in all dimensions and, listening for 'predisposing' factors (e.g. yellow flags, see chapters GE 4.5 to 4.9).

The next thing (and this may link to the yellow flag issues we've just been mentioning), could heightened sympathetic tone be a factor predisposing to an over-the-top swelling response? It's a simple pathway: central stress centre turned up, sympathetic tone goes up, sympathetic outflow goes up, vasoconstrictor tone goes up, and swelling goes up more than it otherwise would! Here's a thought – could anxiety about your swelling keep you swelling? Just like anxiety about your pain can keep your pain 'paining'?

Apologies, but it nicely illustrates the thinking and reasoning that may be required!

The trouble with this type of sympathetic based argument is why don't we see more 'tensed up' super swollen people? On the other hand, I have had so many patients who've responded well physically after being urged to react differently – to wind-down and accept the situation as 'normal', that I believe this sort of 'pathway of maladaptively maintained heightened activity' has to be very, very likely.

Here's the sort of patient...

'I know you twisted your ankle three months ago and you're still worried about the swelling. It'll go eventually – some people are quicker healers than others and sometimes swelling can be around for half a year, even a year, but still there's recovery and it goes. It's slow and it's normal. Now, we may be able to improve the situation and I want you to see how important it is to address the things I've pointed out to you today... Now, to recap on one or two...'

'You're worried about hurting it again – fair enough and as a result you're tense and protecting it all the time. When I managed to get you walking normally and relaxed and trusting the foot just now, you were a lot better – but your face was still screwed up! Screwing your face up means your 'tension' systems are on red-alert and your tension systems slow down your recovery and control systems and make them less efficient. Big lesson for you today – relax your face! Relax your leg! Practice walking relaxed when you're in a place where you feel completely safe, go as slow as you like, then build your confidence by going a little quicker, or by going to slightly less comfortable places. Trust your leg and your foot, smile, flow, soften, chill, go easy, the gradual aim is to get it to a place where you start to stop thinking about it so much... '

If you are able to shift a patient's thinking and they are truly 'structurally', 'pain' and/or 'recovery' reassured, they can often move quickly to a better place. The patient gets the message and they can make dramatic improvements... brilliant!

The above patient divulges, when seen sometime after they're better, 'The best thing you said to me at the last appointment was, 'relax your face and trust your leg'... it was then I realised I was responsible for holding it all back... ' and they have a nice big grin. I had taught them a bit of explicit 'top-down' stuff and they quickly picked it up and understood. As a result they quickly changed their CNS 'threat' settings back to a more adaptive level. It sounds simple to do but there's a great deal of trust to be built up before someone listens, understands and takes it on board. I'm now good at observing this and knowing when to talk to a patient in this way but it's taken me many years to get it just right!

In the next section I return to inflammation and the sympathetic nervous system.

Chapter 12.2:
The Sympathetic system: Variation in inflammatory response

Now, what about variation in the inflammatory response? I'm just touching the surface of the known biology of inflammation in these sections – it is marvelously complicated and generally described in terms of 'pro-inflammatory' markers (chemicals), with very little said about those that may actually do a bit of controlling and dampening down. Again, medical research focuses on what causes pathology and symptoms, not what might actually be controlling it – hence the terrible paucity and imbalance in just about all the pain and inflammation and inflammatory disease related literature.

As I've already stated, if we could only understand the natural controlling mechanisms and what influences them we might be much better at coming up with more efficient management strategies. I guess Rottweiler therapy is always an option for the intolerant-neo-fascist-instant-success-therapist-dictatorship. But seriously, the 'relax your face' illustration used at the end of the last chapter more than likely has a well demarked action pathway(s), for example, via a change in sympathetic tone. Changes could just as easily occur in inflammatory controls – again via sympathetic pathways but also via neuro-endocrine, central processing, psycho-neuro-immune and many others. What I'm getting to is that with those three case histories of Helmut and colleagues – could it be that their normal **inflammatory control systems** were weak or compromised in some way?

As research methods grow in sophistication it is becoming more and more feasible to drag unique and personal therapeutic interactions into the realms of reductionist, measurable and researchable biology (see Benedetti refs).

A mention here, for a moment, on focused or local effects. In the 'relax your face' example I was talking quite generally in terms of increased tension or tone for the patient. But the 'relax your face' effect needed to be local, in terms of the swollen and stiff ankle, and it was! Can the sympathetic system be so focused in its effects? Maybe it can, especially if you consider the 'lateral horn' of the spinal cord (the area where the peripherally coursing pre-ganglionic neurones of the sympathetic system have their origins) to be like the dorsal horn. 'Like it', in the sense of being under the influence of local and remote excitatory and inhibitory controls – Shane and Claudia again! So, here in the lumbo-sacral section of the lower spinal cord, where ankle joint sensory segmental impulse traffic arrives via the peripheral sensory fibres, where somatotopically organised descending fibres with their inhibitory and excitatory commands come to synapse and where motor and sympathetic/autonomic messages relay on to their destinations, there is a hive of integrating and modulating activity!

Oh, the language of neuroscience! That was a rather poetic pile of bull which basically means that there's a junction box in the wiring diagram whose inputs and outputs can be modified! It's just like the dorsal horn. Local inputs cause local outputs – incoming nociceptive inputs give rise to a reflex sympathetic output causing localised peripheral vasoconstriction for example. Loss or lifting of local and descending inhibition leads to a widening of the effect and a more diffuse and expanded area of oedema... recall the discussion on receptive fields in the dorsal horn chapters earlier? In contrast, an increase in inhibitory currents should result in a much more focused and reducing oedema.

To make it simple... the junction box acts like a dimmer switch! ... if it works for sensations and for pain, why not local sympathetic activity too?

What's also important is that inhibition or the lifting of inhibition and instigation of excitation can be influenced by the mood, concern, attributions and well-being of the individual concerned. This effectively becomes a 'top-down' influence on the physiological responses and goings on in the tissues and their processing circuits.

It's always puzzled me how often the sympathetic response is described as 'generalised' yet at times of injury it can be very precise. What about if I'm in a 'fight-or-flight' situation and I'm going to need full power to my legs in order to run, or to my arms if I'm going to stay and fight, doesn't the 'generalised' sympathetic response supplying circulation have some degree of control over where it allows circulation to go?

Maybe the following sheds some light on this...

I've always wondered why when I go running and I'm mentally a bit wound up I really struggle, yet when I'm relaxed my performance is so much better. According to Passatore and colleagues, sympathetic activity produces a 'generalized tonic **constriction** of arterioles, pre-capillary sphincters and venules.' They astonishingly apply this to all sympathetically innervated tissues! Well, that's fine for the guts, the immune system, the reproductive system and the healing and repair system, which you want to shut down, but what about the musculoskeletal system that needs to get physically stuck into dealing with the situation? The circulation here doesn't shut down surely, and if it doesn't why doesn't it? According to these authors, in all active tissues and organs which includes muscle, blood flow will **increase** because the 'tonic sympathetically induced vasoconstriction is antagonized and over-ridden by **metabolite-induced vasodilitation**.

The chemistry in the tissues nullifies the sympathetic antagonism!

It's 'ass-about-tit' as we say here in Cornwall.

Or, as an aside, it's a good example of 'unintelligent' design. For your interest, the recurrent laryngeal nerve is one of the best examples of an 'ass-about-tit' 'design flaw'. Two branches of the laryngeal nerve supply the larynx. The laryngeal nerve is a 'cranial' nerve, so it leaves the brain and travels down towards the larynx. It gives off one branch that goes straight to the larynx and as Richard Dawkins states, 'Much as a designer would have chosen'... the other branch doesn't go straight there though, it wanders down the neck into the chest to about level with the heart, loops round the dorsal aorta before going back up to the larynx – a crazy detour of quite a few inches. Now take a look at a Giraffe's recurrent laryngeal nerve to its larynx – it's about fifteen feet long when it only needs to be an inch or two. Wow!

So what happens is the muscles, heart, lungs etc. get the nod to start working really hard. The SNS in parallel tries to stifle them by strangling their circulatory supply, these tissues then start producing 'activity' chemicals which include powerful enough vasodilators to nullify the SNS and the whole thing cobbles together a good enough response. I hope the reader is seeing great potential here for 'imbalance'! Not enough vasodilators and too much SNS activity equates to insufficient blood supply and stresses the system even more.

I now know why I run so poorly when I'm wound up and how the circulation can be well localised to where it's needed. I also have one good reason why a great many 'problem'/'distressed' patients might struggle to do even the most basic of exercises. If the circulation doesn't meet the needs of the tissues you get relative ischaemia/ hypoxia and then a build up of toxic metabolic by-products. This equates with 'tired and heavy' muscle discomfort. These authors suggest that this may be a mechanism underlying exercise induced muscle inflammation, damage and chronic pain. It's certainly worth bearing in mind and it's worth noting that oxidative stress is held responsible for deposition of connective tissue undergoing fibrotic degeneration in numerous tissues and organs including muscles.

Is this a way of linking ong-oing stress, to increased SNS activity, to yet further detrimental tissue changes? Joint stiffening – like frozen shoulder, OA changes and stiffening in vertebral and peripheral joints, muscle pain syndromes like fibromyalgia etc.etc?

Thornell and colleagues have looked at muscle biopsies of patients suffering from 'trapezius myalgia'. They showed that there are 'ragged red' and 'moth-eaten' fibres present. That are '… typically associated with mitochondrial myopathies, similar to the picture emerging in animal models of ischemic muscles... and also a reduction of relative capillary density...' These authors feel that there is an underlying disturbance in the microcirculation.

Now we can't leave this chapter without some rat experiments! Jon Levine's the big guy here – he was doing loads of experimental arthritis ('EA' as opposed to 'OA'!) research on rats back in the 80's and early 90's.

Believe it or not rats can be bred that are 'hypertensive'. They're super jumpy and flighty and not very good at meditation, watching the clouds go by or taking their time over things, compared to 'normotensive' rats. Inject our seaweed extract/sexy lubricant/joint inflammation promoter, carageenan, into a rat's knee or ankle joint to produce 'EA' and it's noted that the hypertensive rats show a much more severe inflammatory reaction than the normotensive ones. What this is basically saying is that **when there's increased sympathetic tone the inflammatory arthritic reaction is more severe.**

Clinically, this translates into including anything that might reduce stress in the patient's life, when guiding patients through a healing process. It has been mooted that it's the reduction in stress, rather than the medications, that helps hospitalised rheumatoid arthritis (RA) patients get through painful flare up phases of their condition. If, when being in hospital you consider that the patient is taken out of their home environment; for example, a mother with RA may have to care and look after her husband and family, her house and everything else that day to day life throws out her. For some, being in hospital and being fed, watered and cared for may provide just the right environment for the body's physiology to work more efficiently. In the good old days well-to-do patients were sent to the Swiss mountain-air resorts for rest and recuperation. These days it's more likely to be a sojourn on your local 'Liz Siccley' ward at the top of the West Tower Block!

If only nursing and general medicine understood and felt comfortable with this sort of stuff, there might be more effort to create these sorts of Alpine environments in hospital departments! Esther Sternberg's book, 'Healing Places' takes a good look at this and provides some remarkable evidence. Esther is a world authority and researcher on stress.

It's time to come back for a summary and tidy-up inflammation in relation to the SNS and I will just list a few final interesting points.

1. As I've already mentioned, noradrenaline doesn't normally have any effect on nociceptor activity and hence in producing pain. Interestingly, there is some evidence to suggest that sympathetic outflow may even suppress nociceptor activity to acute noxious stimuli. Others have shown that it may even block inflammation. This all makes sense when considering the importance of conserving resources by stopping any healing processes in the presence of acute and threatening stressors. Fight or flight requires all the resources it can muster, so it makes evolutionary sense that a system should evolve that can quickly switch off the healing response – hence switching off the inflammatory component of it. So, if you're suffering too much inflammation... excite your life up a bit... get scared... (I've suddenly and rather naughtily thought of all those puffy swollen post total knee replacement knees lining up for a bungee jump while the surgeon isn't looking... oops!). If your healing isn't happening though, do the opposite... get chilled down... go listen to whales and dolphins talking and let the batteries re-charge.

2. In inflamed tissues, noradrenaline <u>can</u> stimulate nociceptors and cause pain – they've injected it into inflamed skin of human volunteers and it's not nice! You can also get the same effect by stimulating the sympathetic chain up near the vertebral column. The key mechanism related to noradrenaline sensitivity is the presence of active noradrenaline receptors (adrenoreceptors) on the terminal branches of nociceptors.

3. It seems that the sympathetic terminal branches may act as 'docking stations' – bringing together various pre-inflammatory chemical 'products' and causing them to produce active inflammatory 'end products'. Pre-cursor chemicals for bradykinin, nerve growth factor and prostaglandins are thought to rely on this docking process. After the separate components 'dock' they then combine to produce the finished product. This is a seemingly passive process but is reliant on the sympathetic post ganglionic fibres having the relevant 'docking' stations in their cell walls. Neat, I could maybe take my next 'Ikea' flat pack there to be put together!

4. Another weird one is that noradrenaline and substance P released by sympathetic terminals may actually 'dock' back onto the terminals from where they were released and in so doing aid in the production of inflammatory end products! The feature of having an effect on the very structure that releases you is termed 'autocrine' and will be familiar to those who study the endocrine system.

5. Some 'rat' work has shown that the sympathetic system's major effect in inflammation is in the more chronic phase – hence blocking its activity three weeks after injury significantly reduces inflammation (e.g. Sluka et al 1995). SNS activity may therefore be a significant factor in maintaining inflammation as time goes on. The clinician has to make a decision as to whether the inflammation observed is adaptive or maladaptive and if considered maladaptive to then, among many other things.... get a feel for the level of stress and tension in the patient's life and include some means of managing it, if necessary. Relaxation, meditation, mindfulness and even more active relaxation like Tai-chi and yoga may have important roles to play in helping provide better healing conditions.

6. I'm wondering if the reader is starting to get a little confused! For example: we have discussed the role of oedema, or plasma extravasation, in recovery and I argued that it was a good thing. Further, in rat experiments plasma extravasation has been shown to reduce the level of damage from EA (see Levine refs). This suggests that keeping sympathetic tone high, to promote swelling, would be a good thing! On the other hand... EA can be decreased significantly if sympathetic post ganglionic nerves are slaughtered before doing the injection that produces the EA! It can also be reduced if prior to injection the sympathetic outflow from the brain stem is blocked by injecting morphine! If you perform an adrenal 'medullectomy' on a rat prior to injection it also reduces the intensity of the inflammatory arthritic reaction. A medullectomy basically removes the adrenal medulla. The adrenal gland sits on top of the kidney and has two parts – the adrenal cortex that produces 'cortisol' (more on this later in the stress chapters) and the adrenal medulla that produces adrenaline and pores it into the circulation. A medullectomy thus reduces the levels of circulating adrenaline. Since adrenaline can act on adrenoreceptors it may well have a role to play in inflammation. The big consideration here is that carageenan or any other provocative toxic chemical injected into a joint or tissue is just not playing fair. In evolutionary terms this sort of thing just isn't day to day life and therefore hasn't evolved a reasonable counter-reaction – so how can we expect a reasonable reaction in return? A massively sudden and toxic input gets a massive response... including a massive secretion of inflammatory neuropeptides from C fibres and SNS fibres – no wonder blocking, cutting or destroying these fibres quells the reaction.

All this stuff is basically telling us that these systems have a role to play in trying to restore the status quo – give them a break!

7. ... last one here. In humans it's been noted that a stroke prior to the onset of rheumatoid arthritis yields less severe joint lesions on the paralysed side...

What I get from all this is the fact that the nervous system has a very important role to play in healing, for example, steering and controlling inflammation and swelling; chemically supporting inflammation and chemically supporting the control of inflammation. Its roles may be direct or indirect; for example neuropeptides not only exert effects via adding to the inflammatory soup, but also, via action on available immune cells and in turn on their complex physiology and biochemistry. I would emphasise that the scientific evaluation of pain has largely kept the focus of attention on inflammation in its acute phase. Three weeks to an animal researcher is 'chronic' yet for human pain states it may be nowhere near it.

My message is this – think 'dimmer switch'. That all these novel healing processes have evolved to work optimally and largely they do, for the most part we all heal eventually and get on with life; but sometimes they run amok, with too little (dimmer switch turned down) or too much (dimmer up), with some of the dire consequences discussed. Consider the massive whole leg oedema of the RSD patients, or inflammation running out of control and becoming destructive as in rheumatoid or osteoarthritis. The ability to turn a process on and off, or dampen and promote, may be to blame, but in terms of survival, life is all about a need for control of resources to fit with the circumstances we find ourselves in. This is what I believe underlies the promoter and controller aspects in the mechanisms we're discussing.

Section 12
Read what I've read

Benedetti F. (2009) *Placebo effects: Understanding the mechanisms in health and disease.* Oxford University Press. Oxford.

Benedetti F. (2011) *The patient's brain: The neuroscience behind the doctor-patient relationship.* Oxford University Press. Oxford.

Blumberg, H., Hoffmann U., et al., (1994) *Clinical phenomenology and mechanisms of reflex sympathetic dystrophy: Emphasis on edema. In Gebhart G. F., Hammond D. L. and Jensen T. S. (Eds). Proceedings of the 7th World Congress on Pain, Progress in Pain Research and Management.* IASP press. Seattle.

Gifford L. S. (2013) *Topical Issues in Pain 3. Sympathetic Nervous System and Pain. Pain Management. Clinical Effectiveness.* CNS Press, Falmouth.

Hanna K.R., Katz A.J. (2011) *An update on wound healing and the nervous system. Annals of Plastic Surgery. 67(1):49-52.*

Levine J. D., R. Clark, et al. (1984) *Intraneuronal substance P contributes to the severity of experimental arthritis. Science 226: 547-549.*

Levine J. D., Coderre T. J., et al., (1988) *The peripheral nervous system and the inflammatory process. In Dubner R., Gebhart G.F. and Bond M.R. (Eds). Proceedings of the Vth World Congress on Pain. Elsevier Science Publishers.*

Levine J. D., Coderre T. J., et al., (1990) *Neural influences on synovial mast cell density in rat. Journal of Neuroscience Research 26: 301-307.*

Levine J. D., Dardick S. J., et al., (1986) *Contribution of sensory afferents and sympathetic efferents to joint injury in experimental arthritis. J Neurosci 6(12): 3423-3429.*

Levine J. D., Gooding J., et al., (1985) *The role of polymorphonuclear leukocytes in hyperalgesia. Journal of Neuroscience 5: 3025-3029.*

Levine J. D., Reichling D. B. (1999) *Peripheral mechanisms of inflammatory pain. In Wall P.D. and Melzack R. (Eds) Textbook of Pain (4th Ed). Churchill Livingstone. Edinburgh.*

Levine J. D., Taiwo Y. O., et al., (1986) *Noradrenaline hyperalgesia is mediated through interaction with sympathetic postganglionic neurone terminals rather than activation of primary afferent nociceptors. Nature 323: 158-160.*

Levine J. D., et. al., (1985) Hypothesis: The nervous system may contribute to the pathophysiology of rheumatoid arthritis. J Rheumatol 12: 406-11.

Roatta S., Kalezic N., Passatore M.S. (2003) ympathetic nervous system: sensory modulation and involvement in chronic pain. In Johansson H, Windhorst U, Djupsjöbacka M, Passatore M, editors. Chronic Work related Myalgia Neuromuscular Mechanisms behind Work-related Chronic Muscle pain Syndromes. Gävle University Press. Gävle

Sluka K. A., Willis W. D., et al., (1995) The role of dorsal root reflexes in neurogenic inflammation. Pain Forum 4(3): 141-149.

Thornell L-E, et al., (2003) Morphological features related to muscle pain and muscle overload. In Johansson H, Windhorst U, Djupsjöbacka M, Passatore M, editors. Chronic Work related Myalgia Neuromuscular Mechanisms behind Work-related Chronic Muscle pain Syndromes. Gävle University Press. Gävle

Section 13

HEALING AND ADAPTATION

Chapter 13.1
Healing and Adaptation: The Toblerone recovery

In the last two chapters I have tried to give a reasonably light overview of some of the basic tissue mechanisms and their control systems that are involved in tissue injury and the onset of pain during and immediately following the injury. Hopefully I have managed to keep contact with the notion of 'sample-scrutinise-respond' from the cellular level way up to higher brain processing levels. For therapists this has included some body-brain-mind and mind-brain-body pathway possibilities so that links can be made between them. I'm really trying to make a case for how and why physiotherapy and other non-interventional therapies may work – using rational science rather than the pseudo-scientific alternative therapy models we so often encounter and which are actually well represented within the physiotherapy profession. It is also making a case for how conventional and 'proven' interventional medicine works or is 'enhanced' too. The key thing here is that: there's a person involved in every intervention, whether it's an injection, a pill, an operation, a pressure on your head, a motor imagery session, or a rub on the back and that person can have a very powerful effect on what the body's physiology and the brain's processing does with that intervention!

The Toblerone recovery!

In my very early naive days as a physiotherapist, I wanted to get into curing and fixing patient's aches and pains. I wanted to be an impressive operator. I wanted to have a good reputation and I wanted patients to be saying 'I walked in doubled-up and went out straight' or such like. I actually believed that this was what I would be taught and, if I got good at it, this was what would happen. As time went on it clearly wasn't like that at all and to be honest that just wasn't the real me, I'm not a natural show-off and I don't do bull-shit very well either. I changed as I've already described. Knowledge, good rational explanations and sound evidence based reasoning were where I was to feel most comfortable. I simply let me be me.

One day, at the end of a list of patients, I remember sitting quietly writing up my patient notes, but feeling quite uneasy and slightly frustrated. I'd just had a very demanding patient, Tom. It struck me that he epitomised everything about what patients really want. And more importantly what I, my profession and the whole of medicine were really crap at doing – which was giving rational answers to simple questions and making clear what we can and cannot do. I realised right then too, that I was beginning to hate the pressure I was getting from the patients to fix them 'NOW' and the pressure I was putting on myself to produce a result. I ended up with this saying in the end: **Desperate patients lead you to do desperate things.**' It made me realise how dangerous one could be, just because of the pressure to 'do something impressive' and 'get a result'. If the truth be known, a great many patients walked out a lot worse than they came in and I blame the 'myth' of manipulation's powers for a lot of it.

Anyway, back to the post Tom revelation moment. I sat there for a while in that end of day peacefulness and reflected upon my own attitude when I went to the Dr and wasn't feeling well, – what did I want from the Dr? It was simple, almost profoundly simple!

If I went to my Dr with something wrong I wanted the following:

1. *Doc, what's wrong with me?*

2. *Doc, how long does it take to get better?*

3. *Doc, is there anything you can do or
    give me to help make it better quicker?*

4. *Doc, is there anything I can do to help it get better?*

That was back around the time I was beginning to make sense of pain, the early 1990's, and from that day on I vowed to get better at answering my four questions for every single patient who came through the door.

I then thought about it a bit more and for some odd reason I flipped to thoughts of the 'older' generation whose attitude might be a bit different. I'm there sitting imagining an elderly patient struggling into the Drs or my surgery and sitting down describing their trouble and strife. The Dr does all the questions and examination checks and is talking gobble-de-gook at the patient and the old fellow smiles and turns to the Doc and says...

'You know best Doc. I know you'll fix it for me.'

You must know the patient I mean? They simply want you to do something, you can tell them what's wrong and explain it all but they just want you to help them, they're not listening to all that 'education' guff you want to spout, they're glazing over. And further, these folk are not always the old; they can be young, in-between or old!

So, I knew there and then that my attitude to what I expect from my Dr might be a great deal different to that of many others. In a way I thought that my attitude would be the ideal one for the Dr! My priority was the order given of those questions above, others may put the third one as priority and some folks may even slide the fourth above the third.

Back to the bad old days and patient Tom.

So in comes my patient 'Off-to-Hong-Kong-Tom...'

'Hi, I'm Tom... (shakes my hand...), Louis, OK.'

Nods and sits down, frowns and leans forward grabbing his right shoulder.

'I've never had pain like this – it's from here in the shoulder, down my arm to my elbow, I've got this stabbing in my shoulder blade and I haven't slept for three nights. It's driving me mad. The Dr is useless, says I've pulled a muscle and he's given me some anti-inflammatories which are also useless. I've got a very stressful job and I'm travelling to Hong Kong tomorrow. I need this thing sorted quickly.'

He looked at me imparting what I felt as intense pressure. I got on with finding out more about the problem and then doing the physical examination. Back then, as I mentioned just now, when confronted by desperate pain combined with a desperate patient I tended to try desperate things! That, to me, is the ghastly pressure you're under when you view your role as 'curer' or 'fixer' of a given problem... and the patient does too...

So, I spent a good while loosening him up, giving him some bull-shit tale about stuck joints and proceeded to manipulate his neck. There were almighty clicks and cracks and it all felt good.

Impressive problem, impressive therapist, impressive therapy and cross your fingers... impressive result...!

But I felt bad. This wasn't at all good. I was responding to pressure. I knew this wouldn't help beyond the euphoria of having your neck clicked nicely and could even make it much worse, but hey, the guy was off to Hong Kong tomorrow, something was worth a try, shit or bust... I was externally bravado but internally lying and lying badly. This was the stuff of 'burn-out' dreams for me. Others might not give a monkey, I did and I care.

I haven't a clue what happened to him and I've never seen him again, but 'High-Pressure-off-to-Hong-Kong-Tom' changed my clinical thinking and approach forever!

My thoughts now are to ask, whether you have ever felt similar pressure and hated it? Or maybe you like the pressure, you're extrovert and you do all the stuff I've described and more, without one jot of concern or thought?

I reckon all clinicians and therapists who have to 'do something' with horrid musculoskeletal pain states feel some kind of stress and pressure. I think I'd worry about your competency if you didn't.

Are we under the illusion that most patients come in hoping for a rapid improvement in their symptoms and for the most part this expectation and outcome are just not realistic? Are you the clinician deluded about what you think you can achieve and, what you think is the cause of the patient's problem? Hmm!

Maybe we just need to do a very simple thing: ask the patient what their understanding of physiotherapy is and what they wanted from the session with us? Then we could honestly answer their questions.

Yes, you can play with pain – after some nice hands-on or machines, a bit of caring and getting along, maybe a joke or two – the patient walks out cared for, treated and feeling better. But the overall pattern, if you really listen, is that the pain wanders back again later on and the 'natural history' follows its chosen course. The subtle, but good part of 'treatment' making the pain a bit better fairly instantly, is that it shows the patient that their problem can settle, the possibility of pain 'off' is quite credible. This result maybe instils a bit of subconscious confidence in a positive eventual outcome... turning a pessimistic attitude into a more optimistic one! That's good 'top-down' biology in action.

The old saying of get the patient in early so you can take the credit for what would have recovered anyway may reverberate here a bit. Hang around with your therapy long enough and you'll bumble along as the biology does its thing... you'll get the credit and make your money. Yep it's cynical and I was getting more and more cynical back then. I'm not now because I've changed my practice to incorporate good diagnosis, the natural history and healing and the best inputs for the best outcome given the time available and as a result have sometimes turned people's problems, if not their lives, around. For those who were healing anyway I've given them the reality of their situation and acted more as a hands-on-and-off therapist, educator, teacher and supporter through their recovery. A great many just need the knowledge and some advice as to what to do and leave it at that.

I determined there and then, whenever appropriate or necessary, to educate the patient's expectations to a realistic position if at all possible. Yes, even now, I still do the hands-on, machines-on whatever 'treatment' stuff too, but it's in a different context – and a much better one too.

If you're of the 'I only ever want to look, diagnose and fix' disposition – the best thing I can recommend is to retrain as a dentist! They've generally got it made because the problem is visible and the surgery done mostly works well!

The next high-pressure 'Tom' who showed up got a different approach, and the next and the next, until I'd perfected what I was trying to put across and achieve. The end result, I felt far less pressure, I felt honest and the patients often got better faster! Why's that? Well, one thing may be that once you accept the reality of a situation, it becomes less threatening. Another is that reassurance is also incredibly helpful in reducing threat levels. As I've already discussed, reduced threat equates with altered processing and altered processing can reduce pain.

So let's jump forward a few months to high-pressure-Tom number two. I'll call him Dick and might find room for a 'Harry' later on!

Dick is a right in your face black and white thinker, with no time for grey-maybe-this-maybe-that scenarios. If you were to ask Dick with his raging right neck, shoulder and arm pain that's just started and driving him mad at night and through the day... a question like... 'What are you expecting from physiotherapy today...?' He'd answer, 'I want it fixed...' Blunt, terse and no compromising... He's a classic pressure patient who wants the fast fix yet has got a problem that is very likely going to be slow to recover. Deal with that!

Now, a little aside, lean in a minute. I've spent my clinical life hearing and being told by 'cure-all' therapists that they can fix things like frozen shoulders, tennis elbows, sciaticas and nerve root problems in one or two treatments. Therapist after therapist used to come up to me when I was teaching my various pain courses to tell me that their special methods can fix such things and fix them quickly. Look, I started out life thinking the same and suffered the same delusion. When I became more sceptical I learned that I was pretty good at 'playing' with the patient's symptoms – closing the pain-gate for a bit and turning on a bit of 'descending-pain-inhibition' – but found that overall, if you really honestly asked, the patient often felt better for a bit but then the problem came back again and quietly set it's sails on its chosen course. The delusion of 'fix' was masked by the instantaneous improvement in range and pain that came with the instantaneous testing we did. Try this, if you see an improvement on re-test after performing a technique, wait five minutes without doing any more treatment and re-test again? The range flips back to where it was mostly. The reality is that pain can be made to fluctuate quite dramatically for short periods but that miraculous sudden pain cures for these type of conditions just do not occur.

I agree though that rapid changes in some clinical pain states can occur and I'll be giving some examples of this later on.

If you do think you have a consistently reliable and quick one, two or even three, treatment cure for these types of conditions – tell an unbiased researcher and get them to run a trial. If you're right, then you've really discovered something amazing and we all need to know. If you don't and you keep telling everyone that you're getting these fantastic results then I would categorise you as a 'faith-healer.' Be aware that the fantastical claims of cure and recovery by faith-healers are yet to stand up in any well controlled clinical trials (because these people refuse to provide any kind of proof or go anywhere near the 'threat' of a trial). The best observers of faith-healers reveal the use of trickery, skull-duggery and flim-flam – and a great deal of money being made from very vulnerable people. These 'faith-healer' people know that they are frauds. And in America they amass vast tax-free wealth. They are nothing short of disgusting people who prey on the sick and vulnerable (read James Randi[1]).

There's a little caveat 'aside' that needs to be mentioned here however, and I hope you are all thinking this – that changes in belief/confidence/threat/attention and hence **CHANGES IN PROCESSING** can produce dramatic changes in symptoms, changes in tissue physiology and in behaviour. Let's not be in total denial. But let's open our eyes to see what I believe is the 'true' or 'most likely' explanation.

Dick's problem was an acute cervical nerve root – he'd lost his right biceps reflex and had a weak biceps muscle but there was no sensory loss. I have seen many hundreds of these and I have scoured the literature to find a description of a cervical nerve root's natural history. I have found nothing that fits with my observations. I have further found nothing that fits with my observation of the natural history of sciatica and I have found nothing that tells me anything about the natural history of carpal tunnel syndrome, tennis and golfers' elbows, shoulder impingement syndromes, plantar fasciitis, tendonitis and so on and so forth.

I have now a life-time of clinical experience and later in the book I will give a bit more detail of some of my observations about common clinical presentations and their natural histories. You may not agree. Fine, but good research often arises from simple clinical questions and observations. What there is later on, are my observations and nothing more. I would love it if some day some unbiased physiotherapists would get stuck in and do what Patrick Wall wanted us to do – record every single detail about a variety of conditions and follow those details over time. I cannot say it often enough, but our knowledge of recovery times and natural history is abysmal. If the general public were to find out! Ah, but maybe if they knew it would help!

What is described below is what I now do – my explanation of recovery has evolved and changed over time and of course it varies depending on the patient, but the fundamental process is still here. I will use high-pressure-Dick's cervical nerve root

---

1 - *Search James Randi on Youtube and also check his website: www.randi.org*

problem to show you how I get to deal with my four 'What I want from the Dr' questions... Dick, as I've said, had ongoing nasty acute pain down his right arm. He described it as a constant nagging deep 'toothache' pain, being vague and deep, covering not only the arm but also the whole of the right scapular and even radiating into his arm pit. Sometimes waves of aching would run from the medial border of scapular over the shoulder and down the arm. When it was really bad his fingers felt numb and sometimes they were cold for no reason. Dick was constantly restless unable to find any position of ease. He got short periods of relief by putting his hand on his head, other times he swung his arm round and round. Nothing gave anything more than fleeting respite.

The problem had come on during the night about four days before and he was unable to recall doing anything or ever having had it before. Dick was fit and in his mid 40's.

I did a full physical examination. I did it confidently (definitely not cocky-confident) and explained everything as I went along. Dick was a bit of a control freak and I want to keep him informed about what was going on and I wanted him to realise that I knew what I was doing and what was talking about too. There's no room for anything airy-fairy with this sort of patient and there's no room for that feeling of the patient taking over.

His neck movements were pretty good but the whole of the right arm and scapular symptoms could be gradually worsened by rotating towards the side of pain and waiting for about 5-10 seconds. Adding a modest amount of side flexion to this position made the pain even more intense. (Note, not doing this sustained testing often misses this important information.) The pain built up and up the longer the neck remained in the rotated position. Biceps reflex was nil and biceps was weak. Etc...

Now, most therapists confronted with a patient with a frozen shoulder start something like this, 'There's good news and bad news. The good news is... that it gets better... and the bad... that it can take a long time... ' For acute nerve root problems, like Dick's, I often use this approach too, but I sometimes go into a fair bit more detail and it's worth it.

'Dick, I've now had a good look at you and I think you can now see what's going on. I hope you can see that it's coming from a nerve in your neck, that the nerve has been injured slightly – hence your loss of reflex and your weak biceps, as I explained when I tested them.'

'Right, so if you were to go and see an orthopaedic specialist or a neurologist/ neurosurgeon – he would examine you and tell you that you've got a, 'Cervical Nerve Root' problem with damage to the nerve. The pain down your arm is what's sometimes called 'brachialgia' (brachi means arm, algia pain of course). You may have heard of 'sciatica', which is pain down your leg from an irritated nerve in your lower back. Well, this is similar to that, but the pain is coming from your neck and going down your arm. What you have is a 'sciatica' in your arm, if you like. Put simply, its nerve pain or neuralgia.'

Dick's frowning a bit now and looks concerned he might not get a quick fix.

Good.

I don't think it's worth asking him what he's thinking. I'm just going to carry on quietly and confidently with the reality of the situation and then see what he's thinking after.

'Before I do any treatment, or start you off getting you involved in helping yourself, you need to understand two things.'

'One, the good news, it does get better! Two, the bad news, and I know this isn't quite what you want to hear, but this is a condition that sometimes takes awhile – this can be a few weeks to several months or longer – everyone is different and it's impossible to say who will be quick and who slow.'

He's still frowning but he nods.

(An important point here is that as therapists trying to help people get better we are almost indoctrinated with having to give positive 'you'll get better soon' type messages – rather than giving a realistic and honest message. Don't feel guilty, because you'll eventually be respected for the honesty and reality. One of the key things is getting the initial clinical picture assessed and understood correctly. You have to be good at seeing the patterns and good at doing the basic clinical testing too. More later when I discuss the Shopping Basket).

I go on...

'I want to show you how recovery proceeds for normal tissues and then show you how it's different for nerve and I'm going to draw a few graphs. I assume you're OK with graphs?'

He nods...

I get out a fresh piece of paper and draw the two graph axes. The horizontal I label time, the vertical, pain.

I draw a curve on it – sharply up, over the top, then tapering slowly back down to the horizontal axis (figure 13.1).

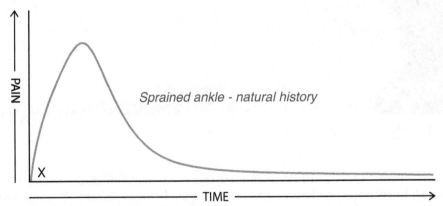

Figure 13.1 Graph of Pain after injury over time.

'This graph represents what happens to pain over time for a pretty straight forward injury – it could be a skin wound, a sprained muscle or a twisted ankle. Let's say it's an ankle. As you can see, the ankle is twisted at point 'X', the pain goes flying up to 'nasty' levels up here, stays there for a day or two then gradually subsides over the next few weeks and it carries on for anything from a month to 6 months or more. But the pain is not that intrusive for those final months – it just hurts if you overstretch it, or stumble or do an awkward movement, or suddenly load it... For the most part the pain becomes pretty much zero after 2-3 weeks or so. Note that I haven't drawn the graph as hitting the zero line. It's just above it, even after six or more months. That is because it heals by scar formation, so it's never quite the same again and in some sprains and strains a little sensitivity may remain, not always, but it does in some people... '

(If there's time and it's appropriate... I may then show him my own ankles which have suffered quite severe sprains in the past – but that they look fine, I can jump up and down, hop, go snowboarding, run, do marathons... but if I really push them into inversion there is still quite a degree of discomfort. I may even show him my pictures (figure 13.2) of how they were. Key message – 'recovery is amazing, but even in a twisted ankle, it can take time....).

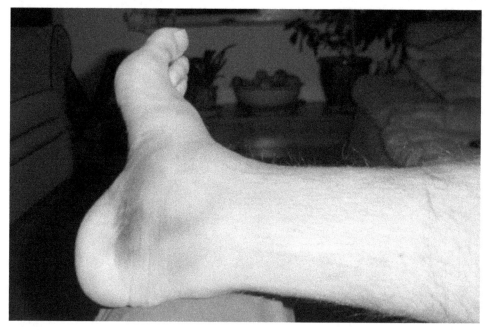

Figure 13.2 My ankle one day after quite a nasty twist.

I go on... (figure 13.3) and I draw another trajectory that's much the same shape but much lower and that doesn't go on for so long before tapering off... and then another, but much higher that goes on for even longer... I continue with Dick...

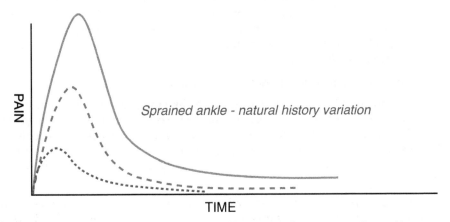

Figure 13.3 Pain and recovery graphs for three different people – some nastier and longer, others shorter and not so bad. Everyone heals at different rates with different amounts of pain.

'These two extra graphs show that some people heal more quickly than others with the same injury and have a lot less pain – that's the lower graph. And also that some have a massive amount of pain and it goes on for ages, but still eventually recover too – that's this higher graph. That's why it is impossible to accurately say how long any injury will take to recover. The important thing with injuries like a twisted ankle is that we know it is safe to start using and loading after a very short period of rest – and that this actually helps a much better overall recovery. That ankle of mine I showed you, I did in November, I played a full round of golf on it two days later and I was back continuing my marathon training within three weeks. I did the marathon the following April. There are absolutely no long term bad consequences of that early movement.'

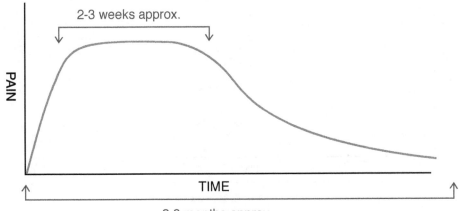

Figure 13.4 Recovery graph showing plateau of symptoms before recovering. See text.

'Now nerve pain is like this too, it's variable – in fact we know that some people can lose reflexes and have weak muscles from nerve injury and have very little pain (I draw an even lower graph now), others have a massive amount of pain (I draw a really high graph). Right, I'm now going to draw two new graphs of what usually happens to people with your problem.'

I do this on another sheet of paper and talk as I draw...

'This first graph (fig 13.4) goes straight upwards like the twisted ankle to nasty high pain, but this time, instead of coming down fairly soon, it carries on at high for a while – this period is usually quite nasty for around three weeks or so before it gradually starts to ease down – becoming much more manageable here – at around one to two months and going to OK'ish or a great deal better by around three months.'

(Note that I could have drawn a gradual increase in symptoms over a week or two or even several months. Some nerve roots do come on very gradually like this – often with just neck pain, or a bit of scapular area pain... and only developing the arm/leg symptoms later... and this can all be discussed and illustrated with the graph if it's appropriate).

Back to Dick...

'You look a bit fed up as most do, hang in there! I'd like to emphasise two things. First that this pain is usually far more variable than the sprain example I gave and second that this graph can stretch out for a year or more too... but in most people if it's managed well early on it gets to a much better state in this 2-3 month period.'

I now draw another graph below the first (figure 13.5) and then another one below that – they're all parallel to the original graph but lower indicating lower symptoms. I draw arrows down from the higher graph to the lower ones...

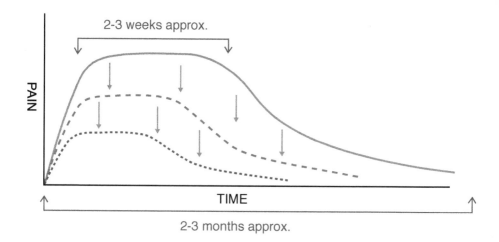

Figure 13.5 See text for full explanation. Shows how reducing pain can quicken recovery time.

'These two graphs represent what we're trying to do to help you get through this better and more quickly. We're going to do anything we can to help get the nerve to shut up and this means doing anything that helps to reduce the pain without any danger of further injuring the nerve.'

I go on...

'Getting the pain down is key to helping pain that comes from nerve. Now, most people at this point go 'I hate painkillers and anyway, taking pain killers and stopping the pain is just masking the problem, it's not fixing it... If you're thinking this I want you to see it this way...'

'Inside your neck is a nerve that's been injured, think of it as being a bit bruised in a small portion of it, but that the bruising has been enough to knock out a very few of the many hundreds of thousands of individual little nerve fibres in it. Those are the fibres that wire you up to your biceps muscle and make it work. They've been knocked out so that the muscle is slightly paralysed! *(Yes, I use pathological language, because it's a hard fact here when a reflex has gone and a muscle is weak)*. As yet medicine has no fix for damaged nerve fibres, just like there's no 'fix' for cut skin, so, they can't be 'fixed', they have to re-grow and mostly they do, and do it very well given time and some encouragement! What's good here is not all of the fibres to the biceps muscle have gone, it's only a few, that's why the muscle still works but it's a bit weak.'

Dick, like many patients then says...

'But what injured the nerve in the first place?'

(Good, he's come down from his 'I WANT A FIX AND I WANT IT NOW' position and starting to seek more information... I may be getting some 'acceptance' going on already...).

I get the model skeleton out (ours, usefully, has plastic nerve roots) and show him the cervical nerve roots coming out of the foramen. I show him how they're stretched, pressured and pinched by normal movements. I show him how much room they have. I show him the little facet joints and the disc... and go on...

'Nerves get pulled and pinched in everyone every minute of the day and night. Sometimes some of the blood vessels to the nerves get pressured and shut off – you may have woken in the night with a 'dead arm'?

He nods and smiles...

'Right, unfortunately nerves get stretched or bruised doing the most mundane things and in a great many people there may be no pain at all. In others, for no known reason, it seems some folk are more prone to this – the nerve gets nasty and starts causing a lot of pain. One other thing is that nerve pain like yours is more common the older you get. It's not common in youngsters unless there's been quite a bad injury to the neck or shoulders. The ones that come on as we get older may be associated with this hole, which the nerve comes through getting a bit narrower. This occurs when the little facet joint here gets a bit enlarged or the disc may bulge a little. This happens in everyone to a lesser or greater degree but mostly is not a huge problem... '

Dick raises a hand... and queries...

'Right, so is it worth getting some kind of scan or x-ray to see what is going on?'

'Good question and the bottom line is that scans and x-rays do nothing to help it get better. They just tell you what it's like in there... and the picture it would show of you, if you had it done right now, would be much the same as it was one year ago, two years ago, even five years ago... unless you've had a bad neck injury recently which you haven't. People who have pain like yours, have a scan which may show a bit less room round the nerve, a bulgy disc and an enlarged facet but still recover in the way I've shown you. A scan won't help you get better here.'

'So you're sure that nothing serious is wrong?'

'Yes, and to reassure you, we are trained to look out for clinical features that suggest something serious is wrong. They're called clinical 'red-flags' and if there are any we send you straight to the Dr for further investigation. You have no red-flags.'

Dick has a hint of a smile now... and a little resigned but with a tinge of humour he says...

'Well, looks a bit gloomy for it getting fixed right now then!'

'You're right, the best thing here is being patient and not getting mad all the time with it. While there's no magic quick-fix, we've still got a lot we can do...'

Dick butts in...

'You know, this constant deep horrid nagging ache and the waves of ache are driving me nuts, especially at night...'

'Right but before treatment and lesson one... I've got one more bit of information about nerve pain that's important to understand...'

'Go on...'

(Note that this is a rather didactic, 'me talking', part of the session, but he's listening, if he was glazing over I'd have simplified it and given far less detail...).

'Back to the graphs a sec. You know I drew the lines on these 'recovery' graphs as straight lines, well there not often straight in most nerve pains, they're up and down and all over the place...'

I now re-draw the graph (figure 13.6) as up and down in a rather haphazard way... saying...

'Look, one minute the pain is 5 out of 10 and not bothering you too much and ten minutes later it's 10 out of 10 and driving you mad... It's up and down all over the place, you may get a few hours when it's good and then it comes back with a vengeance. As time goes on you may get half a day or a whole day where it feels good but later it gives you a ghastly night... Nerve pain is up and down in a crazy way, it has a mind of its own and it's often out of all proportion to the damage done. Nuts and Nasty!'

I superimpose the crazy up and down on the downward recovery section of the curve...

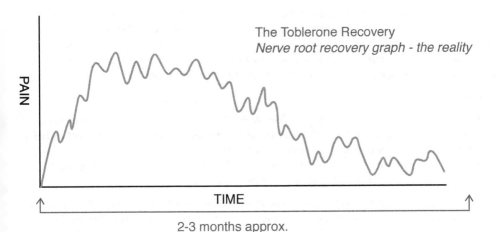

The Toblerone Recovery
Nerve root recovery graph - the reality

PAIN

TIME

2-3 months approx.

Figure 13.6 The 'Toblerone' recovery graph – the reality of most recoveries, particularly nerve root problems.

'This is how most nerve pains like yours recover. One minute you think it might be fixed, then it pops back at you, but over time it gradually gets less and less and settles. We call it the 'Toblerone' recovery! As you can see it's up and down like a Toblerone chocolate on its side!'

There's a story behind why we call it the 'Toblerone' recovery. It goes back to the mid 1990's when Dave Butler and I were giving a five day course in Zurzach in Switzerland. I was up the front teaching the group my way of explaining recovery for nerve roots... similar to what I have just described. I was saying something like this...

'Do you guys ever get a new patient in and you do a bit of treatment and they do quite well, their range of back or neck movement improves and there's a nice drop in the level of pain... the patient kind of looks at you and says 'Wow, that's good, we're getting somewhere...' The patient then goes home and comes back three days later and can hardly walk into your treatment cubicle, they look like death and they're moaning in pain... 'I don't know what you did to me last time but I've never been in so much pain in my life. I haven't slept since I last saw you and I've been back to the Drs... he says that you shouldn't do any more of that manipulation...'

'You feel absolutely shit now and you're wishing you were an office worker drinking a cup of coffee and sending jokes to your mates on the internet. Jesus, what's the guys friggin' Dr going to think of me, my reputation with him has now gone totally tits up.'

I pause and then ask the group...

'Anyone been there? Does it piss you off as much as it pisses me off? Come on hands up...?'

90% of them eagerly put their hands up and there's a babbling, chuckling and nodding of heads...

10% don't put their hands up because they know that they cure everyone and that no one gets worse in their smart-ass clinic. (I wonder to myself that either they're liars or faith-healers or maybe they never really listen to their patients. Or maybe they take no notice when the patient doesn't show up again... Or maybe they're not even listening to my story now, I've totally switched them off!)

I go on...

*'Right, show them this recovery graph and explain that recovery is always up and down... and that up and down is **normal and not to worry... and it's especially up and down when a nerve is involved in the pain scenario...** Since I've been doing my little graph thing with my patients I don't get the nasty reaction that feels like they're blaming you and that you're no good... I get...*

'Louis, I felt really good after the session so I went home and did a bit of gentle gardening and even felt so good that even sex was okay! You know that pain went flying up after but I thought about that graph you showed me and it didn't worry me. I used the TENS and took the tablets like you said and it soon settled down...'

As I was drawing the wavy up and down graph on the board Dave Butler piped up from the back...

'Hey Louis, that's the 'Toblerone' recovery!'

Being Switzerland , the home of Toblerone and Dave being Dave – it got a great laugh. Ever since then the term has stuck and we always tell patients about the Toblerone recovery when appropriate, it takes the pressure off, it stops the patient blaming you for a natural fluctuation in symptoms and it keeps them chill with what is going on – especially if you've given them some kind of 'flare-up' plan should the increase in symptoms get too much for them to cope with.

That's the story!

Back to Dick.

Dick has been listened to, been examined and had his problem explained to him and its recovery pattern.

I've covered my first two questions now:

1. *Doc, what's wrong with me?*

2. *Doc how long is it going to take to get better?*

And I've set the scene for the last two which will be answered later on in the book...

1. *Doc, is there anything you can do or give me to help make it better quicker?*

2. *Doc, is there anything I can do to help it get better?*

I've also helped him understand the natural and normal fluctuations in symptoms that are likely. So that he doesn't get panicked, angry and fed up and go flying off to the

Dr or some alternative therapist who'll spin him some yarn about some abnormality that needs fixing. Hopefully he will go away from treatment understanding the clear logic of my findings, my explanation and my reasoning and be mindful of what I can do to help and what he has to do too.

Here are some clinically important points.

- Note: how I don't say it'll take exactly this long, I give a wide range, 'These nerve problems normally take anything from 8-12 weeks to get better. The bad period is usually the first few weeks but if the pain is managed well they can get better quicker.' I emphasise that I said, 'They 'normally' take 8-12 weeks' and then say, 'That sometimes they take a lot longer and occasionally if we're lucky they can be much quicker.'

- Note: that I emphasise the worst/the bad news, that it could be long, so if it does happen to be quicker, he'll be pleased. 'Dick, I've given you a lot of misery in terms of how long this thing might take? With your sort of problem I've always found it best to give patients the bad news so that they're patient with it. Rather than me telling you it'll get better in a few days or a week or so and it not doing so – leaving you highly concerned that it's something more serious. So, if it gets better quicker than we're saying you'll be nicely surprised and pleased!' (I'm hoping you're a little puzzled and thinking 'Well that's not a very good placebo approach is it... big nocebo if you ask me?' My comment from the clinic is that while you can trick processing for a little while, overall you cannot trick a natural history!)

- Note: that you have to be confident in your diagnosis (more later, in biomedical shopping basket and case histories). As we will discuss, good therapists need to compartmentalise their thinking so that during the initial assessment some time is devoted to what I call 'Thinking like a Dr' would. You need to know and recognise common clinical patterns and their natural history if you are to be confident here.

- Note: that in musculoskeletal injury healing is by scar formation not regeneration and this means that the tissues are never the same again. That doesn't however mean that they can't function well and as good as pain-free, my ankle injury was a good example.

- Note: that to be confident clinically good therapists must be able to differentiate whether the pain problem that they are confronted with is adaptive/useful/proportional to the tissue state, or, whether it's maladaptive/unhelpful/out of proportion to the tissue state. One thing addressing this question gives is increased confidence in the ability to be able to start loading a tissue and reassure the patient that even though it may cause some pain they are very unlikely to be causing more tissue damage or hindering the healing process. In my opinion, therapist-fear of patient's high pain levels and uncertainty over its cause often leads to backing off any physical loading and an inappropriate and unhelpful focus on the pain. Understanding and recognising 'maladaptive pain' is key.

- Note: Dick had 'nerve root' pain. In the nerve root section I discuss nerve root pain and also that I believe it to be maladaptive pain from the very start. It's out of all proportion to the damage done. I will also explain why this designation is important for management!

In the next section I take a closer look at important aspects we need to know about healing.

Chapter 13.2
Healing and adaptation: Some basics that we need to know

In my treatment room I have a white board on the wall and down in the bottom left hand corner is the following

Healing

1. Inflammation: $\uparrow\ {}^{2\text{-}3}/_{7} \longrightarrow\ \downarrow\ {}^{2}/_{52}$

2. Repair/Proliferation: starts ${}^{2\text{-}3}/_{7}$ by $\longrightarrow\ {}^{2\text{-}3}/_{52}$ reaches max

   • Gradually decreases: over months...

3. Remodelling: starts ${}^{1\text{-}2}/_{52}$ ...

   • Needs physical stress
   • Months to a year...

I also have a photocopy of it to give as a handout.

This shows the healing rate of skin – a tissue that we know more about the healing of than any other. It serves very well in the clinic because everyone has visibly witnessed their own skin healing from being cut and everyone knows that for most everyday cuts, you don't need any help from Drs or medicines. It's also pretty self-evident that medicine has nothing to offer to help speed things up either! Most folk don't think about it but they're actually witnessing a wonderfully complex biological process that man actually can do little to help – bar putting on a bit of antiseptic and a sticky plaster.

When I'm talking healing times to patients I start off with the healing times for skin.

It usually runs something like this:

'Right Jock, you've just sprained your back and you probably want to know how long it's going to take to get better?'

'I do indeed Louis.'

'You need to understand normal healing and a good place to start is to look at the timing for skin healing. You've witnessed how a cut heals and maybe noted how quickly it recovers and how soon you actually start using it again and then forget about it; but to start with, for most of us, it is amazingly sore and nasty for several days. Let's say you cut the back of your knuckle. The first thing that happens, as you can see on my little chart here (pointing to my whiteboard), is that you get an **'inflammatory'** phase immediately after all the clotting and the bleeding stops. This is the phase where it's often really sore and very sensitive to touch or move. Most of us find it more comfortable with a nice tight plaster on for a day or two and we tend to be quite careful with it. Inflammation is our body's way of setting the scene for the healing phase proper, but it also brings in a whole pile of white blood cells that fight off any chance of infection. So, as you can see, the inflammatory phase actually builds up over the first two to three days before steadying off and finishing by around two weeks. As most folk know, pain gets worse with the build up of inflammation and it isn't uncommon for an initial modest strain feeling to actually get worse over a few days before steadying out and beginning to settle... '

Notice how I'm taking the pressure off myself already – not to have to fix him and get some miracle result. In my early years of private practice I saw a great many low back problems on the day or the day after the problem had started. I'd do some form of treatment and invariably they'd come back saying they were really sore afterwards – and I didn't like that. The way I'm explaining here is what I now do to get the patient to realise that sometimes the pain does get worse for a few days before it gets better and that their pain has a 'normal' inflammatory component (pah! to the redundant concept that an acute strain pain is purely mechanical – pain mechanisms in the tissue tells us that's impossible).

I go on...

'This second phase (I point to my chart again) is the actual **repair** phase – in biology it's called '**proliferation**'. Because there's a proliferation of fibres that build a net across the wound and then new skin forms on the fibres and it's all neatly put back together. It starts out a bit like a spider's web and eventually becomes very strong. Now, note that this process starts a little later than the inflammation starts and goes along with it, but, as the inflammation settles, so the repair process really gets going reaching its maximum at around two weeks. For most of us who have a minor cut we usually begin using it again pretty quickly – often within the first few days and even though we might make it re-bleed a little , it still heals perfectly well.'

'So, we're designed to heal while we stay on the move and this is important. Most folk think rest is a good thing when there's back pain, or pain from joint strains. And many patients have been told 'If it hurts rest it!' Yet they rarely do this with a skin wound! We mostly just get on with it, curse it when it hurts and weeps a bit and trust it to mend! Right, healing goes on regardless of what we do; but the ideal, is to take it a little easy in those early stages, that's why it's so sore, why it aches and why it hurts a lot if you over-do it. As time goes on it becomes stronger and safer to load and naturally the pain subsides.'

'You'll note that the repair, even in skin which we think of as healing very quickly, keeps on going for many months. If you're surprised by this next time you have a skin wound take a look at it every few weeks, even after its stopped being painful. What you'll notice is that the wound is red for a very long time – that means that there's still work going on in there! Which nicely brings us to the 3rd phase called **remodelling** – this is where all the network of fibres put down haphazardly in the repair phase get their act together and become organised along the usual lines of force. The repair phase is like a big dollop of 'goo' bodging the wound and the remodelling phase is where the dollop is then shaped and neatened up. Big point here is that this phase starts in the first 1-2 weeks and needs movement and physical stress to stimulate the shaping and neatening. Not only that, astonishingly to most, is that remodelling can go on for up to a year – in skin!'

Summary:

- because of inflammation (and the waking and sensitising of the nervous system) – 'sore and achy' may build up for a day or two

  (expect sharp pain with movements that stress the wound, or are about to stress the wound! even here, though repeated movement and the sharp pain often gets less and less, it soon comes back after a period of rest)

- early nice movement even though it might make it a bit sore is OK

- be patient, it takes time and you may get little bits of pain for quite a long time after the wound has been secured

- pain that's driving you nuts is not helpful and needs dampening down (I'll discuss this with you in a moment... see yellow flags and stress sections later)

- skin is slow, ligaments, tendons are even slower, but muscle can be reasonably quick

- there's lots of variation but use the skin healing timetable as a good rough guideline

- remember, just like skin, it's safe to start loading all but the worst injuries (I'm thinking unstable fractures or osteoporotic fractures for example) quite quickly and it's safe to return to normal activities within a few weeks, if you gradually build back up, as I'll discuss later on

- healing is by scar formation – it takes time and is never quite 100% as strong as it was.

  (But on a very positive note, for the most part it is strong enough for the on-going rough and tumble that is our action-filled lives!)

Understanding healing of collagenous musculoskeletal tissues, should give us a jolt of reality to lower and better balance our recovery pacing and eventual outcome expectations. The reality is that healing of collagenous tissue is slow; and ultimately not that good. To expect a 'cure' and hence perfectly recovered tissue after injury is sadly naive and unrealistic. On the other hand, the 'bodge' job that our fantastic repair-yard gives us, for the most part, does the trick and a good many of the worlds injured get back to sometimes quite incredible levels of fitness and activity.

A couple more graphs now that can be useful at appropriate stages of recovery for the injured patient...

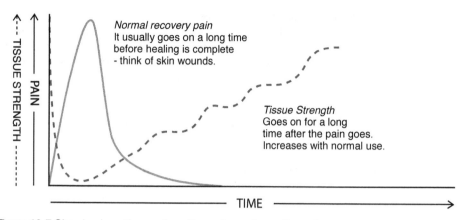

Figure 13.7 Showing how tissue strength continues long after pain goes.

The first graph (figure 13.7) shows how the pain eventually subsides and, for all intent and purpose, goes (think skin again for a minute) – yet the healing plods on for many months after the brain has forgotten about the pain or the incident. Healing plods on and the scar/bodge gets gradually stronger the more it's used until eventually it reaches a peak of strength. Research into skin repair and remodelling tells us that the amount of collagen reaches a maximum between two and three weeks after injury but that at one month the tensile strength is only 40% of the original! Even at the end of remodelling at around one year the scar in the skin only reaches 80% of its previous strength.

What's neat about this graph is that it shows how pain is at its height early on, just when the tissues are at their weakest. Pain changes the injured owner's behaviour in favour of being careful and looking after the tissues when resting or moving about; but later on, with the tissue requirements being more intense movement, the pain usefully subsides at around the right time to allow this to happen. You may recall from earlier that I mentioned pain never really going because the nervous system 'knows' the injury site is never the same again. What I mean is that a degree of protective sensitivity remains, for example pain occurring with threatening stretches or forces, but for the most part where day to day activities and function are concerned, there's no need for pain at all.

This is all very smart and 'adaptive'. Pain to 'slow you up' and 'take care' then later on, a no pain phase (but really with a bit of end range/over-stress sharp sensitivity protection still around)... that feeds the need to get moving and put some good stresses through the system to get it well up to strength.

Actually, I think it is total bunkum that pain is 100% a warning **not** to do something as most pain writers would have us think. Sure, early on, it's not nice and pain makes you care and avoid, but as the healing runs on the pain starts to actually make you want to use it and move it... You know that stiff pain you get and even some sharp pains actually tempt you to 'try me'... 'Test me out a bit'... and get the thing moving. That's 'healing pain' and I'll review it again in the clinical sections of the book later (chapter GE 3.1.)

Let's call it a four phase 'pain-healing-timeline'...

But, look at the second graph (figure 13.8)! This is what happens when things become maladaptive; where pain goes on for too long, preventing adequate movement and loading, which in turn deprives the tissue of adequate remodelling stimuli and leaves the final strengthening of the tissues way short of the mark. This graph is the 'maladaptive' scenario for any clinician who sees patients many months or more on from the original injury and who are typically avoiding movement and are in on-going pain. These patients are our challenge and it seems so common these days that one begins to wonder how our smartly evolved healing programme could desert so many! What's the cause and what's the answer?

One issue may be that we're simply no longer living in an evolutionary environment? (Think 'hunter-gatherer'!). Modern living allows us to rest, to take it easy, to avoid stress and strain for extended lengths of time and with little overall loss; we still can get fed and watered, we don't have to get moving to find food and water to survive, it's all taken care of with a weekly bank draft, the turn of a tap and a home delivery! On top of this we might be given a sick note and told to take pills and rest up for a few weeks by our well-meaning, time strapped and not uncommonly ill-informed medical services. Clinicians whom we seek help from may well be saying... 'If it hurts be careful or don't do it.' They'll certainly say, that if they're unsure what's wrong (because in this day and age), it's always best to 'err on the safe side.' Sadly, erring on the safe side, meaning rest, may be the least appropriate advice to give.

So, here's politically incorrect Louis again, going ... 'Bring back good old hunter-gatherer therapy'. Where your family and tribe will look after you for a day or two but after that they get a bit narked and start grumbling, bringing you meagre scraps and then, oh, they didn't show today... nothing, 'up you get son... time to get moving.' You have to get going and that's just what the situation needs. It seems that our 'sympathy' or 'tolerance' time for anyone close to us who is poorly is well tuned to the normal healing response timetable! I do marvel at evolution sometimes...

A quick point, before a little thought leaves me never to return. I wonder if you've noticed the patient who gets maladaptively stuck in phase three – the 'restless' phase. This patient just can't be still and yet can't keep moving either. One minute they get comfy sitting or lying, five minutes later they have to move, five minutes later they want to sit again. Up, down, up down all the time. Restless Reginald or restless Rosemary, they're pain has got stuck in phase three and gone 'maladaptive' and they're driving themselves and everyone else mad. Many nerve root pains do this.

When you really start to think and recall patients you realise that you can come up with examples of problems that have been maladaptively stuck at any one of all the phases above. You know, Lady Farquar from the castle down the road, twisted her ankle and banged her knee three months ago, hasn't moved it since... stuck in phase two. Then there's Christian who hasn't got any pain at all and hasn't gone back to anything more than a five minute walk just in case the pain comes back... he's stuck in phase four and is going to miss out on adequate loading and repair and good remodelling...

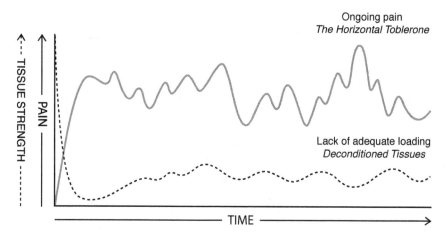

Figure 13.8 The 'Horizontal Toblerone' – the situation in chronic maladaptive pain. Note that because of the level of on-going pain the tissues don't get a chance to be adequately loaded to increase their strength – they become 'deconditioned'.

Think of the phase and then you can see what options might be available i.e.

- get gradually moving and build confidence

- better rest for longer (yes, it does work sometimes – even though it seems counter intuitive, but it's very rare)

- overcoming restlessness (there's often a great deal of tension and pain focus in these presentations), these patients have to pace up being still and pace up normal movement

- better pain control

- a hell of a lot more movement than they're currently doing (sorry, but the patients who are stuck in a phase are usually given hopelessly pathetic amounts of functionally meaningless exercises, and need to build up to one hell of a lot more. It's the therapist fear of movement thing I think?)

- never forget to consider 'yellow flag' issues, they're mostly maladaptive components linked to their situation and history; like fear-avoidance, pain or illness behaviour, the patients understanding and attributions, levels of distress and coping strategies etc.

Chapter 13.3
Healing and Adaptation: Useful Facts – Muscles

Knowing about tissue's healing and adaptation is, in a sense, a forgotten art. Or maybe it's just never been an 'art'? Maybe it's never even been thought of to forget? It's just not out there.

My big gripe is... How can a patient be confident in you if you don't know much about how long it takes an injured tissue to recover or how long it takes to get stronger etc.?

What follows are some facts and features that I've found searching the literature over the years and that I have in my memory bank to use appropriately when explaining things to my patients. If you're keen you'll enjoy doing a current literature search and update what's here! Hopefully there's enough here to be clinically useful.

What also follows from time to time are some really quite simple questions that I would like answers to if I were a patient. I give the answers from what I've gleaned in the literature, but there are also some questions which I haven't been able to find adequate answers for and I mention those too.

Musculoskeletal tissues, especially muscle and bone are wonderful examples of 'sample-scrutinise-responders'; change their environments and they change, if you're not bothered, they're not bothered, if you're bothered, they're bothered – they respond to the changing demands put on them and for the most part they do so remarkably quickly.

I've put the bit for the 'patient' in italics.

Muscle training... rest... and immobility...

This is a bit of 'factoid' thing!

...did you know?

1. That each muscle cell normally lives for the entire life of the individual. New cells are only produced following acute trauma. *Muscles, or at least the bit that does the contracting in muscle, the muscle fibres, are capable of healing by regeneration. They can recover in the same perfect way that a newt's or frog's tail does if you cut it off!*

2. Muscle metabolic turnover rate is rapid, in adult muscle cells the turnover 'half-life' is around seven to fifteen days. No wonder muscle is a very rapid adaptor to new mechanical requirements. Compare this to say the disc, whose turnover is measured in years and years... *Muscle fibres don't take long to regenerate after injury because they are biologically very busy, they have a good blood supply and therefore plenty of nutrients and energy. Compared to say a tendon or cartilage they're streets ahead... weeks versus months or years!*

3. Training – the maximum weight that can be lifted repeatedly during weight training exercises can increase by 100% in twelve months due to two things: first, increased endurance and improved neuromuscular activation/

efficiency – hence increased proportion of fibres that can fire at any one time; and second, hypertrophy. *Muscle is one of the most impressive tissues in the body that responds to exercise and getting fitter. It has a remarkable ability to change – by increasing its own blood supply, by improving the 'factory' work rate and by enlarging and getting more efficient at working.*

4. Inactivity/immobility reduces muscle mass. Within hours a demonstrable decrease in protein synthesis can be demonstrated. Muscles that are immobilised, in a shortened position, decrease in length (the number of sarcomeres diminishes) and in girth, but there's an increase in the relative amount of collagen. The muscle becomes stiffer and less extensible. Complete immobilisation of the leg for six weeks reduces the cross sectional area of the quads by 15-20%. *'You've been advised to rest. I've assessed you and shown you where you need to be careful and I'm also going to advise you strongly not to rest – why? I'll use muscle as an example, if you rest a muscle it's biology slows right up within hours, it starts to get lazy and sluggish, it starts to shorten and lose it's flexibility, it gets rapidly thinner – for example the thigh muscle can lose one fifth of its size in just six weeks... and it takes a long time and a lot of hard work to get back.'*

If you get a 'techy' type patient you may find some of this useful to add...

Observable changes as a result of lack of use and cast immobilisation are most dramatic in muscle tissue. Decreased use of muscle has been shown to reduce the volume and oxidative capacity of myofibre and myofibrils and hence produce a loss of muscle mass and strength. Concomitant with this is an increase in intramuscular connective tissue volume and a decrease in capillary density (Jozsa, 1990). Rigid immobilisation produces far more dramatic changes:

- muscle protein synthesis decreases within six hours of cast immobilisation of a limb (Booth 1987)

- two weeks of cast immobilisation decreases muscle fibre size and causes loss of myofibrils

- mitochondria enlarge, lose their cristae and disintegrate (Cooper, 1972)

- eventually muscle cells contain only amorphous protein, vesicles and fragments of membranes

- as the myofibres degenerate, fibrous tissue and fat become a progressively larger proportion of the tissue

- six weeks of cast immobilisation decrease the weight of cat muscle nearly 25% and after twenty-two weeks muscle weight loss is nearly 70% (Cooper, 1972)

- In humans, six weeks of forearm cast immobilisation reduced the adductor pollicis muscle maximum voluntary contraction by 55% and maximal electrically evoked contraction decreased 33% (Duchateau, 1987)

- length associated changes in muscle may occur within a few hours of a muscle being immobilised; typically the number of sarcomeres decrease if the muscle remains in a shortened position and increase in a lengthened position (Gossman, 1982; Noonan, 1992).

Here is some more on muscle adaptation and fitness...

The specific adaptive changes in response to increased use depend to a large extent on the pattern of use. What is apparent is that initially a muscle responds rapidly to increased use and training, but soon the adaptive rate of change decreases until the muscle reaches a stable state.

- Endurance training, (low-tension high repetition exercise), like walking, running, cycling or swimming, performed for thirty to sixty minutes at a time, increases the capacity of muscle cells for sustained effort. It increases the number and size of muscle cell mitochondria, muscle glycogen concentrations and the proportion of muscle cells identified as having oxidative capacity (Buckwalter, 1995; Morgan, 1971). These changes can double the muscle oxidative capacity.

- Strength training using high tension, low repetition muscle activity increases muscle strength and volume primarily by causing an increase in myofibril numbers and hence cell hypertrophy. I've always been confused, possibly a bit thick about the difference between a muscle fibre and a myofibril! Well, a muscle fibre is the muscle cell and it's full of myofibrils – they're the contractile part of the cell. Myofibrils are the long spaghetti like units in the cell that contains the actin and myosin and that make up the sarcomeres. Sarcomeres are arranged one after another, in series, along the length of the myofibril. How many per cell then? That's my question...? Well I found out and there are thousands per cell. So, when someone starts doing a bit of fitness training, weight lifting etc. the muscle cell samples-scrutinises and responds by producing more myofibrils – hence the cell enlarges and eventually the whole muscle enlarges... until you end up like Mr or Miss Universe!

- Stretching has been shown to accelerate muscle protein turnover and can cause hypertrophy and increased strength (Buckwalter, 1995). Back to the myofibril and it's long series of sarcomeres. Sarcomeres apparently like to have a given length so, if you take a muscle and leave it in a stretched position for a few days it 'samples-scrutinises and responds' and ends up producing more sarcomeres. More sarcomeres equals larger myofibril equals hypertrophy equals stronger! So, a degree of stretching may help improve strength.

As a therapist I've always wanted to know more about the 'dose' of exercise. I must say throughout my whole career I've been totally unimpressed by the 'pathetic' amounts of exercises most therapists give to patients. For example, 10 repetitions three times a day seems to be pretty standard. I don't get this at all. It is just not reality. Reality in human movement repetitions is hundreds, or more realistically, thousands of repetitions per day. For example, fitness studies are urging the lazy Westerner to try and walk 10,000 steps a day! Sounds huge, but if you stick a pedometer on and laze around all day doing next to nothing you'll find you've done around 1,500-2000 steps! The message is that our musculoskeletal tissues, even degenerate ones, are far more capable than most of us think. In the clinic one of my stock phrases with all patients is:-

START EASY BUILD SLOWLY... Of which more, later, when I discuss treatment and management. The point here is that small beginnings, like ten reps three times a day, can be very effective but they must be followed up with FUNCTIONAL REALITY! Generally that is one hell of a lot more than most therapists care to give and most patients thought they could ever do.

The story of Wallace (figure 13.9)

Wallace used to come to me on and off over many years. He's long since dead and I was very fond of him. He taught me a lesson that I'll never forget.

It was usually his back but sometimes his neck and shoulders. He was around 90 years old when he last came. I hadn't seen him for about a year. It turned out that this time he had back and leg pain – he had a bit of what Greg Grieve used to call 'old man's sciatica'. I treated him weekly over about a two month period and symptoms 'Tobleroned' a bit but gradually improved. During the time I gave him various exercises and told him to start easy and build slowly. The exercises were pretty simple for him to do I thought, lying on the floor; knees to chest curls, legs side to side, bridging, active curls of legs (no hands); active straight leg lifts... I also got him doing sit to stand and some step ups and finally standing doing all the standard back movements. Easy! All anyone would ever need to give their back a daily workout.

'Start with 5-10 -15 reps Wallace and see if you can build up from there. I'm going to see how you go for a month and then we'll review you and see how the exercises are going.'

He didn't come back in a month as arranged, something had cropped up and he cancelled. About eight months later he called up and made an appointment.

'I want you to check these exercises and see if I'm doing them OK Louis... '

Three days later in he came...

'How's the back and leg now Wallace?'

'Oh fine, forgotten about it... '

'So what are we looking at then...?'

'Can you check these exercises I'm doing... '

'Sure... '

By then I hadn't a clue what I'd given him and I was fumbling in his notes and chatting away...

'Wallace, easiest thing, why don't you show me what you've been doing...'

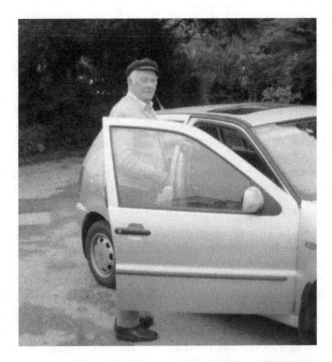

Figure 13.9 Wallace getting into his car after coming for treatment. (With permission)

With that 90 year old Wallace got down on the floor and started doing straight leg raises quite vigorously...

'Looks good Wallace... how many of those are you managing?'

'Hundred.'

'Wow, that's good... Ok, let's have a look at your next exercise...'

He started doing vigorous knees up to chest from crook lying...

'How many here Wallace...?'

'Hundred...!'

I'm thinking, blimey, 90 years old this is bloody amazing... I'm smiling down on him and he's working away...

'Next!' I shout...

He's now bridging away... up and down... effortless...

'Hundred here too Wallace..?'

'Yup...'

The whole thing went on... Afterwards I worked out that he was doing about a thousand repetitions and it all took him about half an hour.

'I'm impressed Wallace, the main thing though is how do you feel doing all that?'

'Never felt better and wouldn't miss it... It gets me going in the mornings.'

That's a story I tell my patients when they're struggling to fit three simple sessions of five mins exercise per day. It's also a story that's testament to the capability and adaptability of even a 90 year old. What are therapists doing giving ten reps three times a day and NOT increasing and increasing and increasing it all? Maybe it's a pathetic sop to how pathetic we westerners have become. Or maybe it has to do with our inbuilt but totally unreasonable fear about the actual strength of the tissues we deal with day in day out. If I'm honest, Maitland's 'SIN', the 'Severity, Irritability, Nature' judgement, gave me the 'fear of structure'; plus no one ever teaching me about tissue strength, healing and adaptation. One word for it: TERRIBLE!

Take a look at this though...

I found a clever bit of muscle research that looked into the contribution of two components of 'strength'. These are: the 'neural' and the 'muscular' components. The contribution of each to increased strength following exercise can be simply computed by recording electrical activity in a contracting muscle (EMG) and measuring the 'maximal voluntary contraction' or MVC of the exercised muscle.

The original experiment was done by Moritani and DeVries back in 1979 (In: Lieber RL 2002). They trained normal young volunteers to do an isometric elbow flexion exercise. All they had to do was produce two-thirds of maximum contraction of elbow flexors with the elbow held in 90 degrees flexion. They were asked to do ten repetitions twice a day and only to do it three times a week for eight weeks! Every two weeks they went into the lab to have their MVC and their EMG's recorded. At the end of the eight weeks the 'trained' arms increased strength by almost 25% (MVC went from average of 58lbs to 79lbs). They also measured the untrained arms as controls – what happened there? Amazingly there was a significant increase here too of 15%, going from 54lbs to 67lbs. The result was totally unexpected and led the two researchers to investigate the contribution of the nervous system to strength.

Their logic for working out the contribution of neural versus muscle factors (e.g. muscle hypertrophy) was this: that if an increase in strength was achieved purely via neural mechanisms then that would register as increased EMG activity in the muscle. On the other hand, if the increase was due to pure muscle factors there would be an increase in strength *without* any change in the EMG. Of course, increased strength is a feature of both factors and they were able to attribute the amount of each component by doing some simple mathematics.

They then repeated the training and noted that in the first two weeks about 80% of the strength change in the trained arm was achieved by increased muscle activation i.e. neural factors. The remaining 20% was due to changes in the muscle itself. From two weeks on, to the end at eight weeks though, the neural contribution decreased and the muscle increased. At eight weeks 95% of the strength change was attributed to muscular factors and 5% to neural.

So early improvements are largely neural, meaning increased muscle fibre recruitment... and those later are muscular.

What a great example of quick response to changing conditions... Plasticity rules OK!

In the untrained arm increases were all neural of course, or were they? Rat studies have shown that electrical stimulation of muscles in one limb led to muscle changes in the un-stimulated contralateral limb muscles. Some unknown trophic stimulation seems to be going on there?

The clinical thing here is of course, that if you ever have to suffer any form of immobilisation you may still be able to maintain some of the strength, if you keep the rest of you fit. And in particular, work the equivalent muscles in the contralateral good limb.

For those who can't even be bothered to do that there's further good news – all you have to do is imagine you're doing exercise and there'll be some improvement!

Yue and Cole (1992) (see p 216 of Lieber 2002) did some clever research on the hypothenar muscles of the hand. They're the little muscles that abduct your 'pinky' – the abductor digiti minimi! They used three protocols: the first where subjects performed active little finger abduction exercises with the hand strapped into an exercise device; the second where control subjects who came to the lab and were just tested; and the third group who were strapped into the same hand exercise device as the 'active' group and told to only 'imagine' they were doing the exercise (they checked participants for hypothenar EMG activity so they knew whether or not they were activating muscles).

Results were very interesting. As you'd expect, the exercisers did the best and showed a 30% increase in strength over a four week period. The control group did the worst but still managed to increase by 3.6% but the 'imaginary' group managed a colossal 22% improvement! The researchers even tested the untrained hand and showed significant increases in the 'exercise' (about 15% better) and 'imaginary' (about 10% better) groups.

The last clever twist to this imaginative bit of research is that they stimulated the ulnar nerve 'supramaximally' at the beginning and at the end of the research in the untrained hand; and showed no change in muscle strength with the same current , thus indicating that the improvement was wholly neural rather than down to any muscle hypertrophy factors.

Messages I use for patients

It takes only two weeks to get significant improvements in muscle efficiency but you need to do minimum of two months to make real changes to the muscle. Best to keep going forever!

It seems that you can get quite marked improvements in strength with minimal exercise! I tend to avoid telling patients any of this... I want them to work a lot harder than ten isometric contractions twice a day three times a week. Let's get real! The point is that the strength increase with minimal exercise is largely neural and not hugely impacting the intrinsic muscle fitness.

I love telling some patients about these experiments, especially those who are being lazy – just because one part of them is immobilised. 'Get the rest of you moving and keep 'you' healthy... and... You'll even help to keep the bit that's being immobilised stronger than it otherwise would be... and when you do exercises on the good side do them mentally on the immobilised side too... '

Muscle repair

The main clinical questions here relate to... 'How long to better?' and 'How safe is it to start loading?'

A good deal of research into muscle injury has been done on rabbits... One of the key things about muscle is that the actual contractile cells have impressive regenerative capability, but unfortunately, some scar also gets in there too! Here are some useful facts to inspire confidence in the clinic... Note the timing and early vulnerability... but note the rapid development of scar too... I've highlighted important findings in bold (i.e. to be learnt of by heart!).

1. In muscle 'tear' within twelve hours of injury, 'myoblasts[1]', the precursors to muscle cell regeneration, may be present. Over the next 1-3 days these cells orientate to the long axis of the broken ends of the muscle fibres.

2. But by 5-7 days fibroblast proliferation is evident and local fibrosis and scarring result. If the muscle is lacerated the healing is by extensive scarring. **In rabbit research by twelve weeks 50% of muscle strength had returned and the muscles ability to shorten had reached 80% of normal.**

3. In more modest injuries, what researchers call a 'strain' injury, the muscle goes through **a 1-2 day phase of rapid loss of power and tensile strength** but thereafter it begins to strengthen. Thus, **after twenty-four hours a strain injured muscle is only capable of contracting to 50% of its normal capability** when its innervating nerve is maximally stimulated. However, by **the seventh day the muscle is capable of a 90% contraction.** Just the ticket and well done evolution for providing such a rapid return to a pretty good level of function! Yes, but... when the researchers test the passive strength of the muscle i.e. they stretch it and stretch it... **it's only got 77% of its previous strength at seven days.** That's still not bad though?

4. In muscle strain injury, **the inflammatory phase is up to four days** and any muscle fibre **regeneration is complete by 10-14 days.**
Again, it's very quick.

---

1 - *Before this you activate satellite cells – these sit in muscle all your life waiting to be mobilised. After damage their phenotype changes and they become the myoblasts – you have a set number predetermined in each muscle and can't make any more!*

---

5. **Overall muscle recovery can take anything from ten days to ten weeks.**
I find this useful to quote in the clinic.

Further useful facts...

6. Repair tissue contains weaker type III collagen for the first week or so but is replaced by stronger type I collagen from the twelfth day on.

7. Contraction of the wound may continue for up to eighty days, but most occurs from day seven, to, day twenty-one. The clinical message is to avoid stretching very early on and then move on to gentle stretching slowly building it up over 3-4 weeks and keeping it going for up to three months or more...

   • because remodelling, like skin, can go on for up to a year

   • and again, just like skin, tensile strength may only reach 80% of pre-injury status.

The literature cautions the use of immediate mobilisation after muscle injury since it may precipitate an increase in scar tissue formation and interfere with the orderly regeneration of myofibres (see Jarvinen, 1993). However, when mobilisation follows a short period of immobilisation a better penetration of muscle fibre through connective tissue is found and the orientation of regenerated muscle fibres is better aligned with the uninjured muscle fibres (Jarvinen, 1993). There are also reports that mobilisation following a short period of rest produces more rapid disappearance of the haematoma and inflammatory cells, more extensive, rapid and organised myofiber regeneration and more rapid increase in tensile strength and stiffness (Jarvinen, 1975; Jarvinen, 1976; Jarvinen, 1993; Lehto, 1986; Lehto, 1985). Importantly and in contrast, prolonged immobilisation following muscle injury produces muscle atrophy and poor organisation of the regenerating myofibres (Jarvinen, 1993; Lehto, 1986; Lehto, 1985).

For the most part our natural tendency is to do just this – take it easy for a couple of days and then start gradually loading and getting moving again. Problems come when various trainers, therapists and Drs put their spanners in the works!

Chapter 13.4
Healing and Adaptation: Useful facts – Bone, tendons and ligaments

'Disuse is catabolic'

Walter Bortz 1984

The facts here are for use in any post-immobilisation/re-activation/rehab situation, but also use to try and get anyone going and be fitter and more active. Even your bones change when you get fit and patients find some of the facts below fascinating and encouraging. There's so much stuff to promote movement and so much to demote immobility!

Bone

Non weight-bearing results in loss of bone mass. After twelve weeks of lying on your back (yes, people volunteer for this)... bone mass is halved and it may take many months of vigorous activity to regain normal bone density – even in children and in some, especially the elderly, it may never return to previous levels. Lack of use, especially immobilisation, causes bone resorption to exceed bone formation and the exact opposite occurs with increased use – it becoming more dense and increasing in volume and strength.

For example:

- if a pig's ulnar is removed so that it is forced to weight-bear on its radius alone, there is a rapid increase in the size of the radius such that its cross-sectional area approaches the combined sizes of the radius and ulnar

- the forearm bones in the dominant arm of professional tennis players have been shown to increase in size and density

- elite weight-lifters have been shown to have very dense vertebrae

- people who exercise regularly have a higher general bone mass than those who do not

- comparing cross-country runners with controls shows that there is increased bone density at all sites – including those of the arms!

- the fit elderly are less likely to suffer fractures – like fractured neck of femur. If you've had a fracture the sooner you can get weight bearing or forces going through the fractured area the better, it stimulates bone growth. Decreased loading slows fracture site healing. If I had a fracture I'd very soon be doing modest isometric contractions to create a bit of a compression stimulus.

Back in 1981, Smith and colleagues rather nicely demonstrated that exercise can actually increase bone mineral content, even in elderly women whose bone mineral content is expected to fall over time.

These researchers took thirty elderly folk with a mean age of 84 and measured their bone mineral contents. They divided the women into two groups that were matched on the basis of age, weight and degree of ambulation. The 'experimental' group participated in a thirty minute exercise programme three days a week for three years. The bone mineral content was then re-measured and compared to the non-exercise group. They found that the exercise group achieved a modest 2.3% gain in mineral content whereas the non-exercisers lost 3.3% content. Not a startling result on the surface, but it's actually quite impressive that the normal slow decline was actually pinned back and some gains were made. Now, if they'd only used the 'Wallace' regime

Another result along these lines was published by Ayalon et al in 1987. These researchers looked at the effects of 'dynamic forearm loading' exercises on post-menopausal women (age range 53-74 years) and compared them to controls. After five months the control group's forearm bone density had diminished whereas the exercisers recorded a 3.8% increase. The exercises consisted of three, fifty minute sessions per week.

Galvanise your patients – you can tell them about this sort of research and the results and you can find out a lot more in books like Adrianne Hardman and David Stensel's book, 'Physical Activity and Health: The evidence explained.

Tendons and ligaments

Fundamentally there is no great difference between the healing of tendons and ligaments. They are both collagenous, poorly vascularised and have a very slow biological turn-over rate and metabolism. Healing is therefore slow, by scar formation and ultimately not likely to be very strong. We could also consider discs in the same breath, but I'll go into a bit more about them in the 'Nerve Root' section later.

Let me get the basics sorted (all from animal observations and sacrifices!): Take a normal looking sheep...cut a tendon through and then keep the ends approximated, observe what happens:

Inflammation starts and lasts three to five days. It seems that blood supply is vital to the amount of inflammation and the speed of subsequent proliferation/repair. So, one of the earliest observable events is a massive vascularisation of the wound area. Vascular buds and capillaries appear and herald the laying down of early 'granulation' tissues around day five to seven. Fibroblasts start to invade and get busy – some are already there, a great many arrive from neighbouring tissues and many start dividing to produce more. The result is type III collagen synthesis starting at the end of the first week and carrying on for a good month. Note: the collagen fibres require physiological loading to orientate correctly. The literature is full of statements like: 'Total rest and immobilisation are clearly contraindicated'... a statement that seems to have fallen on deaf ears, especially in the orthopaedic domain.

So, a big dollop of 'bodge' is produced in the first month and the process of remodelling begins around the second week and may take as much as thirty weeks (that's seven months for our sheep)... What happens is the type III collagen re-orientates along the lines of stress and at the same time gradually converts to the stronger type I collagen. And all this requires loading or the dollop of 'bodge' stays a 'bodge-dollop'. Here you go: loading even alters the rate of repair, three weeks following injury, surgically repaired tendons treated with early mobilisation had twice the strength of repaired tendons treated with immobilisation (see Gelbermann 1982).

It seems that the key is a bit of rest very early but soon getting into graded increase in loading over the following early weeks and months... for up to a year.

The final strength of a scar-healed ligament or tendon may not be that good. For example in a mid ligament tear of knee medial collateral ligament Houglum (1992) reported that the tensile strength of the repair may be 85-95% **below** normal by anything from sixteen to fifty weeks (four to twelve months!). That folks is rubbish and hardly worth waiting around for!

Observations of vascularity in healing ligament reveals high content at three weeks and staying high for seventeen weeks (four months), but by ten months it had returned to normal levels (Bray 1996). Think how long it takes for 'swelling' and inflammation to settle in some knee injuries... this may help make sense of that and reassure you and the patient that it will take time.

In rabbit ligament injury observations myofibroblasts (they're the cells that bridge any wound gap and bring the two gaps together by contracting) have been shown to become abundant between six and twelve weeks after injury.

So here's a chart like the one for skin that you can use:

Ligament and Tendon Healing:

- poor blood supply, a 'white' and gristly tissue – therefore slow to heal. But new blood vessels invade area within about a week and keep growing for quite a long time...

- ****Collagen heals by scar formation,** not by 'regeneration' (which is perfect healing – like bone, liver and some nerve fibres!).

Inflammation:

- slow build up over 3-5 days, may go on for many weeks.

Repair/Proliferation...

- blood vessels start growing in, starts 5-7 days... increases for three weeks and still high at four months but normal by ten months...

- scar starts with weaker fibres around one week and keeps going for a month.

- needs movement and loading to get the fibres aligned and stronger.

chart continued on following page...

...chart continued

Remodelling...

- starts around two weeks and goes on for seven or more months. May be well over one year.

- needs loading to align fibres and stimulate them to convert from weaker to stronger fibres.

Comment on inflammation: I find this five day limit to inflammation hard to believe clinically. Note that skin doesn't subside until around two weeks. For skin, I guess it is important to maintain a healthy immune presence, since any breach to the outside world is a potential invaders route to victory. But still, five days isn't long for such a sluggish tissue and a great many patients show what I consider to be inflammatory signs for many weeks. Perhaps I'm not reasoning it correctly? Chronic swelling and thickening/scarring doesn't mean inflammation, nor does nasty point tenderness.

Why don't surgeons write papers on what they observe when first going in to view and then repair tendons and ligaments? It would be so useful if a surgeon could tell us what they see... 'After exposing the medial collateral ligament of a 45 year old male skier who'd had a problem for six months we noted clear evidence of inflammation in the form of increased vascularity, swelling and significant redness...' Or this: 'After exposing the extensor tendon insertion of Mr 'A', a chronic epicondylitis sufferer, we all thought it looked completely normal (as they invariably do in our experience); there was no evidence of inflammation, swelling or scar tissue, so, rather than the usual excision and debridement we quickly sewed him right back up. All present agreed a pact of silence. He was none the wiser, we told him the operation went well and within a few weeks he was 100%, pain free and back to playing top level tennis again...'

Please don't take it too literally, the messages are important though. The same outcome could have occurred if there was evidence of scarring, inflammation and swelling... and they all just looked at it and then sewed it up... did the pact and fibbed convincingly to the patient. Processing and changing processing as we saw in the placebo chapters can have massive benefits.

A real patient now...

Tracy is 35. She's a regular runner with the local running club and has done several half marathons and a couple of full marathons. She suffered a partial tear of her right Achilles tendon about three months ago and told to stop running and rest it. She was told it would take three or four months.

She made an appointment to see me because progress was so slow, it was still painful and it had a very sore lump on it.

The salient examination finding was that the tendon had enlarged a lot around where the injury was. She also walked flat-footed and leant towards the left. She couldn't walk on tip-toes but going up and down on right and left together tip-toes was possible while holding on.

This was how I explained the situation to her...

'First of all your healing is going fine. I think it worth spending a few minutes explaining tendon healing to you and then you'll be able to see how we can help it along. I'm not sure what you've been told, but it sounds like you're under the impression it should be healed in three or four months. The reality is that tendon healing goes on for seven to eight months and usually well on into a year. Tendons are white cord-like structures, which you may have seen on chicken legs if the feet have been left on! Look you can see mine easily through the skin here round my wrist...'

I flex and tighten my wrist and up spring palmaris longus and flexor carpi radialis tendons. I also get her to pull her toes up hard on her own feet and look at the cords of the extensor digitorum longus tendons on top of her foot. I could have also got her to flex her knee against resistance and feel the hamstring tendons.

'Those are all tendons, they're thick tough and gristly – or fibrous, they have a very poor blood supply and are nothing like as alive and active as say your skin or your lips or your tongue... which bleed easily, but heal pretty quickly too. When it comes to healing, tendons are the opposite, they're sluggish and slow and over months and months they bodge a big lump of scar tissue and that's what you have here on your tendon. The lump you're feeling is the scar forming – it's a good sign! Now, just so you can see what this lump is all about I want you to think of a broken bone and how it heals...'

I now draw a fractured long bone.

'When you break a bone the Drs re-position the bits of bone so they're touching and lined up. If they don't touch they don't heal well at all.'

I now redraw so the bones are touching...

'When the bones are like this new bone starts forming between the broken ends. Lots of new bone gets made and the area becomes much enlarged with what Drs call a 'callus', you may have heard of that?

'Yes I have, but I never realised what it was...'

'I think you can see what I'm getting at... just like your tendon, bone gets a big dollop so it's hugely enlarged with the callus. Once the callus is formed the bone is a lot stronger than it was. From there on as the person uses it and puts weight and forces through it so it gets even stronger... and... it also starts to get remodelled back to its normal shape.'

All through this I've been drawing the callus and then drawing the various stages of remodelling as it reverts to a normal sized bone shaft.

Tracy is nodding her head now...

'So my fat tendon is the equivalent of the bone and its callus?'

'Yes... and now it needs to do a bit more remodelling than it's been doing and that requires we start building up the loading on it...'

'Right... so should I have been loading this a bit more than I have?'

'That's possible, but you haven't and this is where we're starting from and that diagram is where we are trying to get to!' (I point at the sketch that's the perfect shaped bone again). But there's a BUT!'

'What's that?'

'That bone heals by regeneration. If you break a bone and take an x-ray of it say a year later you won't be able to see the join, the bone that's reformed is just like the original bone that was there. Now, with tendon it's made of tough fibrous stuff called collagen and collagen heals by scar formation – that means it's not perfect healing like bone'

'Does that mean it may always be weak?'

'It may, but the big point is that there are a great many folk who have injured the tendon, just like you have and they're fine, they've got back to their former activities and just kept going. I've got many patients who've gone back to running, climbing, skiing and so forth – with no problems. Their secret of success is that they got the tendon strong by gradually increasing loading under my guidance, which wasn't actually much, when they understood the principles. The main thing I want to get over to you today is that you have to accept that it takes time and the remodelling and strengthening process is quite slow... and, that to get this, it needs to be loaded regularly.'

Tracy nods then looks a bit quizzical...

'Have you ever had one of these actually tear again?'

'Smart question! And the answer is yes! But it's not that bad, in the whole of my thirty plus year career of seeing lots of tendon injuries I have only seen two that tore again. Both had a very poor scar, there was very little 'bodge' and you could still feel the thin zone of the tendon where it had torn (I draw another diagram, see fig 13.10). These two patients were eight and nine months down the time scale and it was looking unlikely that they were going to get much further healing anyway. The best way to look at this understandable bit of fear is like this: that if it's going to go again, it'll go! These two patients whose tendons 'went' on them did so just doing a simple movement – hardly any more force than taking a normal step. So, if it does go – it goes and it'll be off to the surgeon to get it stitched back together.'

'So what happens if it goes and you don't have a surgeon fix it?'

'You'll be flat-footed forever if it goes completely – walking with no spring or push off in your stride. If it helps we have had one patient who tore both her Achilles tendons. She was a triathlete and she was around fifty years old. She went to see the foot surgeon and he said she'd be out of running for a year if he were to operate. She started getting going again flat-footed and within about six weeks she was plodding again and then started to be able to run. That was about four years ago. She is still doing triathlons with no problems and if anything she's gained in her running times!'

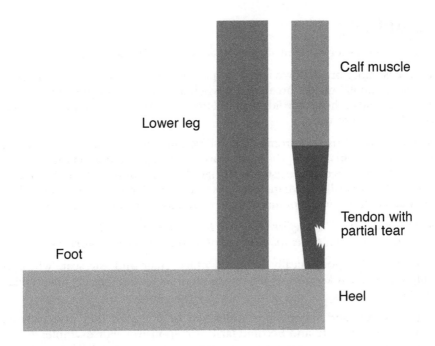

Figure 13.10 Crude drawing of the basic anatomy of an Achilles tendon with sufficient a tear to cause a hollow in the tendon.

I have now...

- set the scene to start a graded loading programme and building confidence, getting her to start walking normally and starting to forget about it...

- I've hopefully got her to understand the amount of time it takes to heal and to accept and adjust to slow progress rather than worrying about it not having mended when 'they' said it would

- I've also hopefully painted a positive picture about what the future holds and what the worst scenario might be – in a positive light!

- I've hopefully decreased her concern about any pain – which may in turn help to lessen it somewhat

- the rehabilitation process was similar to 'Runner Pete' in chapter 14.2.

Underactivity

Way back in 1984 Walter Bortz made a great statement: *'Disuse is catabolic'*

In other words things break down and go to pieces when you don't use them. If you didn't know, catabolic means break down whereas 'anabolic' means build up – as in 'anabolic steroids', those steroids that athletes, body builders and probably many famous cyclists used to use.

Bortz's article 'The disuse syndrome' really stirred me, because he had evolution in mind when he wrote his paper. His incisive article highlighted the fact that for much of the two million years of our existence we have lived as hunter-gatherers, have had to be extremely physically active in order to survive and that it is only in the last two hundred years that our levels of inactivity have greatly accelerated. Let's quote...

'Our ardent pursuit of less effort has led to the wheel, pushbutton tuning, the horizontal escalator and the emobodiment of least effort – the motorized golf cart.'

Let's also add the ergonomically designed office chair and car seat, which are incredibly successful at keeping us happily motionless for biologically unacceptable periods of time.

If biological organs and systems are underused or not used they physically and physiologically degenerate and become far less responsive. For example, animals raised in deprived environments, as contrasted to those raised in enriched environments, solve mazes slower and have smaller brains and sparser dendritic branching (Diamond, 1967). The gut needs to be used to retain its functional capacity; the liver atrophies during starvation; the kidneys when excluded from filtering requirement and the bladder when excluded from storage – will atrophy and lose vitality; and the body temperature falls and circadian rhythms desynchronize with inactivity (for references see Bortz, 1984). Lack of use is probably more detrimental than overuse and misuse and is possibly the most important unsuspected aspect of modern life that has been scientifically passed-by.

I am likely to be booed down but it's my opinion (fascist hat on here) that the average Westerner hasn't a clue what it's like to feel physically 'overused' or physically really and truly exhausted. The very common prescription of giving exercises consisting of 10 reps 3 times a day says it all. Come back Wallace!

Chapter 13
Read what I've read

Ayalon J., Simikin A., et al., (1987) Dynamic bone exercises for postmenopausal women: Effect on the density on the distal radius. Archives of Physical Medicine and Rehabilitation 68: 280-283.

Booth F. W. (1987) Perspectives on molecular and cellular exercise physiology. Journal of Applied Physiology 65: 1461-1471.

Bortz W. M. (1984) The disuse syndrome. Western Journal of Medicine 141: 691-694.

Bray R. C., Rangayyan R. M., et al., (1996) Normal and healing ligament vascularity: a quantitative histological assessment in the adult rabbit medial collateral ligament. J Anat 188(Pt 1): 87-95.

Buckwalter J. A. (1995) Activity vs. rest in the treatment of bone, soft tissue and joint injuries. Iowa Orthopaedic Journal 15(42): 29-42.

Cooper R. R. (1972) Alterations during immobilization and regeneration of skeletal muscle in cats. Journal of Bone and Joint Surgery 54A: 919-953.

Diamond M. C. (1967) Extensive cortical depth measurements and neuron size increases in the cortex of environmentally enriched rats. Journal of Comparative Neurology 131: 357-264.

Duchateau J., Hainaut K. (1987) Electrical and mechanical changes in immobilized human muscle. Journal of Applied Physiology 62: 2168-2173.

Gelberman R.H., Woo S. L.-Y., et al., (1982) Effects of early intermittent passive mobilisation on healing canine flexor tendons. Journal of Hand Surgery 7(2): 170-175.

Gossman M. R., Sahrmann S. A., et al., (1982) Review of length associated changes in muscle. Physical Therapy 62: 1799-1808.

Hardman A.E., Stensel D.J. (2003) Physical activity and health: The evidence explained. Routledge. London.

Houglum P. A. (1992) Soft tissue healing and its impact on rehabilitation (review). J Sports Rehabil 1(1): 19-39.

Jarvinen M. (1975) Healing of a crush injury in rat striated muscle. 2. Histological study of the effect of early mobilization and immobilization on the repair process. Acta Pathologica, Microbiologica et Immunologica Scandinavica 83: 269-282.

Jarvinen M. (1976) Healing of a crush injury in rat striated muscle. 4. Effect of early mobilization and immobilization of the tensile properties of gastrocnemius muscle. Acta Chirurgica Scaninavica 142: 47-56.

Jarvinen M., Aho A. L., et al., (1983) Age dependent repair of muscle rupture. Acta Orthopaedica Scandinavica 54: 64-74.

Jarvinen M. J., Lehto M. U. K. (1993) The Effects of Early Mobilisation and Immobilisation on the Healing Process Following Muscle Injuries. 15(2): 78-89.

Jozsa, L., Kannus P, et al., (1990) The effect of tenotomy and immobilization on intramuscular connective tissue. A morphometric and microscopic study in rat calf muscles. Journal of Bone and Joint Surgery 72B: 293-297.

Lehto M., Duance V. C., et al., (1985) Collagen and fibronectin in a healing skeletal muscle injury. An immunohistochemical study of the effects of physical activity on the repair of injured gastrocnemius muscle in the rat. Journal of Bone and Joint Surgery 67: 820-828.

Lehto, M., Jarvinen M., et al., (1986) Scar formation in a healing skeletal muscle injury: a histological and autoradiographical study in rats. Archives of Orthopaedic and Trauma Surgery 104: 366-370.

Leiber R.L. (2002) Skeletal muscle structure, function and plasticity. The physical basis of rehabilitation. Lippincott Williams and Wilkins, Baltimore.

Morgan T. E., Cobb L. A., et al., (1971) Effects of long-term exercise on human muscle mitochondria. Advances in Experimental Medicine and Biology 11: 87-95.

Noonan T. J., Garrett W. E. (1992) Injuries at the myotendinous junction. Clinics in Sports Medicine 11(4): 783-806.

Randi J. (1989) The Faith Healers. Prometheus. New York.

Smith, E. L., Reddan W., et al., (1981) Physical activity and calcium modalities for bone mineral increase in aged women. Medical Science and Sports Exercise 13: 60-64.

Section 14

PHYSICAL STRESS AND HEALING

Chapter 14.1
Physical stress and healing: Thoughts and some treatment/ management principles

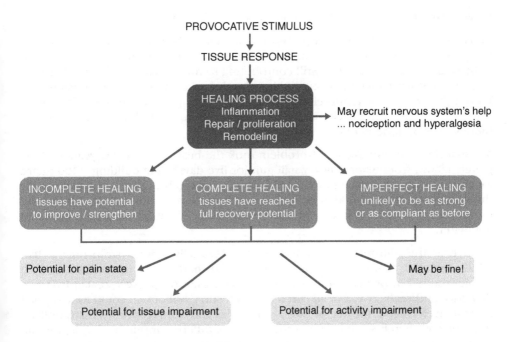

Figure 14.1 Healing outcomes and possible repercussions.

Back in my mid 1990's pain trip, I drew the following diagram (figure 14.1). It was dead simple, provocative physical stimulus (stressor), damages tissues – which in turn kicks off the three-phase healing response. My clinical thought then was how does it all end up? Do tissues always reach their full healing potential? Could one of the reasons why some of the patients I see are still in pain be because their tissues are somehow incompletely healed and have further to go? And that their 'sampling' system's are still registering this and responding by maintaining a level of sensitivity and pain? Could it be that their healing mechanism is being held back in some way? Could it possibly be that processes are still going on in the tissues when, according to healing theory as per the last section (13), they should have stopped long ago? Or, could it just be that the pain and sensitivity has stayed long after healing finished?

Say we got the tissues fitter? Wouldn't that calm the sampling systems unease with the situation and in turn calm the pain response and its pain circuits...? What if we could persuade the patient at the same time that things weren't as bad as they were thinking? Getting the tissues fitter would be a good way of proving to the individual, that even though there was still pain, they were quite strong enough? We could even tell them that getting the tissues fitter was a powerful way of helping the pain to get better, acknowledging that to start with sometimes the pain can get a bit worse...

I thought about what I knew about healing – all the sort of material from the previous chapter. Yet still I saw patients with muscle, tendon, ligament and joint problems that still seemed inflamed and were still highly sensitised way after the 'literature' and the 'research' said it should have completed, or stopped, or 'been fine'. I wanted to write an article: 'The healing time-scale – is it a fairy story?'

I was obviously thinking about centrally maintained maladaptive pain and sensitivity components as possibilities but there was also a part of me that felt there was bound to be some tissue mechanisms still contributing to the scenario. After all there are many musculoskeletal conditions and injuries that take a year or more to get better. Frozen shoulder, some tennis elbows or 'epicondylitis' presentations, tendo-achilles tears and strains, some back pains... and that's without including problems where there's clear peripheral nerve involvement.

My own shoulder impingement problem took the best part of three years and my golfers elbow, from using a heavy nail gun for five days while building a 100 metre long wooden fence, took almost as long to get completely better. I did all the right things, ignored them and kept going, cursed them occasionally, adjusted how I did things a bit, but never rested or avoided using them. They just took their time and got better.

I can hear the murmurs, 'Ah, you should've rested it... put a strap on it... had 'Mulligans' and acupuncture, had your 'AMT' turned inside out... ionto-freeked it, stair-rodded it, or even gone to Australia and then on to New Zealand via San Francisco and yeah... we'd of all cured it'... No, sorry, bollocks, I could have dipped it in the river Thames for free or flown to Lourdes and been ripped for many dollars. It got better when it sorted itself. I tried a pile of different inputs and while they all were beneficial for a week or two... it Tobleroned on and went when it was ready to.

Same old appeal.... Can someone please do the desperately needed research that records natural histories in an unbiased way...? For those of you wanting to do this sort of longitudinal study into natural history/recovery... you need to find people like me who just get a problem, maybe seek a little early advice, adjust a bit and get on with life... and follow them up regularly and find out about all the dimensions, all the physical, the coping, the activity levels and the modifications... all the pain behaviour and behaviour of pain... and keep it going.. . It's a good five year process I reckon... and there will be a Nobel prize at the end of it for sure.

As you can see in the figure 14.1 I divided the end result of healing into three: 'Incomplete healing', 'Imperfect healing' and 'Complete healing' and then thought about it in the light of tissue status and CNS pain mechanisms. Clearly the sensory fibres looking after 'incomplete' and 'imperfect' healing tissues are likely to keep informing the CNS.

... C fibre Numskulls supplying nearly healed tissues talking to CNS and trying to get some attention... 'Oi, you, yes you... you know my tissues out here are not quite 100% don't you... don't you... don't you... don't you...?' Nag, nag and nag.

Well there you go, one person's nervous system may be tuned to go 'Oh you poor dear, I'll tell them up top and we'll see what we can do'... 'Wa-hey, result!' Pain allowed to keep going on and on and on. Or this: 'Look shut up and stop being pathetic, squirt, you'll do as you are, none of us up here are at all interested, pull yourself together and stop pestering... in fact we're going to send down the sweep-up team to sort you lot out...'

Brilliant, gate control centrally and the sweep-up team are going to get down into the moaning tissues and do some further shutting up, gate control in the tissues too!

Back to the diagram... to note that I ended up realising that a pain state is possible no matter what is going on in the tissues. With central mechanisms in mind, that means pain being possible even with nothing at all wrong in the tissues. Remember the amputee's phantom in-growing toe nail pain from section 5?

BUT to my mind, the tissues where the pain is being felt are highly likely to be in an 'impaired' state, simply because having a pain in a tissue that comes on when the tissue is used is likely to lead to it being used in a less than full way, it's protected to a degree; hence, it may well be 'still healing' 'impaired', 'deconditioned' or 'less fit' and have further potential to either get fitter or, complete it's healing and heal better.

Some clinical questions that arise and need thinking about are:

1. Have the tissues that are hurting been injured at some point? (Well they may not have been!). Another question here then is 'What does this pain mean?' 'Is it useful? Useless? Reflect the stage of healing? Totally pointless? Maladaptive? '

Sorry, I'm going to have to have a little wander off the topic a minute...

There's one thing that's really annoying me that I'd like to clear up a little now but which I'll come back to later in the management parts of the book. David Butler and I made the case for bringing 'pain mechanism' reasoning into Mark Jones' clinical reasoning 'hypothesis categories'. So, when confronted by a patient we felt it pertinent to reason whether the pain presentation in front of us could be categorised into 'nociceptive'; 'peripheral neurogenic', 'central', 'affective/psycho-social' or 'output'. I want to deconstruct this a fair bit later on, for now, the part that annoys me is that this continues to be used in a simplistic way. For example when it is said that: a pain that is local and well defined, that behaves in a mechanical way and responds in proportion to the physical stress put through it – is most likely to have a 'nociceptive' pain mechanism and thus, represent some kind of abnormality or fault in the tissue where the pain resides. Also stuff like this: 'central' mechanism pain, is more imprecise, has a mind of its own, is vague and unattached, or less attached in relation to the physical stresses brought to bear. This reasoning is flawed I think. Look, all pains have all the mechanisms, even a cut finger has! From, input to central processing to output inclusive of all the meaning and emotion that the individual has attached and added to it. The key clinical question is to ask yourself whether the pain that you're listening to and assessing seems to be a reasonable representation or requirement of the state of the tissues that hurt. A great many clinical pains are clearly not a reasonable representation – many being way out of proportion to the damage done, the state of degeneration, the stage of healing or the amount of inflammation. These 'out of proportion' pains include a vast spectrum, from the vague and weakly or non-mechanically patterned, all the way through to the precise and clearly mechanically patterned, as far as I am concerned. Can we please drop this narrow way of categorising pain into a single mechanism? The labelling of pain as purely 'central' has led many therapists to plead that because a pain is coming from the nervous system then 'physical' inputs must be irrelevant and therefore that 'physiotherapy' has no place!

What's preferred then? Simple... ask the question: 'Is the pain adaptive or maladaptive in relation to the state of the tissues?' And work from there. The least you can do for anyone who is in pain, is do something helpful for them, that may even improve their pain at the same time. And that is, get them moving and fitter again, and help them get their physical confidence back.

More of this later, let's get back to some clinical questions...

2. How long has it been now since the injury/onset of symptoms? This gives us some guidance as to the stage of healing and hence tissue strength. So if it's a pulled tendon, where there's been more avoidance and care than increasing use... and it's now five months on... we're well into remodelling and it needs loading more... But it certainly won't be as strong as a five month tendon problem that had taken regular loading.

3. So always check: has the person with the problem been using the tissue normally, or are they being wary and protecting it? If there's been any degree of avoidance then the healing tissue hasn't had anything like the forces through it to stimulate adequate remodelling let alone strengthening.

4. If they have been loading it, have they done it minimally or done a lot? Simple thing here is that most patients who've had a problem for many months have actually done a bit of loading but nothing like enough to get it back to where it was originally.

5. Is it time to start loading the tissue? Or building up the loading to one hell of a lot more than what it's currently getting? The answer here, from the tissue perspective is invariably... 'Yes, if at all possible.' But, loading always has to take into consideration the natural history and healing time-frame. My shoulder took only so much loading and I couldn't really push it to doing pull-ups and press-ups for a good few months, but occasionally I'd test it, or do some modified pull-ups or press-ups – which were easy.

6. For the not-too-sure clinician an important question to ask yourself is: 'From my clinical assessment are the tissues strong enough to start loading, to build up loading and to get back normal function?' This is regardless of any thoughts about 'incomplete', 'imperfect' or 'complete'. Every musculoskeletal tissue that is put to work has the capacity to adapt and increase its fitness – a good thing for all these tissue states. As we've

seen, graded loading should start early; and rest of more than a few days is not a good option.

7. Take into consideration the fitness of the person you're dealing with before they had the problem. A lifetime on a couch probably means their tendons aren't that strong compared to someone who's been active. So the couch potato gets an injury on an already weak structure and then does more nothing. The starting point and progress may have to be a very slow incline on the graph.

Clinically what I've found over the years is that focus on pain tends to stymie the process of providing good and adequate loading. This is the antithesis of what I was taught as a manual therapist – where the whole focus was on listening obsessively to pain location, intensity and behaviour and trying to change it, above all else. The approach was unwittingly accompanied by an ingrained fear of doing any sort of loading until the pain had gone, 'until the joints had been cleared' or similar tosh. Even when the pain had subsided, loading was side-stepped rather, just in case the patient messed-up and the pain came back. I think one of the 'not so helpful legacies' of manual therapy was (probably still is) – the 10 reps 3 times a day scenario that I've been harping on about. It's called therapist fear of pain, of making things worse, at the very time when the tissue needs progressive loading and the patient needs to understand the 'Toblerone' recovery journey. The 21st century patient and therapist needs to accept that pain fluctuates and there is no such thing as 'stable' pain or stable pain behaviour/behaviour of pain.

Right, **physical stress** and healing is virtually a must! It's called progressive loading and if there's a great deal of pain preventing loading the skill of the therapist is **to find a way of loading the tissue** somehow. The ideal way is to do it without causing any, or if that's not possible, only a minimal amount of pain, or perhaps more practically, an 'acceptable' amount of pain and an acceptable amount of Tobleroning.

Remember from the last chapter, loading stimulates collagen fibre remodelling and scar strength; it encourages bone repair and remodelling and promotes fibre alignment along the normal lines of stress. Graded loading beats rest and immobilisation just about every time. Well, unless you're an orthopaedic surgeon whose main focus is on not wanting things to come apart that have been carefully sewn or stapled together. We have to respect their concerns I know. But, it may be best to think hunter-gatherer a little more, it's much easier! The trouble is that most of us don't want to upset the orthopaedic or the patient, so we do as we're told.

When the three week old shoulder tendon repair comes to me for, 'passive movements only' for the next five weeks and they ask me whether they can move it a little themselves? I usually wink and say something like 'computer says no!' I'll never forget one of my patients, about six weeks post op, drove himself to his consultant's house for a private follow-up appointment and got such a bollocking. The consultant wouldn't let him drive himself home! The outcome though was the quickest recovery I've ever seen from those ops; no frozen shoulder and the usual, about a year of getting it all back; no massive loss and fibrosing of shoulder muscles and excellent function. If only we could grade active movement very gradually alongside the forceful passive stretching they like us to do! Dream on.

I mentioned loading with no pain just now. This is a huge skill which I'll go into again in the management sections of the book, but it's worth illustrating and discussing now I think.

I also mentioned my shoulder pain that lasted three years and I give the full story in the Graded Exposure introduction chapter (GE 1).

You might be thinking – what a hopeless physio if he can't even get his own shoulder better, but I'm trying to get you to see reality and the time it takes for some things to recover. Now, one simple thing that resulted from my shoulder experience was my slight twisting of a phrase I learnt whilst learning and working with Geoff Maitland. Many of you may have seen it in his old 'Vertebral Manipulation' book (it was in the 1986, fifth edition that I've got!). Geoff used to say 'A technique is the brainchild of ingenuity'... and having watched him many times I'd agree. But, my phrase is more in the spirit of a post-manipulation dominated era, where I think *'An **appropriate exercise** is the brainchild of ingenuity.' Actually, it's not so much the exercise, it's the combination of context, understanding and meaning in which the exercise is done that makes in 'ingenious'.*

You may recall Donald Hebb's phrase '**Cells** that fire together wire together' from back in section 6? It was in a sense a fundamental rule of neurology that he came up with when investigating the neurobiology of learning way back in the late 1940's. Long ago I adapted it for patients to this:

'**Circuits** that fire together wire together'... and I also added another useful gem thanks here to Ian Robertson, the psychology professor from Trinity College, Dublin, who said, '**Cells** that fire apart, depart' when he was discussing forgetting! I hope you have come to realise that if we really want to understand pain going away, we have to consider the physiology of forgetting – at least if we're considering pain from the perspective of central 'memory' type mechanisms. So my clinical phrase from Ian Robertson is of course that '**Circuits** that fire apart, depart.'

I'll give an example of how I use these phrases shortly, but first, my shoulder pain and what I learnt from it all those years ago. I've just thought you might be wondering where I'm wandering off to, that this is supposed to be a chapter about healing and stress...? Yes it still is, right now I'm following on from the last chapter and looking at the importance of physical stress to turning on healing; and producing the best end-product possible and, acknowledging that the patient and their horrid pain response, can get hugely in the way. Even though it would be great if we could just get the pain to go away a-la-manual-therapy... and then start the loading programme, the reality is it just isn't like that.

My early shoulder problem... (an experience that helped change my patient approach for the better and got me to adopt a 'graded exposure' approach whenever possible). When it was acute I was totally unable to actively lift my arm beyond about 30 degrees of flexion or abduction.

One day in the clinic, I was demonstrating bending forward to a patient with back pain and realised when I was down there that I was dangling the bad arm in full elevation... Pleased, I stayed there and thought about it. Stick your hand on your head Louis... done... Now, keep it there and come back up to standing... up I came... hand on head and there I stood arm up and no pain. Tee hee! Down I went, let hand go off head and stood back up arm by side... repeat a few times... nice... Come back up standing with hand on head and think, wonder if I can now lower it from here... Hand off head, arghhhh... the slightest increase in muscular tension and pain blasted back in. Right, this time just slide it smoothly off the head and let it drop... yup, swish... the arm's down and I'm flopping it about with no pain... All fine, unless I contract something. Floppy... nice... lean forward and floppy pendular... nice... (see the full story in the Graded Exposure Introduction chapter later).

The big 'ah-ha' thing for me was that by changing the way I did a movement, by for example changing my starting position, I was able to find a way of getting pain free movement. A classic example from the clinic is the low back pain who can only bend forward 10 degree when standing, yet find relief curled up on their side or in kneeling on the floor.

Clinically I went on to experiment and, yes, 'practise' with my patients! It is now very rare that I cannot find some position or little physical trick that will produce some kind of good quality movement with no or very little pain that's a useful rehab tool for getting going. The really difficult ones are the well entrenched chronic pain disability type presentations, more of which later, or, the ones who seem to have ghastly pain reactivity no matter what stage in the acute-chronic spectrum. But even here I can usually find something that is reasonably productive.

So, I fiddle and grapple with things like: position, speed, muscle tension, gritting teeth, fear... anxiety... concern... long term habits... frowning, holding breath... all the little and big things that unhelpfully feed the task or movement I'm trying to do into the 'threat' and 'pain' processing centres of the patient's nervous system. The aim is to get the movement processed away from the 'threat centres' if at all possible (see sections 16 and 17).

Let's now take a patient example to see how this thing can be set up and then got going. The example is a very localised calf pain in an obsessive runner.

Chapter 14.2
Physical stress and healing: Patient example, 'Runner Pete's' calf problem

The runner is called Pete, he's 38 years old, a big presence in the local running club, normally runs marathons in around three hours and does anything from twenty to forty-five miles a week. Six months ago he was running, tripped and stumbled a little awkwardly but kept going. He felt a pain in his mid right calf a while later, thought nothing of it and kept going for another forty minutes. By the evening he couldn't walk normally and walked flat-footed. After four days he went to his Dr who diagnosed calf strain and told him to rest and take ibuprofen. Ten days later it was marginally better but he was still hobbling and couldn't run. It then became one of those typical calf strains that the patient rests for two to three weeks like the Dr said, then it feels better and then they go and try it out. Two runs, fine, then 'bang' it comes back and they're hobbling again. It really pisses the athlete off and many go on to rest for very long periods and get really run-down and worked-up. Pete had been to two local therapists who'd massaged and ultrasounded. One had manipulated his back and neck and done lots of pressure points in his buttock and upper leg. He said he got better with both but when he ran again it all came back again (so, he didn't really get better even though the therapist probably thought he was better.) Moral: follow your patients up to find out the truth.

What was really getting to him was the prolonged recovery phase before it felt normal after he'd re-strained it; and then the increasing likelihood that it would re-injure and then the whole process starting again. He admitted that he was becoming fearful of it and focused on it when moving around now. Its current status was that he'd exacerbated it about two weeks ago and while it had settled a bit it was still quite nasty. He also said that this time it was quite a lot worse than the previous re-injury flare-ups.

When I observed him he was walking flat-footed and described a bit of a nagging awareness but the main thing was the sharp very local pain in the middle and slightly lateral area of the right calf muscle belly. The whole pain area was about the size of fifty pence piece.

The physical findings were simple:

* localised tenderness right where the pain was now and where it had always been (it was easy to find a lump right where the pain was – but palpating the other normal calf revealed a similar lump, which wasn't painful (like you do, or ahem, should do).

  Patients love you to find painful lumps but they're everywhere. A great many patients have already found the lump and site it as proof of damage. If I can find a similar lump on the other side I try to normalise it for the patient. I have this phrase: **'If you look you will find'**.... that's straight out of my copy of the English version of the Bible of Pain, in the chapter and verse dedicated to physical 'Impairments'. The next chapter is 'Thou shalt make loads of money from those worthy impairments you desire to find'.

* walked flat-footed and couldn't walk on toes and couldn't do a calf-raise on one leg.

- checked knee, hip and back – all fine (I checked mainly because the other therapist had focused on them and given him some concerns).

- checked achilles tendon – palpating to look for any signs of a tear, dips and hollows, lumps and raised areas next to hollows etc. There were none, he had healthy rounded TA's.

  Note that degenerative changes in tendons may be undetectable, being central and deep, so quite often we simply cannot tell if the tendon is degenerate and therefore whether or not it has the potential to tear. The thing I come back to, and you may want to criticise me here, is that if the TA's going to go, it's going to go, there isn't much that anyone can do about it... So, if that's the case let's make that clear and get on! If it goes it's over to the surgeon!).

This is how it went from there on...

'Right, I'm going to do some more things with you now and I want you give me honest answers. My goal is to find a way of getting some good loading without any discomfort if we can, is that OK?'

'Yes, well fine, so long as you don't re-injure it again.'

'OK, before we start I'm going to show you something.'

I went over and pulled out my old edition of Gray's Anatomy and opened it to the page showing the posterior aspect of the lower limb muscles. I pointed to the calf muscle.

'Pete, see here, the gastrocnemius muscle is the outer calf muscle, the muscle underneath it is the soleus. I want you to see that gastrocnemius is huge. Now, I'm going to draw your area of pain onto here. What I want you to take on board is that this small area of your problem is about 3-5% of the total muscle bulk, if that, it's really quite small compared to the whole muscle.'

He nods...

'Also, I want you to appreciate that if I was a surgeon and went in there and cut that bit out there'd still be plenty of muscle left for good function – in fact, once the wound had healed you'd hardly notice the power difference, OK?'

'Yeaaas.'

'I think you can see what I'm coming to and that's that even if this little bit tears completely – the rest of the muscle will be able to cope admirably!'

He's nodding thoughtfully and I go on a bit further...

'Right so to me, the big problem is the recurring pain you're getting with it – far more than being worried about the muscle itself. What you've probably got in there is some scar tissue that's become so sensitised that it's unhelpful. Mind you, when I felt around there I couldn't feel any big mass of scar tissue, though it is a bit knotty as you've noticed. Anyway, it's now six months on and if you carry on the way you're going you're not going to get anywhere. It needs a different approach and we need to get you going and build confidence if we can.' (I'm honest, but I say all this in a very positive way).

I now point to my whiteboard and the healing phases for skin and mention how healing is faster for the belly of muscle than skin, but a bit slower for the tendinous parts, which he can see from the Grays anatomy, they go right up between the two heads of gastrocnemius – the area where his pain is located.

'So, from this healing time scale, it's six months down the track with lots of ups and downs. But, the tendon-muscley bit in there is still in a healing phase, mostly it's 'remodelling'. Which means it needs an increasing degree of easy forces through it to start, then more normal forces and then back to your full-on running forces and any other things you get up to. Remember, tendon changes take time, they don't change and adapt as fast as skin or muscle belly, so that is one reason why it's slow.'

(Note how rather than dismissing the pain as meaningless and being just a 'central mechanism'/self-generating pain/tissue- all-healed-type categorisation (yes it could be...but...). I've given it some tissue credibility... based on sound healing knowledge. But at the same time I've also played down any structural danger by pointing out the area involved is such a low percentage of the whole. If it goes, hey, it goes, so what!).

I go on...

'There are two issues that influence the way the pain is behaving; the first, is that you've been giving it long rests followed by more or less full-on go and it may respond better to gradual increase with a bit of guidance from me. The second is that with the repeated exacerbation of the pain, your pain system may have now become over-sensitised. Another thing you mentioned is that it grabs your attention all the time, and we know that this helps to maintain the pain presence and volume in your mind.'

I go on now with a bit of paper, drawing diagrams...

'It works like this: whenever you get a pain, even a simple pain like a cut finger, damage sensing nerve fibres send electric pulses into your spinal cord and up to your brain that then makes a 'circuit' of nerves fire off and it's this that creates the cut-finger pain. Now, the 'pain-circuit' usually just dwindles away as the skin heals and you hear no more about it. Sometimes though, especially with tissues that take a while to heal and get strong enough again, the circuit has to hang around to offer a bit of on-going protection. Unfortunately the amount a circuit actually fires and then 'plays it's tune' can be variable – it can play too easily or it sometimes may not play at all. Sometimes it's easily set off, other times you can do a great deal and there's no pain. So big question here, have you noticed sometimes that you may have just walked or tip-toed or even run without noticing it – often for quite a while and especially so if you've been busy?'

Pete looks up and nods...

'Well, to tell you the truth two days after I stirred this up again we had a load of sand delivered for the patio pavers and me and two mates spent an afternoon wheelbarrowing it all through to the back yard... and after initially being a bit stiff I forgot all about it... there was loads of banter going on all day which must have taken my mind of it!'

'What was it like later and the next day?'

'I didn't notice it later and the next day it was back to the normal sharp and nag.'

'Sounds like you hadn't made it any worse then?'

'No, not at all.'

'Sounds weird, but this is very common: even obvious and nasty wounds and cuts can be sore one minute and then go unnoticed for a while – without any long-term detriment to the healing outcome.'

Pete looks up...

'Have I been backing off a bit too much do you think?'

'That's hard to say, but what you've done is what a great many others have done too, sometimes it's really hard to know what's for the best. Let's get back to this circuit for a minute then we can get on with doing something and getting you going again – with a better understanding of why we're doing what we're doing.'

(Hebb's rule in practice...)

'In biology, there's a rule for learning that goes... when **circuits** fire together they wire together... *(note the word 'circuits rather than 'cells')*. What this means is that if every time you walk you hurt, or every time you do an exercise you bring on the pain – the circuits for walk or the exercise will wire together with the pain circuit. (I draw the circuits together on a piece of paper, see figure 14.2). The more you do the two together the stronger they become bonded together (1. in figure 14.2) and if it goes on and on for a long time it's very hard for them to separate. They just come on, even if it's all healed up and safe! Don't panic, that's the worst scenario, but you can see how pain can link itself to a variety of activities sometimes. Now, the opposite rule to this one is, that if circuits fire apart, they depart (2. in figure 14.2), meaning if you can do an activity or exercise without any pain and keep doing it then the circuits can abandon, or break, their association. No longer does the pain respond to the exercise or movement trigger and that's our task for you today, to get you doing some exercises that are worthwhile for the tissues, but doesn't attract that pain circuit to get wired in!'

Pete's looking eager... and goes...

'Let's go! ... One thing though, many of my mates succeed by running through this sort of thing, they go through agony, some get a whole lot worse. But I've got two mates, they say while it's always agony, eventually it slowly goes... that doesn't fit with what you're saying quite...'

'No it doesn't, but the opposite of what I'm going to get you to do is called 'de-

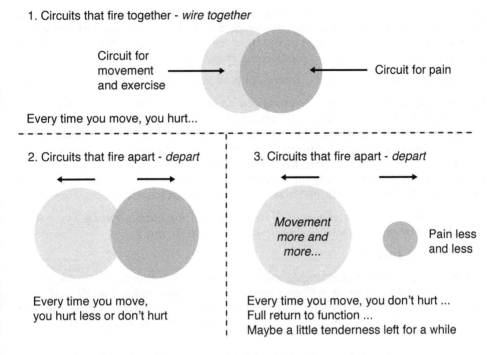

1. Circuits that fire together - *wire together*

Circuit for movement and exercise ⟶   ⟵ Circuit for pain

Every time you move, you hurt...

2. Circuits that fire apart - *depart*

Every time you move,
you hurt less or don't hurt

3. Circuits that fire apart - *depart*

Movement more and more...   Pain less and less

Every time you move, you don't hurt ...
Full return to function ...
Maybe a little tenderness left for a while

Figure 14.2 A useful patient diagram to explain 'circuits that fire apart depart'.

sensitising'. That means going into a pain repeatedly until it goes. Sometimes it can be quick other times it's slow. It's a bit like going in the sea in the middle of winter, if you do it often enough the 'cold' pain gets less with time and repetition and you get used to it, you desensitise! We may come to use that later on, but right now it may be best not to risk flaring the pain up any more than we can help to start with. Why risk sensitising it even more when your system at the moment is highly geared to going that way and then we get you being even more pissed off and totally losing all faith in ever getting anywhere. Your two mates did well, but they were lucky too, I've seen many who've tried what they did and they eventually gave up running.

The plan with you is that we start with fire-apart-depart approach and if all goes well later we start doing the 'nudging into pain' and desensitising... I hope that makes sense?'

'Great, sounds like the wisdom of experience and knowledge to me...' We both chuckle. (And you realise how important a good reputation can be, I've seen plenty of his mates and got them back running again and he knows it.

While he was sitting I got him to cross his legs with his right leg over his left and move the dangling right foot in all directions – it was pain free. 'Right, see how easy it is to find a movement with no pain! A bit pathetic, when you're a marathon runner but let's put that on your list!'

I then got him to start doing calf raises while sitting, with the bad right leg crossed on top of his good left. So, in this cross-legged position, he did up and down with the left heel, pushing the weight of the right leg up and keeping the ball of the left foot on the ground. There was no discomfort at all of course.

'Push it until you feel it's tired... and count how many you're doing' I said.

He was doing it slowly... I got him to speed up heaps. This was his good leg he was working after all. He quickly got to fifty to sixty reps and looked totally un-phased. 'I can feel a bit of 'use' he said, but normally I wouldn't even give it the time of day. I reckon I could do several hundred of those.' I then got him to stop, cross the legs the other way and now compare his bad leg to the good... 'Start counting... I want you to distinguish between anything like the pain you get and simple tiredness in the calf like you had with the left just now... tell me what happens and keep counting...'

He gets to thirty reps and tells me he's tiring, not hurting but it's getting a very slight struggle and by fifty he's feeling muscle-knackered as he put it.

'That one's on your list too...!'

(Let me suggest you try this simple exercise to see how feeble that is – especially if you consider this guy to have been running forty or more miles a week until quite recently! I've just done sixty reps with no problems. I hope you can see the result I got with him is testament to either a processing dysfunction and/or remarkable weakness...!)

I now point out to him how the condition of his calf muscle as a whole has deteriorated and that getting it stronger will protect the little vulnerable bit. It's obvious he's picking all this up anyway...

He's now quite shocked at the level of calf strength.

'No wonder it keeps 'going' on me, it's pathetically weak!'

I then get him up and holding on taking some weight through his arms at the end of my treatment plinth. I ask him to try up and down on tip-toes on both legs all the while pushing through his arms. He does it OK but he's biasing to the left, so I get him to go up high and hold it, sway over to the right and back to the left... I'm watching his face...

'No pain?' I say and he nods.

'Repeat and get used to it... use your arms to take weight if you need to... remember our starting rule – fire apart, depart.'

He nods again. He now does about 1ten reps and he's starting to test it a bit, finding he can go up on the left, stay up evenly on both and then go over and take just about all his weight on the right with no pain. This is classic mechanically patterned behaviour, which gets better/stronger/easier/less discomfort with careful repetition.

'Keep holding on and taking some through your hands and try to get a good tip toe walk on the spot going... with no pain... so adjust the push with your arms...'

He's getting it. 'Fire apart, depart!' I enthuse...

'Got the idea' he's saying...

'Right... you can work the calf sitting – move the foot in mid air, any time you like, lots of up down, let's call it 'a quick thirty to forty', any time you get a minute through the day (he works in the local council offices, mainly computer work). Plus, you can do the sitting cross legged 'work to comfortably tired', plenty of times through the day and let's say three to four times a day to spend four or five minutes on your feet like we've just been doing holding on. If it's going OK after a couple of days, do it more times per day.'

'Circuits, that fire apart, depart – it's NO PAIN and building up to lots of activity ...'

Lastly I ask him to try a modest bike ride to see what that's like on it, same rule applying and my big other rule, START- EASY- BUILD- SLOWLY!

In other words, don't go nuts like an 'Exercise-Jock' and mess it all up.

'Find a sensible baseline, hold back a little to gain confidence then we can build from there. If you get a flare up by doing too much you get put-off doing that activity again and we have to start even more pathetically and take even longer to build back up again!'

SUCCEED-NOT-FAIL...! (Another of my rules I give to patients!).

He gets the message.

To follow this up: I see him again in a week and he comes back having understood the principles and can now 'high' tip-toe walk but still can't go up on one tip-toe and he's still flat footed as a consequence. He looks a bit happier than he did and he's now doing something every hour or so through the day. He's happy too because the bike was fine and he's been out for over an hour three times with no problems.

Good! Even though, this improvement may simply relate to his normal post flare-up recovery period. Thinking sceptically like this is vital! Real progress can't be gauged until he starts running again. What is so important though, is that he's understood some basic rehabilitation issues, that healing is still going on and, he's trying it out and starting to feel he's getting somewhere, safely in his mind, with his own efforts and awareness of his activity gains – in a completely different way to the 'treatment' approach he'd had with its fragile and somewhat shaky hopes of improvement.

It was now time to find a way of getting his calf raises and hence walking going.

I'm hoping that you're maybe thinking there's 101 different ways of getting all this stuff going again? Well there are a few! Remember that this little trip with me is all about getting him back running again and burying that calf-pain circuit and his habitual over-focus on it too. What I'm describing is one way, one logical way I think, of getting it there.

I get him standing by the raised end of my treatment couch with hands ready to take weight through as before.

'Hold on as much as you like and try going straight up on the right tip toe – show me what you can do...'

He pushes through his hands like mad and manages it with a grunt. It's sore.

I then ask him to go up on both tip-toes using as much pressure as he needs to. He does it quickly and with very little pressure. I then get him to go over onto right tip-toe and hold it, there's no pain, good.

'Now just lower the heel straight to the floor.' As I talk I demo what I want him to try. Down he goes, (just like me being able to flop or drop my shoulder down from full elevation) he does it no problem... so I get him to repeat... up on two, over on the right then drop down heel to floor.

'This time Pete, try and slow it down a bit... '

He squirms a little but keeps doing it and it's getting easier.

'Right, go up on two, over to right then down one third then back up again, feel free to use your hands to keep it comfortable...'

He's getting it fine.

'Now half way down and back up again...'

That's good too. He's only using the hands for balance.

'Now walk **low** tip-toe on the spot...'

He's doing that fine.

'Right, off you go round the room, low heel, just off the floor... great... now back here again...'

'This time, I want you to go up left over on the right, then heel right down onto the floor and immediately straight back up again, don't let it relax so you flow straight from down onto heel to right back up... and use your hands if you want...'

He uses his hands the first few times then gets going...

'Now walk away normally, no flat footed...'

He picked it up quickly. Isn't it weird, or more correctly perhaps, evolutionarily very smart. How quickly antalgic gaits can over-ride normal movement patterns and how difficult it can be to get them back sometimes. In my opinion, it's not so much forgotten but inhibited by concern/fear, that's why it's so important to 'set the brain up' before doing any loading! Think about it, you'd hardly want to start putting big forces through something you believe to be weak or likely to give you horrid pain for a long time, set it all back and make things worse again.

I knew Pete understood the significance of my chat about his injury only affecting 5% or less of the muscle and that the rest could easily cope even if it never healed. (He told me six months later when I saw him that, that little perspective on it, was probably the most important thing I had told him). Simple! A simple explanation! Done at the right time and in the right context. So, another little aphorism in the spirit of Geoff Maitland, but certainly something I never heard him do... could be... 'A meaningful *explanation* at the right time is the brainchild of ingenuity!' It changes brain processing; it shifts the symptom or problem from being processed in the threat centres of the brain to non-threat centres, or even to the 'ignore' processing/pain-off gating side of things!

He was now walking well round the room and I then got him to sit. We chatted for three or four minutes.

'Now, I want to see what happens after a spell of resting! Up you get and just try the walking again...'

Then I added with a little smile as he was getting up...

'Curse me if you want!'

My experience with getting something like this moving again is that a typical immediate response to rest after the movement is that all the pain comes back and it stiffens up again – sometimes really nastily! It's usually more the longer you've rested it. Ask your back pain patients who freed up well with your session what they were like getting out of the car after they drove home!

Classically what many therapists might have done at this point would have been to get Pete up on the couch and get their nasty proddy fingers into the spot for a bit and give it some electro-dazzle of some kind and typically after this he'd get up and hardly be able to walk... 'Aahrgh, what the bloody hell have you done... it was fine ten minutes ago...' (OK, often they're freer and better too).

They then blame the machine!

This scenario used to be very common for me when treating acute and subacute low back pains – especially if you'd spent ten minutes or more with them prone on the couch. It's not funny trying to peel someone off the couch and into standing who was really pretty good before they lay down!

I've got fed up with doing that, so I now 'normalise' the post-rest response by resting and then finding out what happens and if it's stiff and sore I do a bit of explaining.

Pete stood up and stopped and smiled... and I winked and said...

'Stiffened up? It's OK it's normal!'

'Bugger...!' he whispered, but he was smiling.

Right, just move about anyway you can, see if it warms up and see if you can get walking well again.'

I got him walking up and down our corridor and within about twenty paces he was getting going again but looking tense.

I then gave him this little routine to do every time he'd rested.

It's called MOVE-BEFORE-YOU-MOVE! (In the clinic we use this little phrase for the routine we give any patient who finds that they get stiff and sore when they go to move after resting. It's a very common feature of patients with problems related to arthritic and degenerative joint changes as well as joint/ligament/tendon injury too.)

For Pete it was simply this:

- cross legs non-weight bearing ankle movements, try 15-20-25 reps and then test to see if it works... and/or...

- do your cross legged calf raises to work the calf... try same reps and test it... and/or...

- just stand and then do your up over and down exercise as we did...

- just walk away slowly hobbling or flat footed but try to get going when it lets you.

Key is to experiment to find the minimum needed, most folk just get used to it and do what I call...

'Curse it and carry on' and within a few paces or a few minutes they've forgotten about it.

So Pete now had:

- move-before-you-move routine anytime needed

- more bike, build slowly but push it a bit and get out for longer

- if walking flat-footed, make sure that every so often you walk normally for 10-15 paces and build up from there... to back to normal (start going for walks and build up to normal speed and build up time too)

- tip-toe high, mid and low, anytime anywhere, round house, up the stairs

- get going with calf raises – use up, over down, then back up if have to, otherwise just start doing it

(test good left side to see how many reps to 'tired' feeling and use this as eventual goal for right; it's good to do alternate sides – up down left, then, up down right, repeat, rather than continually up and down on the one side)

That's how it is with normal gait; we do one side then the other. The muscle gets a quick rest every other step, which allows blood to perfuse into it. On the other hand pushing on the one leg over and over may challenge the circulation to improve.

- *think about your thinking about it and stop thinking about it!*

Focusing helps keep the circuit firing! This is the distraction challenge, and makes folk realise that they've got in the habit of constantly scanning for the presence of the pain – that their attention is habitually drawn to check it all.

- same rules apply, plus a 'don't panic if it flares a bit – that's normal' rule too

If sore, self massage, use ice or heat or spray – anything that makes it feel good. Even try taking anti-inflammatories regularly for a day or two.

The message here is – circuit turned on needs to be turned off as quickly as possible, to stop the circuit getting practiced at staying on. Drown it out! Quieten it down and **keep the plan going if at all possible.** The basic early simple exercises should still be done during the flare. There's no such thing as stopping and resting here, just modifying.

One week later he came back again – much improved: cycled over ten miles twice with ease – plenty of hills and confident out of the saddle. Walking normally now and starting to stop thinking about it. Tip-toeing heaps and feeling ready for a run. Doesn't need to do move-before-you-move, he used it for a couple of days and worked well – then just ignored the bit of stiffness and now it's gone. Going up and down on calf and can do thirty on the right when it's tired, goal is around fifty as measured on the left.

I then quizzed him about how the pain came back on when he had gone back to running in the last few months. What was interesting, and not unusual, was that on the runs where he'd re-aggravated it he started out fine, noticed it a little after about five minutes, stayed with it for another five to ten minutes and then it really worsened. He'd also noticed the same awareness on his 'good' couple of runs but that the awareness just faded and there was no problem after that. On the aggravating runs when the pain became 'bad' and didn't fade he'd stopped and walked home. He hadn't tried to go again to see if he could carry on. As he pointed out, it had become immediately painful to walk let alone run.

This was now our 'joint' plan to get him back to running.

Circuits apart/no pain rule if possible. The schedule below was a 'rough' suggestion, the emphasis to start with was keeping an eye on precise timing, so that if things did go 'bad' he would know what level he was at and what level to go back to. The schedule was also disciplined in the sense that it just didn't let him go 'free', it kept the macho go-for-it maleness in check a bit.

- first 3 days: walk slow 3 minutes: walk faster 3 mins: small jog 3 mins: if OK repeat this 3 times = 27 minutes roughly

- next 3 days: if OK repeat but add 3 mins easy run after each jog = 36 minutes

- next 3 days: leave out slow walk, fast walk 3 mins: increase jog and easy run to 4 mins each. Repeat 3 times = 33mins with 24 mins total of jog/running

- if OK... next 3 days: fast walk 3 mins to warm up: easy jog 5 mins: easy run 5 mins then fast walk 1 minute and repeat 3-4 times = 30-40 minutes jog/running

- keep the cycling going

- see me again in about two weeks to add some more stuff

- ring me any time (the 'never sit at home worrying about it' rule!)

This two week appointment was the last time I saw him – from here on in I told him to phone me from time to time. He phoned once after a month and told me he was back running normally. Eight months later he sent me a Christmas card, 'Did a personal best in New York Marathon – 2 hours 57mins and 17 seconds... couldn't quite beat the world record marathon for a 70 year old, 2 hours 54mins and 48 seconds... still time yet! Thanks for all your help, flying now, Pete.

What we covered in this last session was the graded introduction of faster running, acceleration, hopping on two and one legs and from one to the other. I also asked him to gradually build up changes of direction and some speed work when he felt like it.

The wisdom?

1. Loading tissues is important.

2. Loading them with appropriate 'top-down' processing in place is even better!

3. If you're confident all is OK, normalise reactions to loading, rather than seeing them as a problem

4. Graded Exposure, in the sense of gradually increasing, or exposing the loading and forces on the problem tissues. Not only making them fitter and stronger, but also desensitising their processing circuitry.

Section 14
Read what I've read

Hebb D.O. (1949). The organization of behaviour: a neuropsychological theory. New York, Wiley.

Maitland G. D. M. (1986). Vertebral Manipulation. (5th Edn). London, Butterworth.

Robertson I. (1999). Mind sculpture. Your brain's untapped potential. London, Bantam Press.

Lightning Source UK Ltd.
Milton Keynes UK
UKHW021306150223
417059UK00017B/409